Perspectives on Biomedical Engineering Education

This book presents state-of-the-art pedagogical approaches to biomedical engineering education within a global context. The book also provides practical guides on adapting pedagogies and designing learning activities in the biomedical engineering classroom that suit undergraduate and postgraduate programs.

Perspectives on Biomedical Engineering Education is the first book of its kind to focus on applications of pedagogical approaches for dissecting and examining complex concepts in Biomedical Engineering in today's modern classrooms in higher education. The book first introduces the historical background and development of biomedical engineering. Its second section focuses on leading scholars' knowledge and experience in applying various pedagogies, including biodesign, design thinking, capstones, and prototyping. The final section distills expert insights into practical pedagogical guidelines on biomedical engineering education for university teaching and academic staff and readers alike who are interested in biomedical engineering education.

The book is primarily written for a wide audience from junior to senior biomedical engineering academic staff, who will find new ideas to adapt the relevant pedagogy into their classroom. Industry professionals and any readers interested in biomedical engineering or related fields would also find the material relevant.

Perspectives on Biomedical Engineering Education

Edited by
Socrates Dokos, Chun Chuen Billy Chan,
and Lauren Kark

CRC Press
Taylor & Francis Group
Boca Raton London New York

CRC Press is an imprint of the
Taylor & Francis Group, an **informa** business

Designed cover image: Shutterstock

First edition published 2027
by CRC Press
2385 NW Executive Center Drive, Suite 320, Boca Raton FL 33431

and by CRC Press
4 Park Square, Milton Park, Abingdon, Oxon, OX14 4RN

CRC Press is an imprint of Taylor & Francis Group, LLC

ISBN: 978-1-032-85885-2 (hbk)
ISBN: 978-1-032-85884-5 (pbk)
ISBN: 978-1-003-52031-3 (ebk)

DOI: 10.1201/9781003520313

Typeset in Times
by Apex CoVantage, LLC

Contents

Preface

Biomedical engineering (BME) represents a critical nexus where biological sciences, engineering principles, and medical practice converge to address complex challenges in human health. As BME continues to evolve from its origins into a highly integrative field, the necessity for robust pedagogical frameworks has become ever more pressing. *Perspectives in Biomedical Engineering Education* provides a scholarly examination of this evolution, offering structured insights from leading educators into the historical foundations, pedagogical methodologies, and sociotechnical dimensions that characterize contemporary BME instruction.

This text opens with an examination of the *historical development of BME and its education programs*. In **Chapter 1,** *Paul Junor* traces the origins of BME from 19th-century German biophysics meetings to its formalization in university settings during the 1930s, highlighting the transition from traditional engineering departments to a distinct academic identity. Expanding on this historical context, **Chapter 2,** *by Ziad O. Abu-Faraj and Sandy A. Rihana,* explores *disciplinarity in BME education*. The authors distinguish between multidisciplinary, interdisciplinary, and transdisciplinary frameworks, arguing that such distinctions are essential for designing curricula that effectively synthesize technical engineering rigor with the inherent complexities of biological systems.

In **Chapter 3,** *Brian P. Helmke* and *Renata F. Ramos* discuss the *critical challenges in BME education*, delineating the difficulties in aligning student learning outcomes with a moving clinical and industrial landscape. To address these challenges and ensure global relevance, *accreditation* serves as a foundational pillar for quality assurance. In **Chapter 4,** *Ziad O. Abu-Faraj* examines the role of accreditation bodies in establishing Program Educational Objectives (PEOs) that maintain program excellence while fostering a sense of professional belonging among students.

Central to engineering education—and to BME in particular—is the transformation of abstract concepts into physical solutions. In **Chapter 5**, *Matthew Wettergreen* introduces pedagogical perspectives on *prototyping*, emphasizing its role in fostering hand-eye coordination and knowledge transfer through iterative design cycles. This is further explored in **Chapter 6** by *Mark Seow Khoon Chong, Lyn Denend,* and *David B. Grayden*, who describe the *Biodesign* pedagogical framework originating from Stanford University, prioritizing the rigorous identification of unmet clinical needs before the implementation of technological solutions. In **Chapter 7**, *Jennifer R. Amos, Joe A. Bradley, and Holly McIlwee Golecki* reflect on *BME capstone design courses*, discussing the complexities of balancing team-based and individual assessments while integrating industry standards and cognitive taxonomies.

Active learning methodologies constitute a significant portion of contemporary BME pedagogy. In **Chapter 8**, *Emily Cook, Fiona Truscott, and Jennifer Griffiths* discuss *problem-based learning* (PBL) *in BME*, demonstrating its efficacy in fostering higher-level cognitive skills by challenging students with realistic, ill-structured problems. To bridge the gap between classroom theory and healthcare delivery, **Chapter 9**, by *William H. Guilford, Miiri Kotche, and Rachel H. Schmedlen*, examines *clinical* *immersion programs* as a vital pedagogical strategy. These experiences are defined as sustained, structured engagements within real clinical settings that enable students to observe workflows and interact directly with healthcare professionals, patients, and technologies. To assist educators in program design, a classification framework is proposed on the basis of setting, duration, focus, and level of engagement. The authors also delineate best practices for implementation, emphasizing the necessity of robust institutional partnerships, clear administrative processes, and the integration of structured feedback and reflection to ensure long-term program sustainability.

Complementing these immersions, *David A. Rubenstein* provides a framework in **Chapter 10** for the *practical design of BME laboratory modules*, emphasizing the alignment of experiments with course learning outcomes to reinforce theoretical constructs.

Recognizing that engineering is inherently a sociotechnical profession, this text also addresses ethical and social integration within the BME curriculum. In **Chapter 11**, *Brit Shields, Aria Zheyuan Huang, and Disha Vaswani* advocate for an *embedded ethics approach*, moving beyond standalone courses to normalize ethical reasoning as a standard component of the engineering design process. **Chapter 12**, authored by *Sharon Aris, Daniela Castro de Jong, and Lauren Kark*, proposes a model for fostering a *social disposition* in engineers. This framework encourages students to understand health and disability as multidimensional constructs influenced by social, historical, and economic determinants.

The final section of the book presents empirical case studies illustrating these pedagogical principles in practice. In **Chapter 13**, *Katherine Sammy* and *Matthew Wettergreen* analyze *BME student prototyping solutions*, observing that increased fidelity does not inherently lead to improved functionality. In Chapter 14, *David B. Grayden* presents a case study of the *Biodesign Innovation program at the University of Melbourne*, highlighting the success of multidisciplinary teams that bridge engineering and business administration to achieve high rates of commercialization. In **Chapter 15**, *Jennifer R. Amos, Joe A. Bradley, and Holly McIlwee Golecki* describe a *design continuum at the University of Illinois* that integrates undergraduate, master's, and medical students into teams that mimic professional organizational structures. Finally, **Chapter 16**, authored by *Joseph Tranquillo*, encourages the use of the *United Nations Sustainable Development Goals* as a pedagogical framework. These "super wicked problems" provide opportunities for intellectual cross-training, requiring students to synthesize systems, values, strategic, and future thinking to address complex global health challenges.

Perspectives in Biomedical Engineering Education serves as a comprehensive resource for BME educators, scholars, and practitioners. It is our sincere hope that the various perspectives offered in it will inspire continued innovation in BME pedagogical approaches and help deliver graduates capable of navigating across disciplinary boundaries to advance global healthcare.

Socrates Dokos
Chun Chuen Billy Chan
Lauren Kark

About the Editors

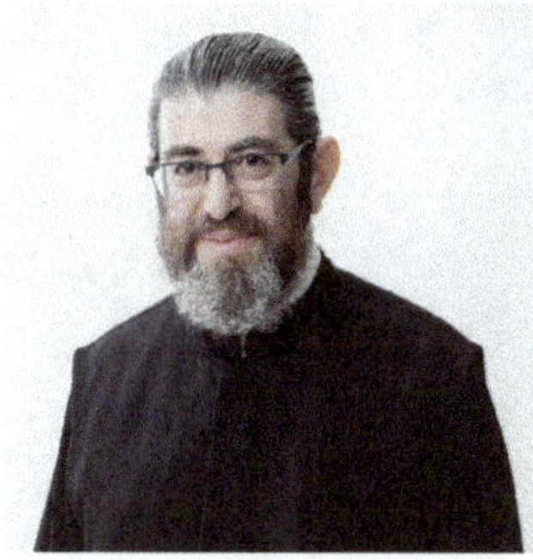

Socrates Dokos is Associate Professor in the Graduate School of Biomedical Engineering, University of New South Wales (UNSW), Australia, where he served as the School's director of teaching and learning for six years until 2021. His research focuses on the development of computational models for various biomedical engineering applications, including neurostimulators, visual prostheses, transcranial electric stimulators, cardiac defibrillators, left ventricular assist devices, and artificial mitral valves. He has collaborated with several medical device companies using computational modeling to better understand and improve their device performance, including Cochlear, Materialise, Tendyne, Bionic Vision Technologies, and Saluda.

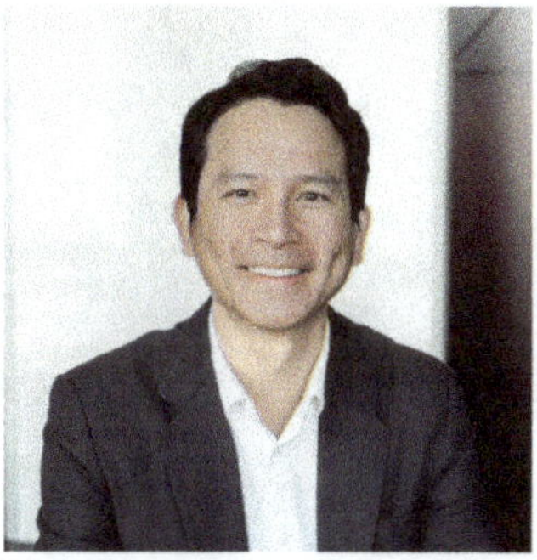

Billy Chun Chuen Chan serves as a lecturer in the UNSW Business School at the UNSW in Sydney, Australia. He earned his PhD in Education from the University of Sydney, where his research focused on exploring the teaching and learning of multimodal argumentation for academic purposes. This involved the use of infographics within an English as a second/foreign language classroom. His primary research interests encompass curriculum and pedagogy in higher education, critical thinking, argumentation, and visual literacy.

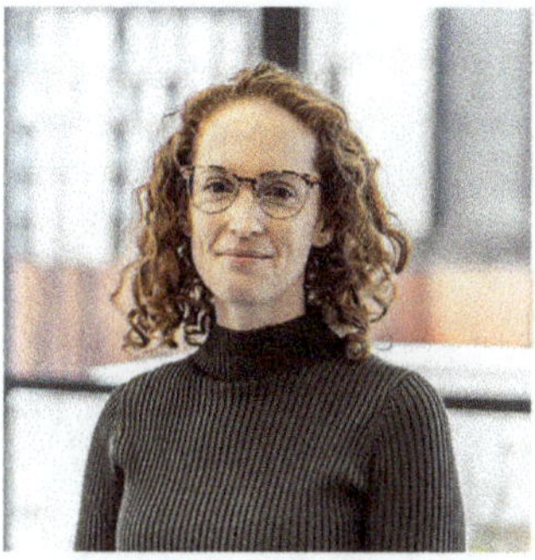

Lauren Kark is Professor and Deputy Head of School (Academic) at the Graduate School of Biomedical Engineering, University of New South Wales. She is an education-focused academic with teaching expertise in biomechanics and assistive technology. Her work integrates technical learning with social impact, informed by her leadership of service-learning programs in both domestic and international contexts. Lauren recently led the development of a new four-year undergraduate degree in biomedical engineering at UNSW. This work reflects her broader academic interests in curriculum design, disciplinarity, and the role of interdisciplinary thinking in engineering education.

Contributors

Abu-Faraj, Ziad O
Mebex Consultants s.a.r.l.
Ghattas Building, Badaro Street, Parc Sector
Beirut, Lebanon

Amos, Jennifer R.
Department of Bioengineering, Grainger College of Engineering
University of Illinois Urbana-Champaign
Urbana, IL, USA

Aris, Sharon
School of Social Sciences
University of New South Wales (UNSW)
Sydney, Australia

Bradley, Joe A.
Department of Bioengineering, Grainger College of Engineering
University of Illinois Urbana-Champaign
Urbana, IL, USA

Castro de Jong, Daniela
School of Health Sciences
UNSW
Sydney, Australia

Chong, Seow Khoon Mark
Department of Biomedical Engineering
National University of Singapore
Singapore

Cook, Emily
School of Science, Computing and Emerging Technologies
Swinburne University of Technology
Melbourne, Australia

Denend, Lyn
Mussallem Center for Biodesign
Stanford University
Stanford, CA, USA

Ditto. Sandy A
Biomedical Engineering Department
Holy Spirit University of Kaslik (USEK)
Lebanon

Golecki, Holly McIlwee
Department of Bioengineering, Grainger College of Engineering
University of Illinois Urbana-Champaign
Urbana, IL, USA

Grayden, David B.
Department of Biomedical Engineering
The University of Melbourne
Melbourne, Australia

Griffiths, Jennifer
UCL Institute for Higher Education Development and Support
and UCL Centre for Engineering Education
University College London
London, UK

Guilford, William H.
School of Engineering and Applied Sciences
University of Virginia
Charlottesville, VA, USA

Helmke, Brian
Department of Biomedical Engineering
University of Virginia
Charlottesville, VA, USA

Huang, Aria Zheyuan
Department of Bioengineering
School of Engineering and Applied Sciences
University of Pennsylvania
Philadelphia, PA, USA

Junor, Paul
Department of Engineering Technologies
School of Engineering
Swinburne University of Technology
Melbourne, Victoria, Australia

Kark, Lauren
Graduate School of Biomedical Engineering
UNSW
Sydney, New South Wales, Australia

Kotche, Miiri
Richard and Loan Hill Department of Biomedical Engineering
University of Illinois Chicago
Chicago, IL, USA

Ramos, Renata F.
Department of Bioengineering
Rice University
Houston, TX, USA

Rubenstein, David A.
Department of Biomedical Engineering
Stony Brook University
Stony Brook, NY, USA

Sammy, Katherine
B.S. Bioengineering Candidate, Department of Bioengineering
George R. Brown School of Engineering and Computing
Rice University
Houston, TX, USA

Schmedlen, Rachael
Biomedical Engineering Department, College of Engineering
University of Michigan
Ann Arbor, MI, USA

Shields, Brit
Department of Bioengineering
School of Engineering and Applied Science
University of Pennsylvania
Philadelphia, PA, USA

Tranquillo, Joseph
Biomedical Engineering Department and Provost's Office
Bucknell University
Lewisburg, PA, USA

Truscott, Fiona
UCL Centre for Engineering Education
University College London
London, UK

Vaswani, Disha
Department of Bioengineering
School of Engineering and Applied Sciences
University of Pennsylvania
Philadelphia, PA, USA

Wettergreen, Matthew
George R. Brown School of Engineering and Computing
Rice University
Houston, TX, USA

Abbreviations

ABET	Accreditation Board for Engineering and Technology
AI	Artificial Intelligence
AICHE	American Institute of Chemical Engineers
AIMBE	American Institute of Medical and Biological Engineering
APACC	Asia Pacific Accreditation and Certification Commission
AR	Augmented Reality
ASCE	American Society of Civil Engineers
ASEE	American Society for Engineering Education
ASME	American Society of Mechanical Engineers
A*STAR	Agency for Science, Technology, and Research
BioTech	Biotechnology
Beng	Bachelor of Engineering
BMC	Business Model Canvas
BME	Biomedical Engineering
BMES	Biomedical Engineering Society
BMET	Biomedical Equipment Technology
BRL	Business Readiness Level
CACEI	Consejo de Acreditación de la Enseñanza de la Ingeniería
CAD	Computer-Aided Design
CAE	Computer-Aided Engineering
CAGR	Compound Annual Growth Rate
CATME	Comprehensive Assessment of Team Member Effectiveness
CBI	Challenge-Based Instruction
CBL	Case-Based Learning
CEAB	Canadian Engineering Accreditation Board
CEEAA	China Engineering Education Accreditation Association
CNC	Computer Numerical Control
DEBUT	Design by Biomedical Undergraduate Teams
DR	Diabetic Retinopathy
EA	Engineers Australia
EAC	Engineering Accreditation Committee
EAMBES	European Alliance for Medical and Biological Engineering and Science
ECG	Electrocardiogram
ECUK	Engineering Council United Kingdom
EHEA	European Higher Education Area
EIA	Environmental Impact Assessment
ENAEE	European Network for Accreditation of Engineering Education (ENAEE)
E-STEAM	Entrepreneurship, Science, Technology, Engineering, Arts, and Mathematics
EUR-ACE	European Accreditation of Engineering Programmes

FDA	Food and Drug Administration
GDPR	General Data Protection Regulation
GFIT	Global Faculty-In-Training
GIST	Global Innovation through Science and Technology
GMI	Global Medical Innovation
HCD	Human Centered Design
HealthTech	Health Technology
HIPAA	Health Insurance Portability and Accountability Act
HPL	How People Learn
IAB	Industry Advisory Board
ICF	International Classification of Functioning, Disability and Health
IDPBL	Interdisciplinary Project-Based Learning
IEA	International Engineering Alliance
IEC	International Electrotechnical Commission
IEEE	Institute of Electrical and Electronics Engineers
IFMBE	International Federation for Medical and Biological Engineering
IPAC	Individual Peer Assessment of Contribution
ISO	International Organization for Standardization
JIT	Just-In-Time
KPI	Key Performance Indicator
LCA	Life Cycle Assessment
LCC	Life Cycle Costing
LCD	Liquid Crystal Display
LCSA	Life Cycle Sustainability Assessment
LED	Light Emitting Diode
MBA	Master of Business Administration
MDPP	Medical Device Partnering Program
MedTech	Medical Technology
MELETI	Medical Engineering Listed Education and Training Information
MENA	Middle East and North Africa
MEng	Master of Engineering
MEMs	Micro-Electro-Mechanical Devices
MIT	Massachusetts Institute of Technology
MOU	Memorandum of Understanding
MSc	Master of Science
NAE	National Academy of Engineering
NBA	National Board of Accreditation
NIBIB	National Institute of Biomedical Imaging and Bioengineering
NIH	National Institute of Health
NSF	National Science Foundation
OEDK	Oshman Engineering Design Kitchen
PBL	Problem-Based Learning
PCB	Printed Circuit Board
PDCA	Plan-Do-Check-Act
PEO	Program Educational Objectives
PhD	Doctor of Philosophy

PjBL	Project-Based Learning
POC	Point of Care
PPE	Personal Protective Equipment
QFD	Quality Functional Development
SAC	Structured Academic Controversy
SBT	Simulation-Based Training
SDG	Sustainable Development Goal
SDH	Social Determinants of Health
SGD	Sustainable Development Goal
SLCA	Societal Life Cycle Assessment
SO	Student Outcomes
STEEPLED	Social, Technological, Economic, Environmental, Political, Legislative, Ethical, and Demographic
STEM	Science, Technology, Engineering, and Mathematics
STT	Sociotechnical Thinking
TA	Teaching Assistant
TBL	Team-Based Learning
TrBL	Triple Bottom Line
TOC	Theory of Constraints
TQM	Total Quality Management
TRL	Technology Readiness Level
TU/e	Eindhoven University of Technology
UAM	Universidad Autónoma Metropolitana
UCL	University College London
UN	United Nations
USA	United States of America
UT	University of Twente
VaNTH ERC	Vanderbilt, Northwestern, Texas, Harvard/MIT Engineering Research Center
VR	Virtual Reality
WHO	World Health Organisation
WW1	World War 1
WW2	World War 2
3D	Three-Dimensional

1 Historical Background and Development of Biomedical Engineering Education

Paul Junor

1.1 A HISTORY OF THE ENGINEERING DISCIPLINES AND THEIR DIVERSIFICATION

Having masterminded the design and construction of the first of the pyramids, prior to 2600 BCE, Imhotep of Egypt is credited as the "first engineer in history" (Cardoso and Chanin 2022). However, the origin of the term "engineer" is explained as originating from the French title "*ingenieur*": one who was skilled in conception, implementation, operation, and maintenance of "engines of war" such as catapults, projectile launchers, and battering rams, in addition to fortifications, barricades, and reinforcements (McDonald 1914). This *military engineering was* considered the product of *ingenuity* (creativity) and well preceded the invention of engines powered by steam and internal combustion.

Hence, Archimedes of Syracuse (287–212 BCE) would be regarded as an engineer of his day, applying his mechanical aptitude and mathematical prowess to devising such contrivances, in defense of Syracuse in Sicily. Likewise, around the turn of the common era (McGivern 1960), military engineer to Augustus Caesar in Rome, Marcus Vitruvius Pollio (around 85–15 BCE), had left a detailed published description of the design structure and operation of some of these "war engines" in the tenth of his series "*De Architectura*" (Vitruvius, Warren, and Morgan 1914). This *military engineering was* considered the product of *ingenuity*—creativity—and well preceded the invention of engines powered by steam and internal combustion.

A number of versatile virtuosos of the Italian Renaissance, renowned equally as master painters, sculptors, and architects, were also noteworthy for their contribution to military engineering. The polymath Leonardo da Vinci (1452–1519 AD) turned his hand to the design of these so-called "war machines." Prior to accepting the role of "*méchanicien du Roi*" (King's Engineer) to the French King Francis 1st, he had been employed by the Duke of Milan as a military engineer; in addition to designing catapults and fortifications, he envisaged the submarine, the army tank, and helicopter-like flying machines of the future (West 2017).

DOI: 10.1201/9781003520313-1

Michelangelo (di Lodovico Buonarroti Simoni, 1475–1564) was an equally famous contemporary and rival of Leonardo; though known more for sculpting and painting, he achieved recognition for his remarkably effective though ill-fated fortification of Florence in 1528–1529, which nonetheless by 1530 succumbed due to starvation by siege (Wallace 1987):

> *In the Renaissance, military engineering was an important aspect of the profession of being an artist. . . . According to Vasari, Michelangelo said that he knew little of painting and sculpture but considered himself an expert on fortifications. Unlike most Renaissance artists and theorists, he had the opportunity not only to design fortifications but to build them, and further, to prove their efficacy in time of war.*

From the Italian Renaissance of the 1400s onward, building design had begun to be acknowledged as including an intellectual artform aspect similar to painting and sculpting, encompassing conceptual aesthetic elements beyond the prevailing "hands-on" stone masonry and carpentry of the master craftsman. This inspired the artist designers of the time to seek acceptance as professionals—architects—and prompted the founding in 1577 CE of the art school "Accademia di San Luca" in Rome (Knoll 1997). For most occupations, consolidation into professionalization involves several key actions: dedicated commitment to required tasks, establishment of training through universities or schools of adequate stature, establishment of local and national professional bodies representing the discipline, licensing (or certification or some form of credentialing), and adoption of a formal code of ethics (Bronzino 2011; Wilensky 1964); by the creation of the Accademia, the first two of these steps had been fulfilled.

Strategic urban design and fortification were often undertaken by Renaissance artistic designers of architecture at the time, due to their drafting and measurement skills, their appreciation of building material and structure, and perhaps their ability to visualize both landscape and human movement.

Military engineering needed to involve not only weaponry and combat but also strategic planning forethought. To be fully effective, this required not only siege craft to mount but also fortification to withstand sieges, pre-emptive defensive strategic town planning, and ingenious building in advance to counteract and ameliorate invasion, and careful consideration of supply chains and for provisioning when under siege.

The fall of Constantinople to the Ottoman Empire in 1453 had illustrated that with the advent of gunpowder, prevailing high but relatively thin stone castle walls, which had hitherto protected city states from breaching by rams and catapults, were vulnerable to cannon fire. The lower but thicker *trace italeane* "star castle" style of fortification layout devised by the Renaissance military architects superseded the older castle structures for security against incursion by invaders (West 2017).

Valleriani (2010) suggests that by the end of the Renaissance, societal changes had necessitated differentiation of multifaceted artist-engineers, such as the ingenious Galileo, into various specializations:

> *engineers, architects, practical mathematicians, military engineers, mechanicians, artists, and shipwrights. . . . Yet until this happened, the situation was so fluid that*

a single person, over the course of his life, might be considered not only as an artist but also as a mathematician or as a military engineer, depending upon the subjects to which he dedicated his time.

1.1.1 Civil Engineering and Its Descendent Specializations

Some buildings, bridges, road making, shipbuilding, and hydraulics (water distribution and drainage) were part of the purview of military engineers, but these activities could equally be undertaken in peacetime by civilians—*civil engineers.* With this blurring between military and civil activity, one might say that civil engineering is what military engineers did peacetime and military engineering is what civil engineers did in wartime. The differentiating title is credited to the English engineer John Smeaton in 1768 (Cardoso and Chanin 2022). The Institution of Civil Engineers received Royal Charter in 1818 CE, and Civil Engineering became recognized as a profession (including building and construction, with later distinctions such as structural engineering and infrastructure engineering).

Further specialization of engineers, in both the military and the civilian spheres beyond warfare, is described by Majoram and Zhong (2010). These new branches of engineering appeared one by one, accompanied by the "constructive disruptions" of technologies largely coinciding with various phases of the industrial revolution, which crystallized each identifiable engineering subdivision.

In the 1700s, *Mechanical Engineering* started to emerge as a specialized discipline distinct from civil engineering. The invention of the printing press in Germany around 1440 had already represented a significant innovation to previously labor-intensive manual work as a forerunner of mass production; previously, distribution of written documents had been limited, but the impact of the printing press on the dissemination of knowledge and consequent multiplier of innovation was not fully apparent till later. In Britain, the mechanization of increasing complexity first produced the spinning and weaving looms of the textile industry; then, steam power that enabled industrial mass-production sewing machines also ushered in heavy railway engines. The Institution of Mechanical Engineers was formed in 1847, a milestone of professional recognition.

Electrical Engineering arose as a specific discipline in the 1800s, with the Society of Telegraph Engineers inaugurated in 1871, and formalized in 1887 by the establishment of the Institution of Electrical Engineers. Observations of electrical and magnetic behavior attributed to Gilbert, Faraday, Volta, Maxwell, Joule, Ampère, Ørsted, and others had paved the way ultimately for the invention of the telegraph, telephone, electric light, and electrical machinery. Importantly, the generation and distribution of electric power for these developments ushered in the third wave of the industrial revolution.

Likewise, *Chemical Engineering* (and *Materials Engineering*) grew from the chemical sciences in the 1900s—the "fourth industrial revolution," responding to needs for economic scaled-up processing and mass production—particularly with the demands in the petroleum industry, and medications/pharmaceuticals in the world wars. The American Institute of Chemical Engineers was established in 1908, and the Institution of Chemical Engineers in 1924.

Having evolved from the originally all-encompassing military and civil engineering, these vocational specialties each have their own discipline-specific identity and body of knowledge. There are shared fundamental common core concepts—mathematics, applied sciences (physics and chemistry), and measurement science—as well as different and often overlapping emphases, outlook, and specific terminologies. Each has relevance to applications in biology and medicine.

1.2 BEGINNINGS OF FORMALIZED ENGINEERING EDUCATION

The previously mentioned rise of formal architecture as a profession provided impetus for the similar professionalization of engineering and the evolution of disciplinary specializations, generally coinciding with phases of the industrial revolution. Likewise, political revolutions also had a profound influence on approaches to education (Cardoso and Chanin 2022; Majoram and Zhong 2010).

The earliest institutions regarded as universities—the Pandidakterion (established in Constantinople in 425 CE), Al Quaraouiyine (Morocco, 859 CE), and Al-Azhar (Cairo, 970CE)—had focused initially on the teaching of divinity/theology, law, and philosophy, as was common in the first and early second millennia. The first university to award degrees, established in Bologna in 1088, acted as a forerunner to those that would come to teach engineering; such early universities in Europe—*universitates*—were in essence guilds or communities of students "contracting" their tuition from selected discipline masters.

The first military engineering education globally was claimed to take place at the Royal Savoy Military College in Turin in 1678, at that time the Duchy of Savoy, now known as part of Italy (Bianchi and Cornaglia 2014). Based on the more limited Prussian Ritterakademie (Academy for Knights) model, an academy of this nature would seem to be tending to not as much a military college but toward a finishing school for the sons of aristocrats: its curriculum *"included physical exercise (dance, vaulting, riding, mock battles and attacks on fortresses) alongside the study of mathematics, and drawing."* Hence, this education, including the *"knightly arts,"* was broader than simply combat; such officer training was consistent with dignified courtly manners amenable to sophisticated society acceptable by the nobility and also fostered appreciation of diplomacy and logistics useful to manage allegiances.

In reclaiming the Netherlands from the Spanish, the Dutch borrowed and adapted insights from the Italian Renaissance military engineers to their largely wetland local geographical environment (Swart 2013), subversively exploiting skills in hydraulics and waterways management. Due to battlefield attrition, there was a pressing need to train replacements for military engineering; this was pragmatically accelerated, efficiently teaching an ad hoc heterogeneous civilian cohort (Lenman 2013). The *Duytsche Mathematique,* a course of instruction substantially for military engineers, was promptly developed in 1599. It was published in Dutch for accessibility by the local population, and formed the basis for a course of instruction, loosely but proficiently delivered through the University of Leiden from 1600 (Krüger 2018).

Scholarship in France had a history dating back to the founding of the University of Paris (the Sorbonne) in 1150, largely as a humanities (or liberal arts) university, as per other European universities of the era, without engineering existing as an academic discipline at that time. In 1671, the Académie Royale d'Architecture was established in Paris, fashioned after the Accademia di San Luca in Rome (Knoll 1997). That same year, largely self-taught military engineer Sébastien de Vauban (1633–1707) had been "loaned" by the French Minister of War to prescribe fortification of Turin in the Duchy of Savoy. During his career, Vauban also led the 1673–1678 campaign for the capture of Maastricht for the Netherlands using his innovative siege craft methods and, importantly, masterminded the "iron belt" of fortresses securing France's borders.

Although there were a number of military schools in France prior to 1700, such military engineering training was limited and largely reserved for the nobility, somewhat along the lines of the Prussian Ritterakademies. In the 18th century, the implementation of separate specialist military engineering academies was preceded by the establishment of specific military corps for civil works, naval construction, and warfare combat. The civil engineering military workforce trained for management of bridges, roads, and water distribution, the Corps des Ponts et Chaussées (bridges and roads), was established in 1716. From 1747, the formal school supporting was the École Nationale des Ponts et Chausseés, which has been suggested was globally the first provider of "*formal engineering education resulting in the title of engineer*" (Cardoso and Chanin 2022). Another part of civil engineering education, the École des Mines in Paris (1783), was modeled after the Frieberg School of Mining and Metallurgy (1702), and the *Bergakademie* (1765), also in Frieberg, Saxony (now Germany).

L'École Royale du Génie de Mézières (Royal Engineering School at Mézières), specifically for instructing the engineers corps of the royal army in defensive work and battlefield preparation, was founded in 1748. This slightly preceded the *École Royale Militaire (Military School)*, set up in 1751 to provide training for general campaign combat strategy and tactics. *L'École des Constructeurs de Vaisseaux*, for teaching naval engineering/architecture innovations in shipbuilding, was founded in 1672. This substantially preceded the civil and defense schools, but due to the success of entrenched traditional shipwright culture, the military engineering education initiative took time and effort to be integrated (Pritchard 1987). As military engineering requirements had become more specialized and complex, these military educational establishments adopted mathematically-based resources, such as de Belidor's (1729) "La Science des Ingénieurs" (Hatchuel 2018).

The 1794 Reign of Terror and subsequent 1798 French Revolution led to an exodus of the aristocracy and a consequent escalating shortage of military engineering officers: hitherto they had been recruited almost exclusively from the nobility. The previous focus of these graduate "King's Engineers" was service for the King; the requirement for the newly developing republic was service for the state. Coupled with the evolving republican ethos for meritocracy rather than birthright, the urgent action required to train replacement officer engineers resulted in accelerated changes for engineering education in France in the late 1700s and early 1800s. Against the turbulent background, Lazare Carnot (1753–1823), a graduate of the Mézières Engineering School, was significantly influential in the mobilization of the population into the armed forces and the concurrent rapid expansion of quality engineering education. The military colleges that had been established, hitherto exclusively for entry by those born into high society, were modified to enable entry for the population at large, based on capability rather than social status. These engineering schools became the educational model of the elite Grande Ecole schools created by and for the state, and were supplemented by the École Polytechnique in Paris, with its rigorous three-year course heavy in mathematics. Having attracted strong applicants and produced excellent engineers, the École Polytechnique model was emulated in Germany and Russia (equally short of capable engineering workforces in the wake of wartime) and also in the United States.

Prior to the 19th century, the geographic region of German-speaking parts of Central Europe that eventually became unified into Germany had consisted of separate independent states occasionally in conflict with each other; engineering (and its education) in these regions was predominantly military engineering (Wollschläger 2013). For some time, engineering education and training remained without formalization, largely apprentice-to-master craftsman style. The closest to formal training were the Ritterkollegien—"colleges for knights" (Keck 2006), better known as Ritterakademies, for the sons of nobles. These provided a form of military training in the so-called "knightly arts," concentrating on "*riding, fencing, dancing, vaulting, and playing all kinds of instruments,*" though perhaps touching on elementary engineering-related topics, "*arithmetic, geometry, mechanics, optics, geography, fortification, architecture,*" designed for state and military service and the cavalier and court functions reserved for the nobility. Military engineering and its education in the 1700s tended to follow French and the Dutch influences; often, such international expertise and training were contracted in as required. In Saxony in 1702, however, the Freiberg School of Mining and Metallurgy (consolidated as the *Bergakademie* in 1765) is credited to represent the first systematic engineering education; additionally, a military academy in Dresden had been established in 1743 with a curriculum of field fortification and artillery, mathematics, architecture, geography, and siege warfare. By contrast, the more extensive and better supported Prussian army had developed a military engineering corps by 1729 which relied on contracted international expertise for training with attention to military strategy and logistics (minimal training in fortification and surveying); it was not until 1810 that the Kriegsakademie ("war academy," or military college) in Berlin was commissioned, this with emphasis on mathematics, topography, fortification, logistics (strategic thinking and staff integration). From 1786 to 1803, the relatively smaller Hanoverian state provided a structured three-part course: first, fundamental mathematics, then military engineering (fortification, artillery, attack and defense tactics), and finally civil engineering. In 1707, nearby Bohemia boasted the relatively early establishment of the Institute of Engineering Education in Prague.

On unification of the separate states, a turning point in engineering came around 1810 with the educational system reforms introduced by Wilhelm von Humboldt, essentially to increase productivity nationally, and based on *Bildung*—a rounded education (character development). The first universities in the Germany region had been Heidelberg (1386) and Munich (1472); these were both preceded by the relatively nearby Charles University (1348) in Prague. Other classical universities followed. The first universities in the Germany region were Heidelberg (1386) and Munich (1472); these were both preceded by the relatively nearby Charles University (1348) in Prague. Other classical universities followed, but those teaching engineering were mostly polytechnics and trade schools in the early to mid-1800s, spearheaded by Humboldtian reforms, produced Universities of Berlin (1809–10), Karlsruhe—polytechnic (1825), Dresden (Technical Institute, 1928), Stuttgart (1829 as a trade school), Hanover (Leibniz University Hannover, 1831), and Darmstadt (1877).

Before the turn of the 18th century, Russian engineering capability was thought by some to have lagged behind that of Europe (Davies 2013). On coming to power, Peter the Great addressed this by hiring the skills of typically Dutch, French, and notably Scottish military engineers, and also foreign educators; this paved the way for an eventual and remarkable catch-up in mathematics, which had hitherto been neglected. The origins of Russian engineering schools in the 1700s, such as those in Saint Petersburg: the Russian (Military) Academy in 1723 and the School of Mines in 1773, are described by Timoshenko (1956). In 1809, the Institute of the Corps of Communications Engineers, influenced by the École Polytechnique in Paris, was also established in St. Petersburg, as was the Technological Institute in 1828, specializing in mechanical and chemical engineering; these were followed by the Technical School in Moscow. Such institutions generally had five-year programs strongly emphasizing mathematics, mechanics, and physics. However, from 1875, polytechnics with four-year programs were established more broadly throughout Russia, and then beyond, to Kyiv and Warsaw in 1898. "Classical" universities had been developed in Moscow (1825) and St. Petersburg (1831), but without engineering courses at the time. Following World War I, merit-based entry to educational institutions was abandoned in favor of seemingly preferential admission for "the proletariat" regardless of capability; academic freedom and self-government were abolished. But because standards declined dramatically, competent engineering graduates came to be in short supply, and consequently, from 1933, those impositions were reversed, returning to previous academic entrance requirements. High standards of mathematics were restored to the curriculum, and five-year courses became the norm; expansion of engineering school enrolment numbers resulted in polytechnics typically being split into separate divisions of specialization.

Notwithstanding the generally low regard internationally for Russian engineering and its education at that time, McGivern (1960) notes the positive impression expressed by early engineering educators from the Massachusetts Institute of Technology (MIT) when attending trade shows and on visiting the Russian Imperial Technical Schools of St. Petersburg and Moscow (Runkle 2022).

The well-known early universities in England, Oxford University (established 1096, formally 1167) and Cambridge (1209), had curricula in "the classics"; engineering education was only introduced, as engineering sciences, in the 1900s (Tryggvason and Apelian 2006). The first engineering education in Britain was in the military engineering context, at the Woolwich Royal (Military) Academy in 1741. This comprised a curriculum of mathematics, scientific principles of gunnery and fortification, bridge building, magazine technique, and artillery work. To reach an acceptable level, the mathematics component went through some arduous evolution (Bruneau 2020). For civilian engineering in Britain, the "Apprentice-to-Master Craftsman" model of engineering education persisted until the 20th century. As in Europe, from even prior to the Italian Renaissance, formal education for the hands-on master craftsmen was essentially non-existent. To bridge this gap, made all the more apparent by the industrial revolution, in the early 1800s, the *Mechanics Institutes* concept was introduced by Professor George Birkbeck:

> *assisting mechanics in understanding the theory which underpinned their work-the understanding of the relationship between theory and practice . . . not to teach them the practical skills of their trade . . . to compensate for any lack of early education amongst mechanics.*
>
> (Scanlon 2023)

This endeavor was initially very popular and became widely established globally, but the original intent of providing education for the working person was diverted into entertainment activities for the more affluent. Other ways of addressing the educational shortfall lay in the creation of institutions such as the Royal (London) Polytechnic (1838) and notably the Woolwich Polytechnic (1890). A post-World War II catch-up in formal engineering education in Britain was possibly prompted by a recognition of the ingenuity and industrial capacity of the United States war machine to "save the day" with its production capability for fighter/bomber aircraft, warships, artillery arms, and ammunition, highlighting the need for a more systematic industrial approach. That the apprenticeship model for engineering training had persisted for so long in the United Kingdom was probably due to the fact that it was successful in the cultural environment of the time.

An overview of the continuously evolving US environment/ecosystem of engineering education responding to societal, political, and economic changes through the 19th and 20th centuries is provided thoroughly by Akera and Seely (2015). Largely following European and British classical (liberal arts) curriculum counterparts, the earliest universities in the United States were arguably Harvard in 1636 and Yale in 1701: these did not have engineering departments per se until the 1870s (Harvard) and 1900s (Yale), but engineering of a sort was taught at Harvard's Lawrence Scientific School from 1849 and from Yale's Sheffield Scientific School from 1852 (McGivern 1960). Although the University of Pennsylvania was established later (1740), this possibly third-oldest university in the United States was soon to commence engineering in 1852. However, engineering practice mostly continued to follow the English craftsman-apprenticeship model of training, necessity being the mother of invention, particularly during times of urgency in the era of expansive wilderness settlement. It was a feature of the fledgling colony to tap the opportunities, the available abundance of natural resources, communities, and availability of labor. The challenges demanded innovation.

As in Europe and Russia, both international and internal political and military events were strongly influential in the development of engineering in the United States. The War of Independence (1775–1783) prompted the establishment of the West Point Military Academy in 1802. The first actual engineering school in the United States, derived from the School for Artillerists and Engineers, was based on the Paris Ecole Polytechnique (Zelbo 2023). It provided a very definite contribution to the growth of civil engineering education at the time, much needed for the rapid generation of vital bridges, railroads, and canals. The next contributors to formalized engineering education in the United States were Rensselaer Polytechnic Institute—1824 (with civil engineering in 1828, and the first civil engineering degree granted in 1835), Norwich University—1819 (initially "Partridge's Academy," providing the first civil engineering *program* in 1821), and Union College—1795 (Jewell, Griggs, and Ressler 2001).

The American Civil War (1861–1865) further underscored the importance of engineering for military hardware and essential infrastructure such as roads and railways. Importantly, the withdrawal of the southern states from the federal legislative process during that time enabled unopposed passage of the 1862 Morrill-Wade Land-Grant Colleges Act, providing opportunity for development of state colleges emphasizing agriculture and "Mechanical Arts" (engineering), though not excluding other studies. Paving the way for the provision of accessible state-based education resulted in a more standardized four-year engineering degree, which highlighted practical skills; the Morrill Act was pivotal to the expansion of engineering in the United States.

Mechanical Engineering was initiated in 1854 at the Pennsylvania State Polytechnic College, at Yale University in 1863, at MIT in 1865, at Worcester Polytechnic Institute in 1868, and at the Stevens Institute of Technology in 1871.

Grayson (1977) observes that mechanical engineering colleges either "*emphasized more of the theoretical concepts in higher mathematics, research, and general science*" or else instead highlighted "*practical shop work producing capable machinists and shop foreman.*" From around 1885, the balance started turning toward didactic classroom teaching of the former, augmented with some laboratory learning, but in the short term, this was by no means implemented uniformly.

According to Terman (1976), the first department of *electrical engineering* was organized at the University of Missouri in 1886, and others at the University of Wisconsin (1891) and Stanford (1892). Under physics at MIT, "*an alternative course in physics . . ." for ". . . Any of the branches of electrical engineering*" commenced in 1882. In 1884, the program (still under physics) was renamed electrical engineering, and in 1902, MIT organized an electrical engineering department in its own right. According to Grayson (1977): "*Electrical engineering followed as an outgrowth of physics departments evolving from the scientific toward the technical rather than in the reverse direction, as did the earlier branches of engineering education.*" Grayson also discusses *Chemical Engineering*, as: "*similar to electrical engineering in that it evolved from a scientific rather than from a technical base.*"

Individual variations in regional and philosophical differences that governed the pedagogical approaches remained throughout the 1900s, with some compromises between "the classroom and the workshop" approach. As Tryggvason and Apelian (2006) have it:

> the theoretical foundation emphasized by the French ecoles and the practical hands-on attitude of the British, permeated across the Atlantic and impacted the development of engineering education in the United States. Although it is possible to argue that the marriage of theory and practice played no small part in the phenomenal successes of U.S. engineering in the 20th century, finding the right mix occupied engineering educators throughout the century.

But by the turn of the 20th century, laboratory instruction had come to predominate, though around this time, prior to World War I (1914–1918), the focus was on innovation driven by scientific progress. Fueled by the improved maritime, burgeoning automotive and nascent aviation industries, inevitably in wartime, improved materials and streamlined production methods, and that led to military weapon and defense capability development, and innovations such as sonar. The World War I period gave rise to radio broadcasting and communication to supplement the telephone.

The 1920s boom decade following World War I saw visits to America and consequent emigration of a number of European luminaries fostering scientific-industrial collaborations and boosting the local science culture (Akera and Seely 2015); these included the famous Hungarian aerospace engineer Theodore Von Karman and Ukrainian mechanical engineer Stephan Timoshenko. However, the mainstream engineering workforce at the time had tended to be more business-oriented rather than technology-oriented, but in the Great Depression of the ensuing 1930s decade, this moderated to a more enlightened management approach. Concurrently, poor employment prospects for engineering graduates resulted in a more than doubling of postgraduate enrolments for some engineering fields, somewhat restoring a scientific focus (Terman 1976).

The war effort surrounding World War II (1939–1945) produced new inventions, such as nuclear weapons, radar, microwaves, control and guidance systems, navigation, and improvements to existing communications. In the wake of the war, the legacies of these innovations were nuclear power, television, and all manner of domestic appliances, as well as further refinements to automotive and aviation transport. The following 1950s and 1960s decades saw satellite communication, commercial/domestic television, semiconductors, computers, and space travel.

Clearly, engineering had a central role in these developments, and the form of supporting education came largely from the mathematical engineering science model, at a higher, postgraduate level. It was here that the research-intensive universities, such as MIT and Stanford, with their substantial industrial affiliations, played a significant part.

1.3 THE ADVENT OF THE BIOMEDICAL ENGINEERING DISCIPLINE

It can be argued that activities in biomedical engineering well preceded the commencement of any formal engineering schools. For example, having accomplishments straddling between engineering, medicine, physiology, and anatomy, the intellectually versatile Leonardo da Vinci could be considered one of the earliest biomedical engineers (West 2017), though education in biomedical engineering (and indeed any formalized engineering training) clearly did not exist in his time. Geddes (1977) lists some 20 or so others, such as Seebeck, Poiseuille, Helmholtz, and Einthoven, who were nominally physicians but provided significant contributions in what can be understood to be precursory biomedical engineering.

The formation of biomedical engineering as a discipline proceeded from Galvani's pioneering electrophysiology experiments of the 18th century, then from the turn of the 20th-century investigations with radiation physics to the more recent applications of computing to intensive care. In the mid-1800s, specific interests in electrophysiology had given rise to biophysics in Germany. The so-called "1847 group" (Geddes 1977), the "Berlin Medical Materialists" (which included Helmholtz), achieved notoriety but had met with stiff opposition to their bold intention: "We four imagined that we should constitute physiology on a chemico-physical foundation" . . . "much more difficult than we had anticipated" (Cranefield 1957). However, along with Helmholtz's ongoing work, that had helped establish biophysics in Germany.

Herman Schwann was a significant identity in the initial establishment of biomedical engineering research and education, first in Germany and later in the United States (Foster 2002). In 1937, he had joined the Kaiser Wilhelm (Max Planck) Institute for Biophysics, associated with the University of Frankfurt, where he completed his PhD on the high-frequency dielectric properties of tissue, particularly blood. One of the German-born post-World War II immigrants, as referred to by Akera and Seely (2015), he moved to the United States in 1947. He states that formal training had existed at the Institute, "where an early Ph.D. program in biophysics was established in the late 30s. Research topics included primarily electrophysiology, ionizing radiation bioeffects, and relevant technologies. No clear distinction existed then between bioengineering, medical physics and biophysics" (Schwan 1991). He had earlier explained, "The meaning of medical physics today is largely restricted to activities concerned with ionizing radiation and, increasingly, imaging techniques . . . The split between biophysics and bioengineering first occurred after 1957" (Schwan 1984). The first use of the actual term *bioengineering* was claimed to be by Heinz Wolff in 1954 (Overy and Tansey 2016).

The term "biomedical engineering" had started to appear in the literature around 1960; according to Brown (1991), it was claimed to have been firmly defined in that decade: "Otto Schmitt and I . . . tried every combination of medical, clinical, and biological terms with engineering, and finally decided that the field was most suitably named 'biomedical engineering,' because it represented most of the identified interests."

Geddes (1977) had elaborated on definitions:

> *Biomedical engineering is concerned with the use of engineering principles and practices in the search for new knowledge of life processes that have application to the cure and control of disease and to the support of life if there is a deficit after the disease process has been arrested. Biomedical engineering activities are therefore linked with and supportive of human and animal medicine and can be found both in a college of engineering and a clinic or hospital"* whereas *"Bioengineering deals with the application of the tools and analytical techniques of engineering to the investigation of living processes . . . Bioengineering activities exist in both engineering and life-science institutions and need not, in general, involve a close contact with human or animal patients.*

Differentiation of the overall generic term is also provided by Bronzino (2011): "consider the terms biomedical engineering, bioengineering, biological engineering, and clinical (or medical) engineer . . . bioengineering is usually defined as a basic-research oriented activity . . . The term biomedical engineering appears to have the most comprehensive meaning." Bronzino further explained, "When a biomedical engineer works within a hospital or clinic, he or she is more properly called a clinical engineer," but appeared to hint at ambiguity between "clinical engineer" and "medical engineer."

The National Academy of Engineering (NAE) (EBM Training Committee of the NIH, 1972) definitions distinguishing these subspecialties are reported by Shaffer (1985): "medical engineering (developing and designing the devices in the industrial environment)" and "clinical engineering (servicing and supporting the devices in the hospital)." Shaffer indicates that they understate the scope of clinical engineering, which extends well beyond corrective and preventative maintenance (under direction and supervision by graduate clinical engineers) to *Planning, Purchasing, New installations, Orientation/in-service training, Evaluation, and Design,* into more sophisticated technology management and design (recently, it has come to have involvement with information technology convergence, device interoperability, and electronic medical records). "Clinical" engineering and "industrial medical engineering" historically share common skillsets, body of knowledge, and body of practice, particularly in technical fundamentals as well as in areas of performance and regulatory standards, and risk and quality management (Pallikarakis et al. 2017); in that sense, the two could be regarded as being along a compatible continuum.

Although not appearing as a biomedical engineering subspecialty in the 1972 NAE list, Rehabilitation Engineering is another such important subdiscipline within Biomedical Engineering (Szeto 2005); its presence is said to have been proposed in the United States around 1970. Paraphrasing the Engineers Australia National Committee for Rehabilitation (2020),

> A rehabilitation engineer is a professional engineer applying informed theory and practice, often in collaboration with a multidisciplinary team, including specialised knowledge and application of technologies to safeguard and improve the quality of life of people who use or would benefit from Assistive Technology.

In many countries, rehabilitation engineers and clinical engineers are not yet required to be registered or licensed to practice, but are globally recognized as identifiable vocations.

Referring back to Figure 1.1, which depicted the traditional engineering subdisciplines, electrical, mechanical, and chemical engineering, the biomedical engineering subdisciplines, clinical engineering, rehabilitation engineering, and bioengineering can be visualized through a similar lens (Figure 1.2). Clinical engineering can be considered to have developed from electrical engineering, rehabilitation engineering to have derived from mechanical engineering, and bioengineering to have originated mostly from chemical and materials engineering. Note the possibility of overlap where there is interaction between subdisciplines, or shared features, for example, all three subdisciplines require a common core knowledge of physiology/life sciences in addition to mainstream engineering common core concepts.

Newer specialized domains in biomedical engineering (Figure 1.3) are depicted by Bronzino (2011), commenting: "The field has moved significantly from being

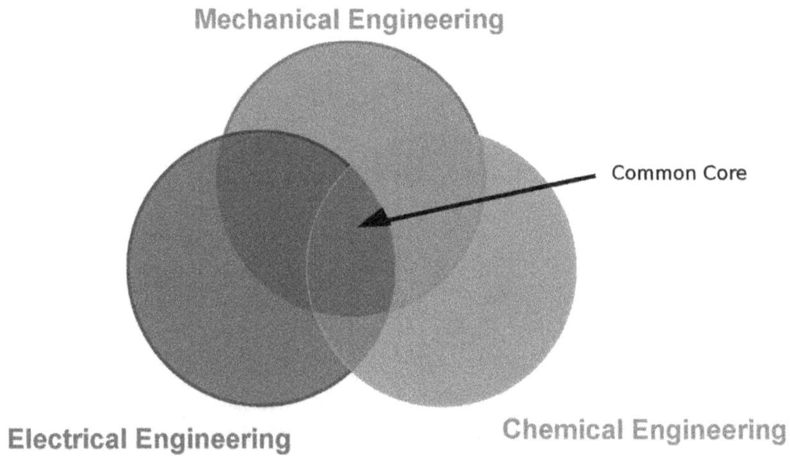

FIGURE 1.1 Disciplines evolved from civil engineering.

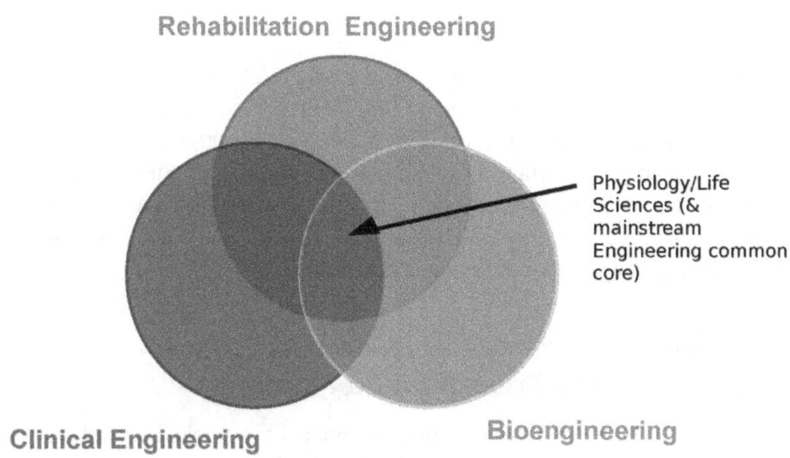

FIGURE 1.2 Biomedical engineering subspecialties.

concerned primarily with the development of medical devices in the 1950s and 1960s to include a more wide-ranging set of activities . . . biomedical engineering now includes many new career areas."

To some extent, these different specialized domains can be classifiable into groups corresponding to the biomedical engineering subdisciplines defined earlier (and with possible reference to their core originating traditional engineering subdisciplines). For example, biomechanics and prosthetics have their origins in mechanical engineering and thus could fall under rehabilitation engineering. Clinical engineering can include biomedical instrumentation and biosensors, having their underpinnings in electrical engineering, although sensing has been a major topic for bioengineering,

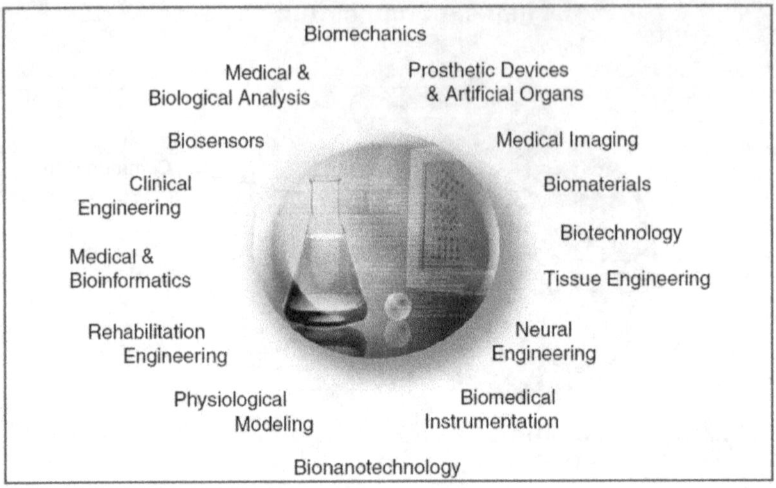

FIGURE 1.3 "The world of biomedical engineering" (Bronzino 2011).

as well as being used in rehabilitation. Likewise, we might suggest that biomaterials, biotechnology, tissue engineering, neural engineering, and bionanotechnology fall into the bioengineering classification (Desai and Magin 2001), though neural engineering would also be important for rehabilitation engineering. Such subdisciplinary clustering of the specialized domains within the greater Biomedical Engineering landscape may provide economies, vocational identity and visibility, and convenience in employment, credentialing, and education.

1.3.1 The Evolution of Biomedical Engineering Education and How It Has Traditionally Been Taught

Biomedical engineering and its educational support have tracked with the evolution of other engineering disciplines. Just as the US blend of theory and practice set the standard for engineering in general, so it may also be said that the United States has proven to be the lead yardstick in setting the running for biomedical engineering and its teaching, providing scholarship in its teaching and research.

1.3.1.1 Biomedical Engineering Education Globally

The World Health Organization (2017) has provided a review of the education and training of Biomedical Engineers globally, with some new insights. Core curriculum and elective specialization are listed for a number of countries within the Americas (27 countries), Africa (25 countries), the Eastern Mediterranean (12 countries), Europe (40 countries), Southeast Asia (10 countries), and Western Pacific (15 countries).

Unsurprisingly, the United States dominates the listings for the Americas: quoted figures for 2015 (see Table 1.1) are 157 undergraduate, 139 master's, and 126 PhD

TABLE 1.1
Countries reporting biomedical engineering programs active in 2015, in order of GDP per capita, and their different biomedical engineering education programs

Country	2015 Approximate Population (millions)	Program			
		Bachelor	Masters	PhD	Other (e.g., BMET)
Switzerland	8.3	–	2	1	–
Norway	5.2	–	1	–	–
Ireland	4.7	–	3	–	–
United States	321.4	157	139	126	11
Australia	24.0	7	6	4	1
Singapore	5.6	2	–	–	6
Denmark	5.7	1	3	1	–
Iceland	0.33	1	–	–	–
Sweden	9.8	1	3	1	–
Netherlands	16.9	1	4	2	–
United Kingdom	64.7	3	13	3	–
Austria	8.5	3	5	1	–
Canada	35.9	11	15	15	9
Finland	5.5	1	5	2	–
Germany	80.7	32	32	1	–
Belgium	11.3	1	4	1	–
New Zealand	4.5	1	1	–	–
France	64.4	–	4	1	–
Israel	8.1	3	3	4	–
Italy	59.8	13	14	10	6
Spain	46.1	–	5	5	–
Slovenia	2.0	–	–	1	–
Portugal	10.3	1	2	1	–
Greece	11.0	2	2	0	–
Czech Republic	10.5	4	4	3	–
Trinidad and Tobago	1.4	1	–	–	–
Estonia	1.3	–	2	2	–
Slovakia	5.4	2	2	1	–
Uruguay	3.41	–	–	–	1
Lithuania	2.9	–	1	–	–
Argentina	43.4	10	1	–	1
Chile	17.9	2	1	–	–
Latvia	2.0	1	2	2	–
Panama	3.9	2	–	–	–
Poland	38.6	1	1	1	–
Hungary	9.9	–	1	–	–
Croatia	4.2	1	1	–	–

(Continued)

TABLE 1.1 (Continued)
Countries reporting biomedical engineering programs active in 2015, in order of GDP per capita, and their different biomedical engineering education programs

Country	2015 Approximate Population (millions)	Program			
		Bachelor	Masters	PhD	Other (e.g., BMET)
Türkiye	78.7	4	6	2	–
Venezuela	31.1	1	2	–	–
Malaysia	30.3	2	1	–	–
Mexico	127	28	2	4	–
Russian Federation	143.5	3	–	–	–
Romania	19.5	–	1	–	–
Brazil	208	8	4	3	–
China	1376	153	108	92	–
Cuba	11.4	2	3	3	–
Bulgaria	7.1	1	1	1	–
Colombia	48.2	10	1	1	–
Belarus	9.44	2	2	2	–
Peru	31.4	1	1	–	–
South Africa	54.5	2	3	3	–
Serbia	8.9	–	–	1	–
Iran	82.6	6	6	3	–
Jordan	7.6	1	–	–	–
El Salvador	6.1	1	–	–	–
Armenia	2.9	1	2	1	–
Indonesia	257.6	4	5	1	–
Bolivia	10.7	2	–	–	–
Nigeria	182.2	6	–	–	6
Moldova	4.1	1	1	–	–
Ukraine	44.8	3	2	–	–
Ghana	27.4	2	–	–	2
Kenya	47.9	–	–	–	3
Cameroon	23.3	1	2	–	2
Zambia	16.3	–	–	–	1
Senegal	14.4	–	–	–	1
Benin	10.6	–	–	–	1
Tanzania	51.5	–	–	–	2
Uganda	39	1	–	–	1
Ethiopia	99.4	2	1	–	3
Rwanda	11.4	–	–	–	1
Burkina Faso	18.1	–	–	–	2
Mozambique	26.6	–	–	–	1
Madagascar	24.2	1	–	–	1
Malawi	17	1	–	–	1

Source: adapted from World Health Organization (2017)

programs, with 11 further programs listed as "other," likely mostly biomedical equipment technology (BMET) level. Countries such as the United States, Switzerland, Ireland, the Netherlands, and Germany tended to be those that are home to multinational biomedical companies and, to some extent, exhibit a greater proportion of higher degrees in their program offerings; developing countries tended to have more commitment to biomedical technologist/technician programs, to support local maintenance of equipment rather than necessarily replacement.

1.3.1.1.1 BME Education in North America

1.3.1.1.1.1 BME Education in the United States Schwan (1984) contended that the first biomedical engineering program was at the Ostwalt Institute for Physics in Medicine, where he had been based in Germany, in conjunction with the University of Frankfurt:

> a doctoral program leading to a Ph.D. degree in biophysics was in existence by the late 1930's . . . directed primarily toward physicists and engineers. A mathematical training . . . and a solid elementary basis in physics were coupled with selected courses in engineering and physics at a more advanced level, chosen to adjust to the individual thesis intended.

Albeit somewhat loosely structured, apparently, there was a level of formality, though presumably tailored to the particular student:

> A variety of biophysics courses was offered which had to be taken by every student . . . reflected the material of primary interest in the Institute"—"biological effects of X-rays, electrical properties of tissues and cells and applications to medicine such as ultrashortwave diathermy, electrical accidents, and electrocardiography.

In 1947, Schwann relocated from Germany to the United States, where he established a doctoral biomedical engineering program (thesis, and coursework in medical electronics and physiology) at the University of Pennsylvania, in collaboration with Johns Hopkins University and the University of Rochester; this was implemented in the second half of 1961 with funding support of the US public health service and the National Institute of Health (NIH). Carstensen et al. (1963) describe the curriculum of the programs offered by the three universities: available preexisting life sciences courseware material supplementing a standard solid undergraduate engineering degree (thus retaining a strong engineering context), amenable to incremental adjustment, and enabling graduates to exit to broader mainstream careers if desired. The contributing universities set the time commitments in the various subject areas (with some individual variations) to approximately 35% mathematics, physics, and engineering, 30% research, 20% special courses in biomedical engineering, and the remaining 15% natural sciences (chemistry, biology, and physiology); in addition to substantial research work, the delivery to relatively small groups was mostly traditional face-to-face didactic mode. Master's by research programs (particularly for industry-employed candidates) and an undergraduate program in 1973 were also instituted (Schwan 1991).

Concurrently, a master of science course in medical instrumentation at Drexel University was also funded by NIH (Le Croissette 1961; Sun and Schwan 1990; Sun 1991). This was for medical graduates (to undertake mathematics, physics, electrical circuits, and electronics), and engineering graduates (to study anatomy, biology, and biophysics), prior to jointly undergoing courses in medical physics, electronics, systems engineering, radioisotope methodology, physical chemistry, data handling, medical instrumentation, biophysics, and a thesis (generally in a hospital setting). The description of the cohort sizes (e.g., two medicos and four engineers), and that they were even listed by name, suggests that in the very early runs of the program, the delivery method of teaching would likely be self-study and tutorial style, if not one-to-one. As the intake size grew, in later years, this very likely would have changed to a more didactic lecture approach.

In addition to noting the master's degree program at Drexel University, Nebeker (2001) mentions two other biomedical engineering education programs in the mid-1950s, for which the details are elusive: a doctoral-level "medical engineering" set up by R. Stuart Mackay at the University of California, and a master's degree at Iowa State University. Nebeker (2001) had previously mentioned that there were 40 universities in the United States with biomedical engineering programs in 1965, and 180 by 1971, when undergraduate programs had started to become popular. However, from a poll of 251 universities in 1979–1980, Potvin et al. (1981) found there were only 126 universities offering "degree and minor or option programs in biomedical engineering (including clinical engineering)"—41 undergraduate programs including those that were yet-to-be accredited by the US Accreditation Board for Engineering and Technology (ABET) (only six were actually accredited at that time), as well as 41 PhD and 48 masters.

An appraisal of biomedical engineering programs over the period 1995–2000 at undergraduate, master's, and PhD levels is found in Harris, Bransford, and Brophy (2002). This includes discipline definitions, trends in program details, and enrolment numbers. It lists 11 areas for attention, which had been determined from a review of programs by the National Science Foundation-sponsored VaNTH ERC in Bioengineering Educational Technologies (Vanderbilt, Northwestern, Texas, and Harvard/MIT Universities consortium Engineering Research Center). Insightful forward-thinking enhancements of curriculum and delivery of content using innovative teaching and learning approaches and emerging educational technology were presented, and some potential challenges specific to biomedical engineering were outlined. A Whitaker Foundation Summit identified appropriate key content areas: *biomechanics, bioinstrumentation, biosystems, cell/molecular engineering, biomaterials, functional genomics, biomems (biosensors), cell/tissue engineering, computational biology, and bioimaging.* Slightly subsequently, Linsenmeier, Harris, and Olds (2002) presented an update on the VaNTH project, providing a revised list of core content topics: *physiology, signals and systems analysis, instrumentation and electronics, imaging, chemical physics and thermodynamics, materials, mechanics, fluid mechanics and transport, and particular applications of mathematics (statistics and modeling).*

Linsenmeier (2003) has described the implications of further work of the VaNTH project; at the time of his writing, the number of accredited undergraduate programs had risen to 24. In the context of the number of proliferating programs at various stages of accreditation, under various disciplinarity names and different emphases, he also provided further confirmation of the biomedical/bioengineering terminology precedence:

> The term "bioengineering" was once interchangeable with "biomedical engineering," but its meaning may be evolving to describe a new biology-based discipline. . . . Humans are the system that is critical to biomedical engineers, while ecology and plant physiology are more likely to be the province of traditional biological engineers.

A further contribution from Linsenmeier was the identification of graduate employment destinations: in the early 1990s, biomedical engineering graduates went into medical schools (70%), industry (10%), or further graduate study (15%). By the early 2000s, the projected cohort intentions had changed—medical schools (21%), industry (42%), and further studies (36%); this indicated that because both further graduate study and medical school required less preparation, the industry sector should be the major employment target.

With the Whitaker Foundation soon to be wound up, Katona (2006) described the successes derived from its philanthropic contributions to biomedical engineering programs from 1976. This generosity had enabled the interactions between engineering and life sciences education to evolve from having been rather arm's length in the 1960s–1980s, through to various degrees of early introduction and merging of content in the programs, similar to integration strategies used in medical education (Brauer and Ferguson 2015).

McCally (2005) describes a Master's Degree Program in Applied Biomedical Engineering, intended specifically for part-time students, which commenced at Johns Hopkins University Applied Physics Laboratory in 1993. The detailed curriculum was unambiguously focused on bioengineering as we have seen it defined, involving courses in biomaterials, molecular, cellular, tissue, and neuroengineering and a significant amount of imaging. Students were required to undertake ten single-semester courses over five years and an optional thesis. Program enrolments appeared to vary between 60 and 130 students.

An account by Hart (2015) of the period from 1975 to 2015 reports that in the 1970s, there were seven accredited undergraduate programs, some of which evolved from electrical engineering departments. In the 1980s, there were 13 new accredited programs, some of which derived from mechanical engineering or materials engineering. Accreditation flattened out during the 1990s, with only four new programs being accredited; this was followed by an uptick with a linear increase in student enrolments over the next 15 years, reaching to over 25,000 by 2013. There were 51 new programs accredited between 2000 and 2009, notably with tissue engineering as a feature, from a chemical engineering-derived base. At the time of a 2006–2007 census, 41% of graduates went into industry, 35% went on to higher degree studies, and16% went into medical school. By 2015, there were 320 engineering schools offering undergraduate biomedical engineering compared with 120 medical schools. The ongoing support of the Whitaker Foundation was noted.

Linsenmeier and Saterbak (2020) then followed up with a very comprehensive and thorough historical review of BME education in the United States over the half-century since inception. They noted that as of 2017, there were 118 active accredited undergraduate programs (roughly one-third of the number for mechanical or electrical engineering, and two-thirds of chemical engineering). This suggests that the total as reported in World Health Organization (2017), 157, might have included as-yet unaccredited programs.

The 2000–2020 growth of this education sector was not constant: between 1970 and 2000, the expansion had been two new accredited programs every five years; from 2000 to 2012, the rate skyrocketed to around eight per year. They comment that while mechanical, electrical, and chemical engineering were driven by industrial needs, "biomedical engineering started in academia when engineers within 'traditional' departments became interested in biomedical problems." However, it could also be argued that as the technology of hospital equipment became more sophisticated, clinical markets stimulated the need for biomedical engineering in the form of clinical engineering. The authors list drivers for curriculum change over the most recent period, such as stronger incorporation of practical skills, a global outlook, and active learning (e.g., flipped classrooms and PBL). They also included the introduction of engineering ethos early in the courseware, for example, embedding "Washington Accord" professional/personal engineering competency attributes (ethical conduct, oral/written communications, teamwork, independent problem-solving, and lifelong learning). Among academics in the field, consensus on curriculum maintenance in the light of 2019 data indicated that the core curriculum previously identified in 2004—*Introductory Engineering; Circuits, Senior Design, Instrumentation, Physiology, Computing; Additional Biology, Statistics, Mechanics, and Materials*—needed extension to include *Transport* and *Signal Analysis*. Further topics are often constructively implemented by electives such as "advanced physiology, cell and/or molecular biology, bioinformatics, tissue engineering/regenerative medicine, and applications of immunology, neural engineering, and nanotechnology." For graduate employment destinations, the authors do not refer at all to vocational employment in rehabilitation engineering or clinical engineering. An originally envisaged rule of thumb that one-third of graduates would be admitted to medical school, one-third would proceed to higher degrees, and the remaining one-third would be employed in industry, occurred only in 2010. The proportion steadily changed over the period from 1990 to 2020 and, most recently, was more like 10% into medical school, 25% pursuing higher degrees, and 60% in industry. The authors conclude by referring to the 225 national and 479 international programs as indices of the success of undergraduate biomedical engineering education.

Underscoring changes in focus, a new paradigm for bioengineering, "BME 2.0," was recently introduced by Miller et al. (2023). This highlights newly available imaging techniques and data science and would seem to be an evolution of precision bioengineering:

> BME programs that grew historically out of founding faculty trained in ChE may more quickly embrace aspects of the molecular focus, just as those BME programs founded by those trained in EE may more quickly embrace the centrality of biomedical data science for all BME students.

It is interesting that of the *Nature Biomedical Engineering* topics list, the authors omit clinical engineering, but retain rehabilitation engineering, orthopedics, and prosthetics.

1.3.1.1.1.2 BME Education in Canada Although the World Health Organization (2017) had stated, "In Canada there are 36 universities offering BME degrees, but only two offering MSc programmes in clinical engineering," they had listed only 18 universities, and six non-university programs, most likely of a Biomedical Engineering Technology nature. Earlier on, concern had been raised of a forthcoming need for clinical engineers in Canada to address a perceived looming increase in healthcare demand; Scott (1979) expressed uncertainty as to what biomedical engineering education program should entail, though the desirability of including a clinical internship or residency was noted. Programs available at the time in nine of the ten Canadian provinces were listed, mostly flexible extensions from traditional engineering disciplines, or MSc by research. Noteworthy programs were the Master of Engineering (M.Eng.) degree in Clinical Engineering offering from University of Saskatchewan, and those with some structure and potentially viable enrolments: McMaster, the University of Toronto, and the University of Montreal.

According to Knowles and DeCoito (2018), the first Canadian undergraduate biomedical engineering program to be accredited was at the University of Ottawa in 2009; there are a total of eight accredited programs of various forms, including multidisciplinary and mixed biomedical engineering with electrical or mechanical engineering.

1.3.1.1.1.3 BME Education in Mexico The first biomedical engineering courses in Mexico began in 1973 at the Universidad Iberoamericana as an outgrowth of an established electronic engineering program, and in 1974 at Universidad Autónoma Metropolitana (Azpiroz-Leehan et al. 2023). The initial interest had been research-oriented programs in engineering and mathematics applied to physiology, but from 1980, the focus switched to streams of biomechanics, medical instrumentation, or clinical engineering, particularly for providing technical support to healthcare facilities (Licona et al. 2014). From the mid-1990s, attention moved to signal and image processing, but after 2005, attempts were made to redress the apparent overweighting in the electrical engineering flavor, which had become at the expense of emerging topics such as biomaterials, tissue, and neuroengineering.

In the meantime, freshman capabilities had declined, while student intake had been politically encouraged, and by 2015, there were 50 undergraduate biomedical engineering programs in Mexico (Azpiroz-Leehan et al. 2015); by 2023, that figure had swelled to over 60. At this stage, the authors stressed the importance of capstone projects as essential for realistically acceptable programs, and more strongly the need to include courses focusing on quantitative physiology, tissue engineering, and cell and molecular biology—much along the lines of Miller's BME2.0 (Miller et al. 2023).

1.3.1.1.2 BME Education in South America

A survey, which was suggested to represent over 95% of the biomedical engineering programs in South American countries along with their educational providers (Azpiroz-Leehan et al. 2017), corresponds reasonably with the World Health Organization (WHO)'s listing for Argentina, Brazil, Bolivia, Chile, Colombia, Cuba, El Salvador, Panama, Peru, Trinidad and Tobago, Uruguay, and Venezuela (World Health Organization 2017).

Some details of the history are difficult to confirm, but we can accept that early programs were commenced in Argentina by 1985 (Valentinuzzi 1986; Valentinuzzi et al. 2010), Brazil by 2001 (da Ana and Lombello 2023), Colombia in 1999 (Soto Castaño 2009), and Chile by 2000 (Allende et al. 2007; Azpiroz-Leehan et al. 2023). These programs typically stemmed from electronic engineering, and there was an awareness that other emerging areas had been neglected (Azpiroz-Leehan et al. 2020; Gehlot 2009). By 2017, there were around 12 undergraduate programs in each of Colombia and Brazil, seven in Argentina, and two in Chile and Bolivia. There was one in each of Honduras, El Salvador, Peru, Cuba, Venezuela, Paraguay, and Ecuador, though there were also quite a number of Master's degree programs suggested (World Health Organization 2017): Brazil (4), Cuba (3), Venezuela (2), and one each in Argentina, Chile, Colombia, and Peru.

1.3.1.1.3 BME Education in Europe

The trajectory of biomedical engineering and its education in Europe are both summarized in an abstract from Edrich (1993): it

> started in Europe at approximately the same time as in the United States. . . . it grew at a slower pace, and its undergraduate and graduate programs, its research orientation, and its relationship with industry and hospitals developed differently, exhibiting even less uniformity than in the United States.

Notwithstanding the contributions of Herman Schwan and his contemporaries in Germany before and during World War 2, Meyer-Hartwig and Bleifeld (1978) contend that prior to support from the Volkswagen foundation in 1969, biomedical engineering was largely unheard of:

> Only clinical physicists in the radiological departments were well established. Hospital maintenance was performed by craftsmen or engineers from the ship building industry . . . Maintenance of equipment was performed by manufacturers or not at all. In the years prior to 1969 and for several years after, knowledge in biomedical engineering was acquired autodidactically by single engineers cooperating in research groups with physicians. Some research workers completed their training as engineers.

Pallikarakis (2022) provides a description of the early postgraduate programs in Europe as being research-based activities from the 1960s. In 1987, a collaborative graduate MSc program in Biomedical Engineering common to universities in European countries was conceived: a basic solid engineering foundation topped up with biology, anatomy, and physiology. This ran in the 1990s, influenced by the 1989 European Credit Transfer System for student mobility and the 1990 Bologna Process for standardization of tertiary education tiers. According to Pallikarakis et al. (2017), by 2000, there were 26 undergraduate programs across Europe, and by the end of 2012, 85 undergraduate programs in addition to 160 at master's and at 65 PhD level.

1.3.1.1.3.1 BME Education in France A very comprehensive account of the biomedical engineering education possibilities available in France from the early 1970s was given by Watteau (1978). This outlined the entry levels for these pathways, and institutional providers with some sketches of the curricula at the time, and their intended target markets. Another undergraduate program was described by Butterlin et al. (2007); this remarkably innovative three-year program was effectively embedded in a biomedical industrial and hospital cluster, capitalizing on the region's heritage in microtechnology.

1.3.1.1.3.2 BME Education in Italy An interview with Riccardo Pietrabissa (President of Italy's National Bioengineering Group) by Reynolds (2015) provides an accessible account of the history of biomedical engineering education in Italy, commencing in 1968 with classwork supporting research at the Polytechnic University in Milan, and then in other large Italian cities. From the first undergraduate programs at the Polytechnic of Milan and the University of Genova in 1995, by 2014, in Italy, there were 13 (three-year) undergraduate programs and 14 master's degree (five-year) programs in biomedical engineering.

Baselli and Cerutti (2011) elaborated on the history and interdisciplinary nature of Milan Polytechnic's Bioengineering Department, describing its teaching and research and design directions, and how it interacted and articulated with the departments of other disciplines. Baselli (2009) had presented a history of the development of the initial BME education programs at Milan from 1971: courses within mechanical engineering and electrical engineering in 1975; a doctorate in bioengineering in 1983; and in 1990, a two- or three-year diploma in BME in addition to the previously established five-year engineering programs. The relative merits of transitioning from an earlier five-year program to a 3 + 2 "double cycle" Bachelor's and then Master's program, aligning with the Bologna protocol, were discussed; the rationale of careful compromises was viewed by the authors as positive opportunities rather than restrictions. The two-year master's degree is provided in four separate tracks: Clinical Engineering; a "Biomechanics/biomaterials" track that encompasses most Rehabilitation Engineering topics; a "Biotechnolgies" track that corresponds with Bioengineering as we have described it earlier, and a fourth track largely congruent with "Medical Engineering" as described by Shaffer (1985) apparently following mostly electrical engineering with biomedical options. Outlines of the courses/subjects in the curriculum are provided in detail, and the phasing of mathematics and sciences in the three-year program is described, along with well-staged engineering and applied biomedical topics.

1.3.1.1.3.3 BME Education in the Netherlands Bekkering (1972) describes how medical physics in the Netherlands arose from the Dutch Biophysics Foundation (established in Delft in 1932) and from 1938 was championed by Hans Burger, somewhat akin to Hermann Schwan's involvement with the Frankfurt Institute for Biophysics. Biomedical engineering education was delivered via the Delft University of Technology, the Eindhoven University of Technology (TU/e), and the University of Twente (UT). The individual contributions of these have been described by Uijt de Haag et al. (2002) as Biotechnology at Delft, Biomedical Engineering at TU/e, and Biomedical Technology at UT. A detailed description of the two programs offered at Eindhoven has been outlined by Slaaf and van Genderen (2009): both were three-year bachelor's degree programs leading into two-year master's degrees; one simply titled "Biomedical Engineering" was more research-based, and the other, termed "Medical Engineering," was intended for clinical/industrial application.

1.3.1.1.3.4 BME Education in Scandinavia Scandinavia has had a rich history in biomedical engineering. In Sweden, Henry Wallman arrived from MIT (United States) in 1948 to the Chalmers University of Technology, Göteborg, established in 1937 (McKelvey and Saemundsson 2025); his important developments in clinical devices and medical imaging signaled the potential advantages of having engineering expertise in hospitals. Kadefors (1977) describes the introduction of biomedical engineers in Swedish healthcare, noting that the engineering activities initially undertaken were in essence medical electronics. At that time, there were four regional educational centers, each with their slightly different emphases, located at Göteborg (Chalmers Institute of Technology), Lund (Lund Institute of Technology and University of Lund), Stockholm (Royal Institute of Technology and Karolinska Institute), and Linköping (University of Linköping). Kadefors also notes biomedical engineering programs in Denmark (Copenhagen, Aalborg), Finland (Helsinki, Tampere), and Norway (Trondheim). Dremstrup and Elberg (2008) describe the five-year program at Aalborg in Denmark. PBL, long championed at Aalborg University, is featured strongly throughout all years of the program. The first three years of the program are basic standard material packaged around PBL projects: first semester "Pilot project" a Health Technology Assessment, second semester "Interpretation of biological signals," third semester "Recording & presentation of biological signals," fourth semester "Processing biological signals," and the fifth and sixth semesters, in the third year, are undertaken in a hospital/clinical environment: "Analysis of health technology in hospital settings" and "Design of biomedical systems." The seventh and eighth semesters are in the specializations (*Medical Systems, Medical Informatics, Biomechanics,* or *Drug Delivery* and *Tissue Technology*). The ninth and tenth semesters occupy the Master's thesis project. This partially embedded program has been extremely successful, producing versatile job-ready biomedical engineers.

1.3.1.1.3.5 BME Education in the United Kingdom (England, Scotland, Wales, and Northern Ireland) In the United Kingdom, as was the case for Germany, the early trajectory of biomedical engineering was somewhat blurred by the contribution from medical physics. Gergely (1979) observed:

> use of x-rays for medical diagnosis led to the employment of physicists in hospitals in the early part of this century . . . the workload of physicists increased and Departments of Medical Physics were established. It was therefore a quite natural development for many of these departments to accept responsibility for the new electronic equipment. . . . Consequently, a new area of specialisation evolved called Medical

> Electronics . . . many of the old Departments of Medical Physics now include the word "Bio Engineering" in their new title.

Heinz Wolff, the "father of bioengineering," observed

> at one time hospital physicists were almost entirely oriented toward radiotherapy, but there is now a tendency for them to take up bioengineering, and concern themselves with the maintenance and design of instruments for use in medical research and treatment.
>
> (Wolff 1970)

The earliest acknowledged biomedical engineering programs established in the United Kingdom were at Imperial College London in the 1960s, the University of Strathclyde, Glasgow, in 1962, and the University College London (UCL) around 1990. After having hosted postgraduate level research, these institutions ultimately initiated undergraduate programs: Imperial College in 2002, Strathclyde in 2012 (with a coupled B.Eng./M.Eng.), and UCL in 2014 (listings of the current curricula of these universities can be accessed at their websites). The acceptance of British BEng programs for chartered status under the Washington Accord was complicated by their usually three-year duration for admission to the incorporated engineer (technologist) level: to achieve chartered status typically calls for topping up with a one-year master's degree, and sometimes a period of industrial experience.

Other undergraduate-level programs had been implemented earlier. Gergely (1979) presents a reasonably detailed course plan of a four-year "sandwich degree" in biomedical electronics that was offered at Lanchester Polytechnic in Coventry. The curriculum and timeline involving 68 weeks of practical training with a company or hospital are presented. For the duration of the program, life sciences units were integrated throughout for the biomedical track, while a parallel mainstream engineering track took conventional options. According to Gergely:

> Someone working in the field of biomedical electronics has to be a good electronic engineer first and foremost, and not someone with an insufficient knowledge of two or more subjects who is unable to do useful work . . . An understanding of the basic processes of biology and physiology and of the elements of anatomy is also important. An appreciation of the language, methodology and thought processes of doctors and biologists is a similarly important aid in the establishment of the good communications between the two groups, which is so necessary for their successful cooperation.

Another such program, "Electronics with Medical Instrumentation," which commenced in 1978 at the University of Sussex, is described in Jones (1980). Having evolved from "Physics with a Minor in Medical Physics," the proffered curriculum bore strong similarities to Gergely's program at Lanchester Polytechnic. It is noteworthy that although biomedical engineering is no longer offered as an undergraduate program at Sussex per se, there is now a one-year (full-time) Master of Science program in place; the final year project that was previously stewarded by the University's Graduate Division of Biomedical Engineering is generally now hosted by the collaborating Brighton and Sussex Medical School.

In 2009, Joyce (2009a) surveyed "medical engineering" programs in the United Kingdom that had "significant medical engineering components" and hence were eligible for accreditation by the Institute of Mechanical Engineers. Of the 14 such programs available in the United Kingdom, seven had a strictly mechanical engineering core for the first two years, with no biomedical engineering or physiology options. Four were four-year undergraduate biomedical engineering programs, and others were three undergraduate years plus one-year master's degree programs: in essence, the three-year undergraduate programs required a further one-year master's degree to qualify for accreditation as chartered engineering qualifications. For a companion survey of mechanical engineering-based medical engineering *master's* degree programs, Joyce (2009b) followed up with 19 UK-based institutions in 2008, noting that accreditation of many of these was now being provided by the Institute of Physics and Engineering in Medicine. Detailed curricula of both the undergraduate and postgraduate programs are provided.

1.3.1.1.4 BME Education in Africa

According to the World Health Organization (2017) survey, undergraduate biomedical engineering education for Africa is offered in Nigeria (six programs), South Africa (two programs), Ethiopia (two programs), and Ghana (two programs), with Cameroon, Madagascar, Malawi, and Uganda offering one program each. Additionally, Master's degree programs are offered in South Africa, Cameroon, and Ethiopia. PhD programs are offered by three universities in South Africa; all other African countries listed so far also offer programs listed as "other" (presumably BMET category).

1.3.1.1.4.1 BME Education in South Africa In 1974, an independent Department of Bioengineering at the University of Cape Town Medical School was formed from the earlier Department of Medical Physics and Bioengineering (Davis and Jaros 1988). This worked in conjunction with the Groote Schuur Hospital to provide support to patient care in rehabilitation and physiological monitoring, to develop medical devices, and to educate biomedical engineers (Douglas 2012). Postgraduate (honors, master's, and PhD) academic programs, tailored from various courses to individual students, were offered to suitable candidates, including medical graduates.

Since then, the University of Stellenbosch has also offered postgraduate only biomedical engineering programs, though the University of Witwatersrand in Johannesburg provides undergraduate biomedical engineering, and the University of Technology in Pretoria offers undergraduate clinical engineering in addition to master's and PhD (World Health Organization 2017).

1.3.1.1.4.2 BME Education in Nigeria For the very populous country Nigeria, there has been an imperative of necessary support for medical and clinical devices; the challenges have been responded to pragmatically, strategically, and systematically, with clinical engineering in the first instance. The first undergraduate biomedical engineering program, commenced in 2007 (Nkuma-Udah et al. 2015), was, in fact, a Bachelor of Technology. According to Oyejide et al. (2025), at the time of their writing, there were seven active undergraduate degree programs, as well as master's degrees from the University of Lagos (from 2013 to 2014) and University of Ibadan (from 2017); curriculum sketches are provided.

1.3.1.1.5 BME Education in the Asia-Pacific

An overview of the BME programs in ten Asia-Pacific countries has been given by Lin et al. (2016), contrasting such features as comparative resourcing, student throughput, and graduate destinations, though brief on curriculum information. Several of the programs related to Clinical Engineering and their implementation generally lagged well behind those of the United States. The background to the biomedical industry in Japan and the relatively late commencement for its education programs is described by Tamura (2015), along with some curriculum details.

The list of participants of Lin et al.'s survey included China, Hong Kong, Indonesia, Japan, Korea, Malaysia, Mongolia, Singapore, Taiwan, and Thailand, but omitted Australia, Indonesia, and New Zealand, whereas the World Health Organization survey lacked data from Japan, Hong Kong, Korea, Mongolia, Taiwan, and Thailand. For those countries in both surveys, Lin's figure for the number of universities with BME programs roughly corresponds with the World Health Organization (2017) listings of the number of undergraduate programs for that particular country, giving partial confidence with the figures.

China's delayed start into the sector, and how it has been catching up to cater for its very large population, is discussed openly by Weng, Niu, and Fan (2009); 153 undergraduate, 108 master's, and 92 PhD programs (WHO 2017). With a population approximately one-fifth that of China's, Indonesia's four undergraduate, five master's, and one PhD program are disproportionate (likewise Malaysia's two undergraduate and one master's program are better, but still not proportionate).

Singapore has two undergraduate and six non-degree programs; the curriculum of the National University of Singapore's (NUS's) exemplary four-year accredited undergraduate program, featuring tailored career pathways, industry placement, and overseas exchange opportunities, is described in Toh (2016). The balance is perhaps similar for New Zealand (one undergrad and one master's program).

Australia has seven undergraduate, six master's, and four PhD biomedical engineering programs, and with a (2015) population of 24 million, seems to be comparatively well accommodated. The history, recent background, and current status of Australian biomedical engineering education are reviewed succinctly by Dokos (2015), in particular detailing the Graduate School of Biomedical Engineering at the University of New South Wales (UNSW) (Farrell, Flicker, and Svensson 1983).

1.4 SUMMARY

The history of the development of biomedical engineering and how it has been taught has been presented in the context of the biomedical engineering discipline and subdisciplines.

Initially, engineers were military engineers who did civil engineering in peacetime, or civil engineers who did military engineering during times of war. As technology advanced, most strikingly with phases of the industrial revolution, the specializations of mechanical engineering, electrical engineering, and chemical engineering evolved.

Engineering schooling initially took place "on the job," master and apprentice, though the classroom afforded some economies of time and resources. But that didn't suit everybody, and gave rise to "theory versus practice" tensions. Ultimately, "the workshop vs. the classroom" became "the workshop *and* the classroom."

Applying engineering methods to different problems in biology and medicine gave rise to a new "body of knowledge and ways of doing," which worked best if there was some understanding of biological processes, and mutually understandable language for communication with biologists and clinicians. Including those capabilities, biomedical engineering became recognized as a distinct discipline. Depending on the nature of the "different problems in biology and medicine," a solution using mechanical engineering, electrical engineering, or chemical engineering might be more appropriate; rehabilitation engineering largely spun out of mechanical engineering, clinical engineering from electrical/electronic engineering, and bioengineering from chemical/materials engineering.

Biomedical engineering and its educational support have tracked with the evolution of other engineering disciplines. Education specific to biomedical engineering and how it has been adapted for some different sample regions has been highlighted, typically following the path of engineering development through Europe to the United States and illustrating how it moved on from there.

REFERENCES

Akera, A., and B. Seely. 2015. "A Historical Survey of the Structural Changes in the American System of Engineering Education." In *International Perspectives on Engineering Education*, edited by S. Christensen, C. Didier, A. Jamison, M. Meganck, C. Mitcham and B. Newberry. Cham: Springer.

Allende, R., D. Morales, G. Avendano, and S. Chabert. 2007. "Biomedical Engineering Undergraduate Education in Latin America." *Journal of Physics: Conference Series* 90: 012019.

Azpiroz-Leehan, J., F. Martínez-Licona, E. G. Urbina-Medal, M. Cadena-Méndez, and E. Sacristán Rock. 2015. "Critical Assessment and Outlook for the 50 Biomedical Engineering Undergraduate Programs in Mexico." In *Annual International Conference of the IEEE Engineering in Medicine and Biology Society (EMBC)*, 3973–76. https://doi.org/10.1109/EMBC.2015.7319264

Azpiroz-Leehan, J., F. Martínez-Licona, E. G. Urbina-Medal, M. Cadena-Méndez, and E. Sacristán Rock. 2017. "Biomedical Engineering in Latin America: A Survey of 90 Undergraduate Programs." In *VII Latin American Congress on Biomedical Engineering CLAIB 2016*, edited by I. Torres, J. Bustamante and D. Sierra. Bucaramanga, Santander, Colombia, October 26–28th, 2016. *IFMBE Proceedings*, vol 60. Springer, Singapore. https://doi.org/10.1007/978-981-10-4086-3_27

Azpiroz-Leehan, J., E. Sacristan-Rock, G. Urbina-Medal, and F. M. Martinez-Licona. 2020. "Updating the Biomedical Engineering Curriculum in Latin America: Moving from Management and Maintenance to Design and Development of Medical Devices." In *42nd Annual International Conference of the IEEE Engineering in Medicine & Biology Society (EMBC)*, 6028–31. https://doi.org/10.1109/EMBC44109.2020.9175362

Azpiroz-Leehan, J., E. Sacristan-Rock, G. Urbina-Medal, and F. M. Martinez-Licona. 2023. "Fifty Years of Biomedical Engineering Undergraduate Education in Mexico and Latin America: Results, Reflections and Perspectives." In *45th Annual International*

Conference of the IEEE Engineering in Medicine and Biology Society (EMBC), 1–5. https://doi.org/10.1109/EMBC40787.2023.10340115

Baselli, G. 2009. "Biomedical Engineering Education at Politecnico di Milano: Development and Recent Changes." *Proceedings of the Institution of Mechanical Engineers. Part H, Journal of Engineering in Medicine* 223: 399–406. https://doi.org/10.1243/09544119JEIM511.

Baselli, G., and S. Cerutti. 2011. "20 Years of the Bioengineering Department at the Politecnico, Milano, and Beyond." *IEEE Pulse* 2 (3): 12–15.

Bekkering, D. H. 1972. "Invited Paper: The History of Biomedical Education in the Netherlands." *Medical & Biological Engineering* 10 (5): 579–83. https://doi.org/10.1007/BF02474161.

Bianchi, P., and P. Cornaglia. 2014. "A Cultural Crossroads Between the Court and the City. The Case of the Royal Academy of Turin, the Capital of the Savoyard State." In *International Conference on Urban History, Lisbon, 3–6 September, 2014*. https://iris.unito.it/retrieve/eda20bf2-86e9-4e2e-b671-77a91d6fb8c4/P.Bianchi_Lisbona%20 2014.pdf

Brauer, D. G., and K. J. Ferguson. 2015. "The Integrated Curriculum in Medical Education: AMEE Guide No. 96." *Medical Teacher* 37 (4): 312–22. https://doi.org/10.3109/0142159X.2014.970998.

Bronzino, J. 2011. "Biomedical Engineering: A Historical Perspective." In *Introduction to Biomedical Engineering*, edited by J. Enderle and J. Bronzino. Elsevier Science & Technology.

Brown, J. U. 1991. "A Personal View of Biomedical Engineering." *IEEE Engineering in Medicine and Biology Magazine* 10 (3): 34–37. https://doi.org/10.1109/51.84184.

Bruneau, O. 2020. "The Teaching of Mathematics at the Royal Military Academy: Evolution in Continuity." *Philosophia Scientiae* 24 (1): 137–58. https://doi.org/10.4000/philosophiascientiae.2212.

Butterlin, N., G. Soto-Romero, J. Duffaud, and O. Blagosklonov. 2007. "ISIFC—Dual Biomedical Engineering School." In *2007 29th Annual International Conference of the IEEE Engineering in Medicine and Biology Society, Lyon, France,* 3098–101. https://doi.org/10.1109/IEMBS.2007.4352983

Cardoso, M., and R. M. Chanin. 2022. "The History of Engineering Education: Learning from the Past to Design the Future." *Research, Society and Development* 11 (11): e364111133606. https://doi.org/10.33448/rsd-v11i11.33606.

Carstensen, E. L., D. W. Healy, P. Schwan, and S. A. Talbot. 1963. "Curriculum Development in Biomedical Engineering." *Journal of Engineering Education* 53 (7): 446–52.

Cranefield, P. F. 1957. "The Organic Physics of 1847 and the Biophysics of Today." *Journal of the History of Medicine and Allied Sciences* 12 (4): 407–23. https://doi.org/10.1093/jhmas/xii.10.407.

da Ana, P. A., and C. B. Lombello. 2023. "Biomedical Engineering: History and Areas of Expertise." In *Current Trends in Biomedical Engineering*, edited by C. B. Lombello and P. A. da Ana. Cham: Springer.

Davies, B. 2013. "Military Engineers and the Rise of Imperial Russia." In *Military Engineers: The Development of the Early Modern European State*, edited by B. P. Lenman. Edinburgh University Press.

Davis, B. L., and G. G. Jaros. 1988. "Biomedical Engineering at the University of Cape Town and Groote Schuur Hospital." *Engineering in Medicine* 17 (1): 37–9. https://doi.org/10.1243/emed_jour_1988_017_010_02.

Desai, T. A., and R. L. Magin. 2001. "A Cure for Bioengineering? A New Undergraduate Core Curriculum." *Journal of Engineering Education* 90 (2): 231–8. https://doi.org/10.1002/j.2168-9830.2001.tb00597.x.

Dokos, S. 2015. "Biomedical Engineering Education 'Down Under': The Australian Experience." *IEEE Pulse,* March/April 2015. https://www.embs.org/pulse/articles/biomedical-engineering-education-australian-experience/

Douglas, T. S. 2012. "Biomedical Engineering at UCT—Challenges and Opportunities." *South African Medical Journal* 102 (6): 456. https://doi.org/10.7196/samj.5553.

Dremstrup, K., and P. B. Elberg. 2008. "Five Year Biomedical Engineering Curriculum: Experiences and Results from the First Eight Years." In *14th Nordic-Baltic Conference on Biomedical Engineering and Medical Physics*, edited by A. Katashev, Y. Dekhtyar, and J. Spigulis. *IFMBE Proceedings*, vol 20. Springer, Berlin, Heidelberg. https://doi.org/10.1007/978-3-540-69367-3_110

Engineers Australia National Committee for Rehabilitation, Engineering. 2020. *Rehabilitation Engineering in Australia: Discussion Paper.* Engineers Australia.

Farrell, P. C., W. Flicker, and N. L. Svensson. 1983. "Biomedical Engineering Teaching and Research at the Centre for Biomedical Engineering, University of New South Wales, Kensington, Australia." *Engineering in Medicine* 12 (4): 201–4. https://doi.org/10.1243/EMED_JOUR_1983_012_055_02.

Foster, K. R. 2002. "Herman P. Schwan: A Scientist and Pioneer in Biomedical Engineering." *Annual Review of Biomedical Engineering* 4: 1–27. https://doi.org/10.1146/annurev.bioeng.4.092001.093625.

Geddes, L. A. 1977. "Historical Background of Interdisciplinary Engineering." In *The Practice of Clinical Engineering*, edited by C. A. Caceres, 15–30. New York: Academic Press.

Gehlot, N. S. 2009. "Recent Developments in Biomedical Engineering Education and Research in Brazil." In *Annual International Conference of the IEEE Engineering in Medicine and Biology Society,* 5862–65. https://doi.org/10.1109/IEMBS.2009.5334542

Gergely, S. 1979. "A BSc Level Option in Biomedical Electronics." *Journal of Medical Engineering & Technology* 3 (1): 24–9. https://doi.org/10.3109/03091907909161599.

Grayson, L. P. 1977. "A Brief History of Engineering Education in the United States." *Engineering Education* 68 (3): 246–64.

Harris, T. R., J. D. Bransford, and S. P. Brophy. 2002. "Roles for Learning Sciences and Learning Technologies in Biomedical Engineering Education: A Review of Recent Advances." *Annual Review of Biomedical Engineering* 4: 29–48. https://doi.org/10.1146/annurev.bioeng.4.091701.125502.

Hart, R. T. 2015. "Biomedical Engineering Accredited Undergraduate Programs: 4 Decades of Growth." *Annals of Biomedical Engineering* 43 (8): 1713–15. https://doi.org/10.1007/s10439-015-1319-2.

Hatchuel, A. 2018. "Ecole des Mines de Paris: A Few Lessons from a Long History." In *Engineering a Better Future*, edited by T. Odumosu, J. Y. Tsao and E. Subrahmanian, 21–32. Cham: Springer International Publishing.

Jewell, T. K., J. Griggs, and S. J. Ressler. 2001. "Early Engineering Education in the United States Prior to 1850." In *International Engineering History and Heritage, Improving Bridges to ASCE's 150th Anniversary.* https://doi.org/10.1061/40594(265)41

Jones, N. B. 1980. "A First-Degree Course in Electronics, with Medical Instrumentation as a Background Topic." *Journal of Medical Engineering & Technology* 4 (1): 7–11. https://doi.org/10.3109/03091908009161080.

Joyce, T. 2009a. "Currently Available Medical Engineering Degrees in the UK. Part 1: Undergraduate Degrees." *Proceedings of the Institution of Mechanical Engineers. Part H, Journal of Engineering in Medicine* 223 (4): 407–13. https://doi.org/10.1243/09544119JEIM455.

Joyce, T. 2009b. "Currently Available Medical Engineering Degrees in the UK. Part 2: Postgraduate Degrees." *Proceedings of the Institution of Mechanical Engineers, Part H: Journal of Engineering in Medicine*: 415–23. https://doi.org/10.1243/09544119JEIM456.

Kadefors, R. 1977. “Medical Engineering Education in Sweden with Reference to Other Nordic Countries.” *Journal of Medical Engineering & Technology* 1 (4): 199–202. https://doi.org/10.3109/03091907709160642.

Katona, P. G. 2006. “Biomedical Engineering and the Whitaker Foundation: A Thirty-Year Partnership.” *Annual Review of Biomedical Engineering* 34 (6): 904–16. https://doi.org/10.1007/s10439-006-9087-7.

Keck, R. W. 2006. “Ritterakademie (Academy for Knights) (CT).” In *Brill's New Pauly Online*. Brill.

Knoll, M. 1997. “The Project Method: Its Vocational Education Origin and International Development.” *Journal of Industrial Teacher Education* 34 (3): 59–80.

Knowles, N. K., and I. DeCoito. 2018. “Biomedical Engineering Undergraduate Education: A Canadian Perspective.” *International Journal of Mechanical Engineering Education* 48 (2): 119–39. https://doi.org/10.1177/0306419018791526.

Krüger, J. 2018. “Un journal mathématique néerlandais au XVIIIe siècle—Le Passe-Temps mathématique (1754–1769).” *Images des Mathématiques, CNRS*. https://doi.org/10.60868/4a7c-he97

Le Croissette, D. H. 1961. “Bio-Medical Engineering Program at Drexel Institute of Technology.” *IRE Transactions on Bio-Medical Electronics* 8 (4): 227. https://doi.org/10.1109/TBMEL.1961.4322919.

Lenman, B. P., ed. 2013. *Military Engineers: The Development of the Early Modern European State*. Edinburgh University Press.

Licona, F. M., J. Azpiroz-Leehan, E. G. U. Medal, and M. C. Méndez. 2014. “Biomedical Engineering Curriculum at UAM-I: A Critical Review.” In *36th Annual International Conference of the IEEE Engineering in Medicine and Biology Society*. Chicago, IL, 1801–04. https://doi.org/10.1109/EMBC.2014.6943958

Lin, K.-P., M.-F. Chen, C.-L. Tsai, and K. Tsai. 2016. “Status of Biomedical Engineering Education in the Asia Pacific.” In *XIV Mediterranean Conference on Medical and Biological Engineering and Computing 2016. IFMBE Proceedings*, vol 57. Springer, Cham. https://doi.org/10.1007/978-3-319-32703-7_256

Linsenmeier, R. A. 2003. “What Makes a Biomedical Engineer?” *IEEE Engineering in Medicine and Biology Magazine*: 32–8.

Linsenmeier, R. A., T. R. Harris, and S. A. Olds. 2002. “The VaNTH Bioengineering Curriculum Project.” In *Second Joint 24th Annual Conference and the Annual Fall Meeting of the Biomedical Engineering Society and the Engineering in Medicine and Biology Society*. Houston, TX.

Linsenmeier, R. A., and A. Saterbak. 2020. “Fifty Years of Biomedical Engineering Undergraduate Education.” *Annual Review of Biomedical Engineering* 48 (6): 1590–615. https://doi.org/10.1007/s10439-020-02494-0.

Majoram, T., and Y. Zhong. 2010. “What Engineering Is, What Engineers Do.” In *Engineering: Issues, Challenges and Opportunities for Development*, 24–6. Paris: UNESCO Publishing.

McCally, R. L. 2005. “The Master's Degree Program in Applied Biomedical Engineering.” *Johns Hopkins APL Technical Digest* 26 (3): 214–18.

McDonald, H. 1914. “The Origin of the Word ‘Engineer’.” *Scientific American Supplement* 1914: 294–5.

McGivern, J. G. 1960. *First Hundred Years of Engineering Education in the United States (1807–1907)*. Spokane, WA: Gonzaga University Press.

McKelvey, M., and R. J. Saemundsson. 2025. “Pairing Engineering with Medicine: Building and Maintaining Academic Engagement in Biomedical Engineering at Chalmers University of Technology 1948–2022.” *Management & Organizational History*: 1–23. https://doi.org/10.1080/17449359.2025.2513692.

Meyer-Hartwig, K., and W. Bleifeld. 1978. "Education and Professional Training of Biomedical Engineers in West Germany." *Journal of Medical Engineering and Technology* 2 (2): 62–6. https://doi.org/10.3109/03091907809161757.

Miller, M. I., A. O. Brightman, F. H. Epstein, K. J. Grande-Allen, J. J. Green, E. Haase, C. T. Laurencin, E. Logsdon, F. Mac Gabhann, B. Ogle, C. Wang, G. R. Wodicka, and R. Winslow. 2023. "BME 2.0: Engineering the Future of Medicine." *BME Frontiers* 4: 0001. https://doi.org/10.34133/bmef.0001.

Nebeker, F. 2001. "The Emergence of Biomedical Engineering in the United States." *Icon* 7: 75–94.

Nkuma-Udah, K. I., E. E. C. Agoha, K. Ejeta, and G. I. Ndubuka. 2015. "Biomedical Engineering in Nigeria: A Developmental Overview." In *World Congress on Medical Physics and Biomedical Engineering, Toronto, Canada, June 7–12, 2015*. https://doi.org/10.1007/978-3-319-19387-8_400

Overy, C., and E. M. Tansey. 2016. "Technology, Techniques, and Technicians at the National Institute for Medical Research (NIMR) c.1960–c.2000." In *Wellcome Witnesses to Contemporary Medicine*. London: Queen Mary University of London.

Oyejide, A. J., O. D. Abodunrin, E. O. Atoyebi, B. Oni, J. E. Idoko, A. A. Adeyemi, G. Akindele, and S. A. Adedayo. 2025. "Landscape of Biomedical Engineering and Technology in Nigeria: A Perspective." *Biomedical Engineering Education* 5: 203–14. https://doi.org/10.1007/s43683-025-00187-5.

Pallikarakis, N. 2022. "Biomedical/Clinical Engineering Education and Certification: Fifty Years of Actions." *Health and Technology* 12 (3): 671–8. https://doi.org/10.1007/s12553-022-00664-9.

Pallikarakis, N., R. Magjarevic, L. Pecchia, and A. Dermitzakis. 2017. "Biomedical Engineering Education: Need for Harmonisation." In *International Federation for Medical and Biological Engineering (IFMBE)*. Tampere, Finland.

Potvin, A. R., F. M. Long, J. G. Webster, and R. J. Jendrucko. 1981. "Biomedical Engineering Education: Enrollment, Courses, Degrees, and Employment." *IEEE Transactions on Biomedical Engineering* 28 (1): 22–8. https://doi.org/10.1109/TBME.1981.324841.

Pritchard, J. 1987. "From Shipwright to Naval Constructor: The Professionalization of 18th-Century French Naval Shipbuilders." *Technology and Culture* 28 (1): 1–25. https://doi.org/10.2307/3105474.

Reynolds, P. 2015. "An Italian Education." *IEEE Pulse* 6 (4): 58–60. https://doi.org/10.1109/MPUL.2015.2428831

Runkle, J. D. 2022. *The Russian System of Shop-work Instruction for Engineers and Machinists*. Legare Street Press.

Scanlon, L. 2023. *An Oasis in the Wilderness: The Foundation Years of the Sydney Mechanics' School of Arts*. Sydney: Halstead Press.

Schwan, H. P. 1984. "The Development of Biomedical Engineering: Historical Comments and Personal Observations." *IEEE Transactions on Biomeical Engineering* 31 (12): 730–6. https://doi.org/10.1109/TBME.1984.325328.

Schwan, H. P. 1991. "Organizational Development of Biomedical Engineering." *IEEE Engineering in Medicine and Biology Magazine* 10 (3): 25–9. https://doi.org/10.1109/51.84182.

Scott, R. N. 1979. "Education and Certification of Biomedical Engineers in Canada." *Journal of Medical Engineering & Technology* 3 (4): 180–3. https://doi.org/10.3109/03091907909161672.

Shaffer, M. J. 1985. "Clinical Engineering Cost-Effectiveness Measurements in the USA." *Medical & Biological Engineering & Computing* 23: 505–10. https://doi.org/10.1007/BF02455303.

Slaaf, D. W., and M. H. P. van Genderen. 2009. "The Fully Integrated Biomedical Engineering Programme at Eindhoven University of Technology." *Proceedings of the Institution of Mechanical Engineers. Part H, Journal of Engineering in Medicine* 223 (4): 387–97. https://doi.org/10.1243/09544119JEIM498.

Soto Castaño, J. M. 2009. "Ingeniería biomédica: Historia en construcción." *Revista Ingeniería Biomédica* 3 (5): 28–30.

Sun, H. H. 1991. "Biomedical Engineering: Drexel University-Pioneer in a Formal MS Degree Training Program for Doctors." *IEEE Engineering in Medicine and Biology Magazine* 10 (3): 44–6. https://doi.org/10.1109/51.84187.

Sun, H. H., and H. P. Schwan. 1990. "Some Early Program in Biomedical Engineering." In *12th Annual International Conference of the IEEE Engineering in Medicine and Biology Society (EMBC)*. Philadelphia, PA, 46–46. https://doi.org/10.1109/IEMBS.1990.690939

Swart, E. 2013. " 'Qualifications, Knowledge and Courage': Dutch Military Engineers, c.1550–c.1660." In *Military Engineers: The Development of the Early Modern European State*, edited by B. P. Lenman. Edinburgh: Edinburgh University Press.

Szeto, A. 2005. "5—Rehabilitation Engineering and Assistive Technology." In *Biomedical Engineering, Introduction to Biomedical Engineering*, 2nd ed., edited by J. D. Enderle, S. M. Blanchard and J. D. Bronzino, 211–54. Academic Press.

Tamura, T. 2015. "Biomedical Engineering Education in Japan." *IEEE Pulse*, May/June 2015. https://www.embs.org/pulse/articles/biomedical-engineering-education-in-japan/

Terman, F. E. 1976. "A Brief History of Electrical Engineering Education." *Proceedings of the IEEE* 64 (9): 1399–407.

Timoshenko, S. P. 1956. "The Development of Engineering Education in Russia." *The Russian Review* 15 (3): 173–85. https://doi.org/10.2307/125587.

Toh, S. L. 2016. "Revamped Biomedical Engineering Curriculum for Future-Ready Graduates." In *XIV Mediterranean Conference on Medical and Biological Engineering and Computing, IFMBE Proceedings*, vol 57, Springer, Cham. https://doi.org/10.1007/978-3-319-32703-7_251

Tryggvason, G., and D. Apelian. 2006. "Re-Engineering Engineering Education for the Challenges of the 21st Century." *JOM* 58 (10): 14–17. https://doi.org/10.1007/s11837-006-0194-6.

Uijt de Haag, M., O. Rompelman, J. Uyt de Haag, and B. Manhire. 2002. "Engineering Education in the Netherlands." In *2002 American Society for Engineering Education Annual Conference & Exposition*. Montreal, Canada. Chemie Ingenieur Technik – CHEM-ING-TECH. 76. https://share.google/wztJTK2NVsLOpLg9v

Valentinuzzi, M. E. 1986. "The Bioengineering Program of the Universidad Nacional de Tucuman (Argentina, 1974–1985)." *IEEE Engineering in Medicine and Biology Magazine*: 21–5.

Valentinuzzi, M. E., B. S. Zanutto, M. E. Torres, and R. Spelzini. 2010. "The Development of Biomedical Engineering." *IEEE Pulse Magazine*.

Valleriani, M. 2010. *Galileo Engineer. Vol. 269, Boston Studies in the Philosophy and History of Science*. Dordrecht: Springer.

Vitruvius, P., H. L. Warren, and M. H. Morgan. 1914. *Vitruvius, the Ten Books on Architecture*. Cambridge, MA: Harvard University Press.

Wallace, W. E. 1987. ""Dal disegno allo spazio": Michelangelo's Drawings for the Fortifications of Florence." *Journal of the Society of Architectural Historians* 46 (2): 119–34. https://doi.org/10.2307/990181.

Watteau, J. P. 1978. "Biomedical Engineering Education in France." *Journal of Medical Engineering and Technology* 2 (4): 178–81. https://doi.org/10.3109/03091907809161790.

Weng, X., W. Niu, and Y. Fan. 2009. "Educational Development of Biomedical Engineering in China." In *World Congress on Medical Physics and Biomedical Engineering*, Munich, Germany, September 7–12. https://doi.org/10.1007/978-3-642-03893-8_29

West, J. B. 2017. "Leonardo da Vinci: Engineer, Bioengineer, Anatomist, and Artist." *American Journal of Physiology—Lung Cellular and Molecular Physiology* 312 (3): L392–L397. https://doi.org/10.1152/ajplung.00378.2016.

Wilensky, H. L. 1964. "The Professionalization of Everyone?" *American Journal of Sociology* 70 (2): 137–58.

Wolff, H. S. 1970. *Biomedical Engineering*. Weidenfeld & Nicolson.

Wollschläger, T. 2013. "Military Engineers and the Development of the Princely State in Germany." In *Military Engineers: The Development of the Early Modern European State*, edited by Bruce P. Lenman. Edinburgh: Edinburgh University Press.

World Health Organization. 2017. "Human Resources for Medical Devices: The Role of Biomedical Engineers." In *WHO Medical Device Technical Series*. World Health Organization.

Zelbo, S. 2023. "The Role of the United States Military Academy at West Point in the Formation of America's Engineering Profession (1802 to 1850) | 2023." *Histoire & Mesure* XXXVIII (2): 217–40. https://doi.org/10.4000/histoiremesure.20113.

2 Integrating Disciplinarity in Biomedical Engineering Education

Ziad O. Abu-Faraj and Sandy A. Rihana

2.1 UNDERSTANDING DISCIPLINARITY IN BIOMEDICAL ENGINEERING

Biomedical Engineering (BME) stands at the forefront of transformative progress in healthcare, uniting the analytical rigor of engineering with the complexities of biological systems to develop solutions that enhance human health and well-being. As global health challenges become more intricate, the role of biomedical engineers expands beyond traditional disciplinary boundaries. This expansion demands not only technical proficiency but also ethical judgment, regulatory awareness, and societal responsiveness.

In this context, the structure and substance of BME education take on strategic importance. Cultivating graduates who can navigate this evolving landscape requires more than the accumulation of knowledge; it demands intentional integration across disciplines. The conceptual frameworks of *multidisciplinarity*, *interdisciplinarity*, and *transdisciplinarity* offer essential lenses through which to design, evaluate, and advance biomedical engineering curricula. Understanding how these approaches differ and how they converge in educational practice forms the basis for fostering innovation, collaboration, and relevance in both academic and professional domains.

2.1.1 Definitions and Distinctions: Multi-, Inter-, and Trans-Disciplinarity

Although multidisciplinarity, interdisciplinarity, and transdisciplinarity are broad concepts applicable across many fields, the following definitions and examples illustrate their particular relevance to biomedical engineering.

Multidisciplinarity refers to the involvement of distinct disciplines working in parallel, where each retains its own methodologies. For example, in BME, engineers may design medical device hardware, clinicians specify functional requirements, and pharmacologists contribute insights into drug delivery. Although collaboration occurs, each discipline operates within its own framework, and their methods are not integrated (Choi and Pak 2006).

DOI: 10.1201/9781003520313-2

Interdisciplinarity goes a step further, involving the integration of concepts, methods, and knowledge from different disciplines to address complex problems. For instance, in BME, computational models that simulate physiological processes require expertise in mathematical modeling, software engineering, and biology. This integration leads to innovative solutions that cannot emerge from a single discipline alone (Klein 2005).

Transdisciplinarity extends beyond academia to incorporate societal, ethical, and legal dimensions. In BME, this is crucial for developing healthcare technologies that are not only innovative but also socially responsible. For example, wearable health monitors must balance technological accuracy with patient privacy and regulatory concerns. Transdisciplinary approaches ensure that these technologies are grounded in real-world applications and align with broader societal values (Montesinos et al. 2023).

These three approaches—multidisciplinarity, interdisciplinarity, and transdisciplinarity—work together to drive BME forward, combining specialized expertise, fostering innovation, and ensuring that developments are socially responsible.

2.1.2 Curriculum and Professional Relevance of Disciplinary Integration

BME education must prepare students for careers requiring both technical expertise and collaboration across disciplines. As healthcare challenges grow, curricula must integrate multidisciplinarity, interdisciplinarity, and transdisciplinarity to equip students for medical device design and healthcare innovation. Abu-Faraj (2008) stresses that BME curricula should combine scientific rigor with career readiness, ensuring students can address healthcare needs while considering ethical implications. Curricula should include hands-on experiences in medical device innovation, diagnostic technologies, and emerging fields such as artificial intelligence (AI)-driven diagnostics and robotic-assisted surgeries, with core topics such as biomechanics, biomaterials, and medical imaging ensuring comprehensive knowledge.

As BME programs evolve, collaboration with industry stakeholders ensures that curricula remain aligned with technological advancements and market needs (Prestigiacomo, Chan, and Kark 2024). Incorporating global perspectives helps BME programs address healthcare disparities and regulatory challenges across regions, preparing students to design culturally sensitive, sustainable, and legally compliant technologies. Integrating multidisciplinarity, interdisciplinarity, and transdisciplinarity into BME education ensures that graduates can navigate complex healthcare landscapes, develop innovative technologies, and contribute to global health advancements.

2.2 EVOLUTION AND INTERDISCIPLINARITY IN BIOMEDICAL ENGINEERING EDUCATION

2.2.1 Historical Development and Interdisciplinary Foundations

Biomedical engineering (BME) has evolved significantly since its inception, shaped by interdisciplinarity and global impact. Studies by Harmon (1975), White and Plonsey

(1982), Harris et al. (2002), Abu-Faraj (2012a), and Linsenmeier and Saterbak (2020) document its milestones and expansion. The first US BME program began at Drexel University in 1959, followed by doctoral programs at Johns Hopkins and the University of Pennsylvania (Abu-Faraj 2012a). By 2012, over 700 programs existed worldwide, reflecting rapid growth (Abu-Faraj 2011). As curricula diversify, integration across multiple disciplines fosters innovation, ensuring that the whole exceeds the sum of its parts (Abu-Faraj 2012b).

Guided by frameworks such as Vanderbilt, Northwestern, Texas, Harvard/MIT Engineering Research Center's (VaNTH-ERC's) learning technologies, the Whitaker Foundation's integration of life sciences and engineering, and ABET EC2000's outcomes-based accreditation, BME exemplifies interdisciplinarity. This section examines how disciplinarity shapes BME education, exploring trends, challenges, and strategies for preparing industry-ready graduates through innovative curricula.

2.2.2 BME Growth, Market Trends, and Future Outlook

Driven by medical advancements and global healthcare demands, BME is projected to grow. The U.S. Bureau of Labor Statistics (2024) anticipates a 7% employment increase for biomedical engineers from 2023 to 2033. Market value is expected to rise from \$268.5 billion in 2023 to \$591.25 billion by 2029, with a compound annual growth rate (CAGR) of 12.3–13.1% (Grand View Research 2023; The Business Research Company 2025). Growth is fueled by aging populations, emerging healthcare economies, and technological innovations. Banks (2024) suggests reversing traditional innovation pathways to enhance affordability and accessibility.

Future projections outlined by Abu-Faraj (2008) span 20 interdisciplinary areas, as summarized in Table 2.1, reflecting BME's dynamic evolution. These categories were conceived as broad, integrative domains that continue to serve as umbrella frameworks within which emerging disciplines have steadily evolved. Their sustained relevance over time highlights the adaptable and forward-looking nature of biomedical engineering, where technological and scientific innovations consistently emerge within and across these foundational areas.

TABLE 2.1
Major umbrella areas and emerging disciplines in biomedical engineering

Index	Biomedical Engineering Major Umbrella Area	Emerging Disciplines
i	Artificial Organs	Organ-on-a-Chip, Bioartificial Organs, 3D Bioprinted Organs
ii	Bioelectromagnetism	Non-Invasive Neuromodulation, Bioelectronic Medicine, Electrostimulation Therapy, Magnetogenetics
iii	Bioethics	AI Ethics in Healthcare, CRISPR Ethics, Personalized Medicine Ethics, Ethics of Digital Twin Technologies

(Continued)

TABLE 2.1 (Continued)
Major umbrella areas and emerging disciplines in biomedical engineering

Index	Biomedical Engineering Major Umbrella Area	Emerging Disciplines
iv	Biomedical Engineering Education	AI and Machine Learning in BME Education, Global Health Engineering, Biomedical Entrepreneurship, Digital and Remote BME Learning, XR (Extended Reality) in BME Training
v	Biomaterials	Stimuli-Responsive Biomaterials, 3D-Printable Biomaterials, Smart Polymers, Hybrid Biomaterials for Tissue Regeneration
vi	Biomechanics	Computational Biomechanics, Wearable Biomechanics, Soft Tissue Biomechanics, Biomechanical Digital Twins
vii	Bioinstrumentation	AI-Driven Diagnostics, Smart Biosensors, Point-of-Care Devices, Wearable Medical Devices, Medical Device Lifecycle
viii	Bionanotechnology	Nanotheranostics, DNA Nanotechnology, Nanoengineered Drug Delivery, Nanoparticle-Based Biosensing
ix	Biorobotics and Biomechatronics	Surgical Robotics, Neural-Controlled Prosthetics, Soft Robotics, Biohybrid Robotics, Neurobiomechatronics
x	Biosensors	Wearable Biosensors, Microfluidic Biosensors, Implantable Biosensors, Point-of-Care Biosensor Chips (aka Lab-on-a-Chip Biosensors), Electrochemical Biosensors
xi	Biotechnology	Synthetic Biology, Organoid Technology, Biomanufacturing, Gene Circuit Engineering
xii	Clinical Engineering	Digital Health, Telemedicine, Healthcare Cybersecurity, AI-Driven Hospital Automation
xiii	Medical and Bioinformatics	AI in Bioinformatics, Multi-Omics Data Integration, Computational Genomics, Federated Learning in Bioinformatics, Neuroinformatics
xiv	Medical and Biological Analysis	High-Throughput Screening, Lab-on-a-Chip, Single-Cell Analysis, AI-Driven Pathology
xv	Medical Imaging	AI in Radiology, Functional Imaging, real-time fMRI, Quantum Imaging, Photoacoustic Imaging
xvi	Neural Engineering	Brain–Computer Interfaces, Neuroprosthetics, Optogenetics, Spinal Cord Stimulation for Neural Regeneration
xvii	Physiological Modeling, Simulation, and Control	Digital Twins, Computational Physiology, Virtual Patient Models, AI-Powered Physiological Simulations
xviii	Prosthetic-Orthotic Devices	Neural-Integrated Prosthetics, Smart Prosthetics, Sensory Feedback Systems, 3D-Printed Smart Orthotics
xix	Rehabilitation Engineering and Assistive Technology	Robotic Rehabilitation, Virtual Reality Therapy, Assistive Exoskeletons, Brain-Responsive Neurorehabilitation
xx	Tissue Engineering and Regenerative Medicine	CRISPR-Based Regenerative Medicine, 3D Bioprinting, Scaffold-Free Tissue Engineering, Organoid Bioprinting, Self-Healing Artificial Tissues

Today, advances in biomedical instrumentation drive medical device design, regulatory frameworks, and sustainability, improving patient care while addressing environmental concerns. AI-driven diagnostics, smart biosensors, and wearable devices are poised to transform healthcare. Purposeful innovation remains central to addressing immediate needs and anticipating future challenges. As academia and industry collaborate, interdisciplinarity, societal impact, and lifelong learning will continue to shape the next generation of biomedical engineers.

2.2.3 Applied Interdisciplinarity in Biomedical Engineering

Building on its interdisciplinary foundation, biomedical engineering applies integrated approaches from engineering, biology, and medicine to solve complex healthcare challenges. It draws on core engineering disciplines while requiring sensitivity to ethical, legal, and societal factors. Saltzman (2015) highlights that BME education equips students with knowledge of molecular and cellular biology, biomechanics, bioinstrumentation, bioimaging, biomaterials, and tissue engineering, preparing them for careers in biotechnology, medical devices, regenerative medicine, and personalized healthcare. This balance between engineering rigor and human health complexities fosters collaboration across disciplines and ensures graduates are industry-ready.

Ethical and legal considerations are integral, as BME technologies directly impact human lives. Engineers must navigate patient privacy, healthcare equity, informed consent, sustainability, and regulatory compliance, including health insurance portability and accountability act (HIPAA), food and drug administration (FDA) medical device regulations, and intellectual property (IP) laws. Emerging technologies—AI in healthcare, bioprinting, synthetic blood, neuroprosthetics, gene editing, and precision medicine—underscore BME's evolving interdisciplinary nature. Educational programs must prepare students to lead advancements while emphasizing adaptability, continuous learning, and ethical responsibility. Abu-Faraj (2008) emphasizes curricula merging engineering and life sciences while addressing industry demands. Collaborations with industry partners, internships, and real-world projects enhance career readiness. The 2019 coronavirus pandemic accelerated digital innovations in BME education, incorporating online platforms, virtual labs, and AI-driven feedback systems. Programs now emphasize biosensors, Internet of Things (IoT)-enabled devices, and personalized healthcare technologies, equipping students to advance patient care while navigating regulatory and data privacy challenges. Interdisciplinarity remains central to BME's evolution, ensuring future engineers drive purposeful innovation with societal impact.

2.2.4 Global Perspectives on Disciplinarity in BME Education

Biomedical engineering education has expanded globally, emphasizing interdisciplinarity and standardization to address healthcare challenges. In the United States, Linsenmeier and Gatchell (2006) highlight a 75% overlap in core courses across 37 ABET-accredited programs, ensuring foundational knowledge while allowing specialization. In Europe, the Bologna Process harmonizes biomedical engineering education, fostering collaboration and quality assurance within the European Higher Education Area (Nagel et al. 2007). The BIOMEDEA project exemplifies these efforts by establishing accreditation criteria for BME programs and clinical engineering training, enhancing global competitiveness.

Beyond the United States and Europe, interdisciplinary teaching models are crucial for addressing healthcare challenges (Abu-Faraj 2012b). In Australia, initiatives like the Medical Device Partnering Program (https://mdpp.org.au) integrate academia and industry to drive biomedical innovation. China's rapid expansion in BME education aligns with industrial growth, balancing technical training and interdisciplinary integration (Weng, Niu, and Fan 2009). Japan prioritizes health technologies, including molecular biology, medical imaging, and regenerative medicine, to address an aging population (Kikuchi 2007). In India, academia-healthcare collaborations enhance BME programs, focusing on regional healthcare needs (Hassan, Zahra, and Bajpai 2019). These global efforts reflect the discipline's critical role in advancing healthcare through research, international collaboration, and responsive educational frameworks.

2.3 TEACHING APPROACHES TO DISCIPLINARITY

Biomedical engineering education integrates multidisciplinary, interdisciplinary, and transdisciplinary approaches to address real-world challenges. These strategies enhance knowledge integration, collaborative problem-solving, and adaptability, fostering innovation in education (Feng et al. 2023).

2.3.1 Multidisciplinary and Interdisciplinary Approaches

Multidisciplinary teaching merges engineering, biology, chemistry, physics, mathematics, and computer science to solve complex problems. It encourages students to connect diverse fields, fostering adaptability and problem-solving skills. Interdisciplinary approaches further integrate foundational sciences with engineering, developing critical thinking. Structured learning modules, including PBL, project-based learning (PjBL), case-based learning (CBL), and team-based learning (TBL), bridge theory with application and promote teamwork, communication, and critical thinking (Martínez-Ávila et al. 2023; Rodríguez Dueñas and Ríos Rincón 2018).

2.3.1.1 Parallel Instruction and Cross-Departmental Collaboration

Parallel instruction, such as combining human physiology with computational modeling, fosters a unified understanding of complex subjects. Faculty collaboration ensures pedagogical coherence, highlighting interdisciplinary connections and enhancing problem-solving (Feng et al. 2023). In the context of course development, this approach allows for the blending of different disciplinary perspectives, enhancing the curriculum's depth and fostering a more holistic educational experience. Cross-departmental collaboration integrates expertise from mechanical engineering, biology, computer science, materials science, and health sciences, breaking down academic silos and ensuring courses align with educational goals and industry trends, promoting open communication and holistic education (Smith 2024; LaFrance et al. 2019).

2.3.2 Integrating Core Disciplines

Integrating core disciplines—biology, chemistry, mathematics, physics, and engineering—fosters a comprehensive understanding of biomedical principles. This cohesive curriculum prepares students to address complex biomedical challenges by emphasizing connections rather than isolating disciplines, fostering both technical proficiency and collaborative problem-solving skills. Tripp and Shortlidge (2019) stress that interdisciplinary frameworks enhance undergraduate education, equipping students with the expertise and collaborative mindset needed for biomedical innovation.

2.3.3 Collaborative Learning Modules and PjBL

Collaborative learning modules and PjBL extend the integration of core disciplines. These group-based projects, encouraging teamwork across biology, chemistry, engineering, and physics, promote technical expertise and soft skills such as communication and leadership. Rodríguez Dueñas and Ríos Rincón (2018) highlight the role of active learning in fostering communities of practice, while Krishnan (2013) advocates for the stepwise integration of interdisciplinary PjBL in medical device development. Singh et al. (2018) emphasize clinical immersions as a means to enhance adaptive learning and problem-solving, preparing students for interdisciplinary collaboration in biomedical engineering. Active learning in these settings strengthens creativity and adaptability, ensuring that students are prepared for real-world biomedical challenges.

2.3.4 Transdisciplinary Models in Teaching

Transdisciplinary teaching integrates engineering, healthcare, social sciences, ethics, and law to solve global challenges. This model fosters inclusivity, adaptability, and systems thinking, preparing students for health issues such as inequities and sustainable healthcare. Baturalp, Bozkurt, and Baldock (2024) assert that transdisciplinary models equip students to design solutions that are technologically advanced, socially responsible, and ethically sound. Montesinos, Salinas-Navarro, and Santos-Diaz (2023) advocate for transdisciplinary experiential learning, bridging theory and practice to enhance skills, critical thinking, and innovation while addressing global health disparities. For instance, AI-driven diagnostic tools require expertise from multiple disciplines to create impactful solutions.

2.3.4.1 Addressing Complex Health Challenges and Ethical Considerations

Addressing evolving health challenges such as aging populations and chronic diseases requires transdisciplinary collaboration. Curricula integrating biomedical engineering, healthcare, and social sciences prepare students for these issues. Lawlor et al. (2015) and Montesinos, Salinas-Navarro, and Santos-Diaz (2023) highlight the importance of transdisciplinary collaboration, ensuring solutions remain technologically advanced, socially responsible, legally compliant, and ethically sound. Courses such as *Bioethics* and *Legal and Regulatory Aspects*, and *Societal Impacts* in *Senior Capstone Design* help students navigate the ethical, legal, and societal dimensions of healthcare, fostering systems thinking and responsible innovation. The Interagency Working Group on Convergence (2022) emphasizes that transdisciplinary learning enhances students' ability to innovate responsibly while considering broader legal, societal, and ethical impacts.

2.4 CHALLENGES AND SOLUTIONS IN IMPLEMENTING DISCIPLINARITY

The integration of disciplinarity in Biomedical Engineering (BME) education faces significant challenges, including institutional barriers, resource allocation, and faculty development. Collaboration between engineering and biological sciences is vital to preparing students for the complexities of the field. Additionally, enhancing student engagement and optimizing assessment methods are essential for improving learning outcomes. Addressing these interconnected challenges offers opportunities for advancing BME programs.

2.4.1 Institutional Barriers and Resources

Integrating non-engineering students into BME graduate programs poses challenges, particularly concerning professional recognition and regulatory compliance. Some institutions admit students without ensuring foundational engineering knowledge, raising concerns in countries with strict licensure requirements. Without clear policies, non-engineering graduates may face ethical, legal, and career challenges. To mitigate potential gaps in foundational preparation, particularly in programs oriented toward professional licensure or engineering-intensive outcomes, BME departments may consider admission pathways that assess or support foundational engineering knowledge. This can include offering remedial courses in engineering principles and mathematics where appropriate. In contrast, programs with a stronger orientation toward bioengineering or life sciences may prioritize flexibility in admissions while addressing preparedness through tailored academic advising, bridge modules, or interdisciplinary course sequencing. Coordinating such pathways requires careful curricular planning and administrative alignment to ensure that all students are equipped to meet the program's academic and professional objectives.

Resource allocation remains another challenge, particularly within larger engineering departments where visibility and access to specialized funding are limited. Insufficient institutional support hampers faculty development, interdisciplinary collaboration, and research infrastructure. Institutions should allocate dedicated budgets, prioritize faculty training, and foster industry-government collaborations. Tripp and Shortlidge (2019) emphasize the need for program leadership to advocate for flexible academic frameworks and resource allocation to ensure the sustainability of BME programs in a rapidly evolving global landscape.

2.4.2 Faculty Development and Interdisciplinary Collaboration

A significant barrier to interdisciplinarity within BME programs is the lack of faculty incentives for cross-disciplinary collaboration. Promotion criteria often prioritize disciplinary achievements, limiting faculty involvement in collaborative efforts. Program leadership should incentivize collaboration through competitive research grants, interdisciplinary metrics for promotion evaluations, and recognition awards. Shared teaching assignments and interdisciplinary seminars can further foster collaboration, creating a culture of interdisciplinarity that benefits educators and students alike.

Additionally, faculty may lack training in interdisciplinary pedagogy. Leadership should establish professional development programs, including workshops and mentorship, to equip faculty with effective interdisciplinary teaching methodologies. This is crucial for sustaining interdisciplinarity in BME education. Research from Universidade Católica Portuguesa underscores the benefits of faculty participation in learning communities, where educators collaborate across disciplines to refine teaching methodologies (Soares et al. 2024).

2.4.3 Coordination Between Engineering and Biological Disciplines

Fragmented curricula across engineering, biology, chemistry, physics, and ethics present persistent challenges in BME education. Interdepartmental conflicts, stemming from differing pedagogical priorities and resource competition, often lead to content duplication and misaligned learning outcomes. Structured coordination mechanisms, such as joint curriculum committees and formal memorandum of understanding (MOUs), are essential for aligning disciplines and creating a cohesive curriculum. Interdisciplinary workshops and co-taught courses further foster collaboration. As Quon and Low (2024) note, robust interdepartmental coordination is crucial for aligning educational objectives and enhancing program coherence.

2.4.4 Student Engagement and Assessment

Student engagement in interdisciplinary BME education can be challenging, often due to difficulties in connecting course content to real-world applications and the diverse motivations of students (Rooney et al. 2025). To address this, BME programs should integrate real-world projects, such as prosthetic limb design, that require both biological understanding and engineering mechanics of materials. These projects foster collaboration and help students develop the skills needed for multidisciplinary teamwork. Program leadership should prioritize PjBL, in collaboration with industry and healthcare partners, ensuring projects reflect practical challenges.

Developing effective assessment methods is equally important. Traditional exams may not assess interdisciplinary competence. Holistic assessments, such as capstone projects where students propose solutions to experts from both fields, measure both technical proficiency and the integration of engineering and biological principles. Fasco et al. (2024) stress the importance of leveraging active learning techniques, technology, and personalized education to enhance student engagement and foster a collaborative learning environment.

2.5 CASE STUDY: INTEGRATING TRANSDISCIPLINARITY IN A BME CURRICULUM

Biomedical engineering spans diverse areas such as biomedical instrumentation, biomechanics, biomaterials, organ investigation, and biomedical imaging, each requiring a blend of engineering and life sciences expertise. The Medical Device Lifecycle curriculum stands out as an exemplary case for integrating disciplinarity due to its need for collaboration across research, design, ethics, regulation, and patient-centered implementation. Several undergraduate biomedical engineering programs have adopted medical device–centered frameworks that span concept development, regulatory compliance, and post-market evaluation. For example, the University of Michigan's undergraduate BME track emphasizes medical device design, safety, and regulatory affairs as part of its Product Development concentration (University of Michigan n.d.). Similarly, the UC Davis Quarter at Aggie Square provides an immersive undergraduate program structured around the full lifecycle of medical devices, from user needs to clinical translation (UC Davis College of Engineering 2022). These examples demonstrate that lifecycle-based approaches are not only viable at the undergraduate level but already guiding BME curricular design at leading institutions. This section explores how a curriculum focused on the medical device lifecycle fosters multidisciplinarity, interdisciplinarity, and transdisciplinarity, preparing future biomedical engineers to navigate the complex intersections of healthcare technology and societal needs.

2.5.1 Overview of the Curriculum Context

Biomedical engineers operate at the intersection of engineering, medicine, technology, and society. A transdisciplinary BME curriculum prepares them to develop, evaluate, and regulate health technologies with technical excellence, regulatory adherence, and ethical responsibility. The Medical Device Lifecycle curriculum exemplifies multi-, inter-, and transdisciplinarity by integrating engineering principles, clinical needs, regulatory requirements, and ethics. Anchored in the biodesign process, it complies with accreditation requirements by integrating college-level mathematics and basic sciences, along with relevant experimental experiences. It aligns with engineering topics, including engineering and computer sciences, engineering design, and modern engineering tools. A broad education component complements the technical curriculum, ensuring consistency with accreditation standards and the program's educational objectives. As shown in Table 2.2, the undergraduate curriculum integrates multi-, inter-, and transdisciplinary elements, providing a comprehensive education that prepares future biomedical engineers for the complexities of the medical device lifecycle. This four-year curriculum demonstrates disciplinarity by integrating foundational knowledge in mathematics, basic sciences, and engineering principles, ensuring mastery of core concepts. It advances interdisciplinarity through specialized courses in bioengineering, computer science, and regulatory affairs, while promoting transdisciplinarity by incorporating ethics, societal impact, and hands-on industry experiences. The curriculum also emphasizes accreditation compliance, regulatory and industry standards, and prepares graduates with the technical, ethical, and practical expertise to navigate the medical device lifecycle and contribute to societal well-being.

TABLE 2.2
Cross-disciplinary integration of the medical device lifecycle curriculum

Cross-Disciplinary Integration	Course Name	Credits
Multidisciplinarity	**Mathematics**	**21**
	Calculus I, II, III	9
	Discrete Math, Linear Algebra, Differential Equations	9
	Probability and Statistics	3
	Basic Sciences	**30**
	Engineering Physics, General Chemistry, Organic Chemistry	12
	Biochemistry, Cellular and Molecular Biology, Genetics	10
	Anatomy and Physiology, Quantitative Physiology	8
Interdisciplinarity	**Engineering Core**	**39**
	Circuit Analysis I and II, Digital Circuits	12
	Digital Signal Processing, Computer-Aided Design, FabLAB	7
	Signals and Systems, Control Systems, Bioinstrumentation	11
	Medical Device Lifecycle	3
	Capstone Design I and II	6
	Medical Device Lifecycle Electives—Select 5 Courses	**15**
	Wearable Medical Devices, Regulatory Affairs for Medical Devices, Medical Robotics, Medical Imaging	12
	Healthcare Data Analytics, Post-Market Surveillance and Risk Management, Biosensors, Clinical Engineering	12
	Computer Science	**11**
	Programming I and II, Artificial Intelligence	11
	College Requirements	**12**
Transdisciplinarity	**Humanities and Social Sciences**	**9**
	Regulatory and Ethical Aspects of Medical Devices	**3**
Co-op Experience	**Professional Training Experience I and II**	**2**

2.5.2 Challenges Encountered in Designing and Implementing a Disciplinary Framework

Developing a transdisciplinary curriculum within the Medical Device Lifecycle involves balancing foundational sciences, engineering design, and human-centered engagement while integrating emerging fields such as digital health, AI, and health informatics. A significant challenge is bridging analog and digital medical device development while maintaining flexibility within regulatory constraints. This approach distinguishes multidisciplinary, interdisciplinary, and transdisciplinary learning. Foundational sciences provide core knowledge, interdisciplinary courses facilitate cross-domain synthesis, and transdisciplinary elements—such as humanities and law—enhance ethical and civic competencies. Sustainability and patient-centered care align with Healthcare 5.0's vision for equitable, personalized healthcare (Kolasa 2023). By fostering a systems-oriented mindset, students evaluate technologies beyond functionality, ensuring sustainability, accessibility, and societal impact. Accreditation in biomedical engineering ensures curricula meet academic and industry demands, aligning PEOs with institutional goals and integrating cutting-edge technologies through continuous feedback, enhancing program quality and adaptability (Abu-Faraj 2025).

2.5.3 Pedagogical Innovations for Transdisciplinary Competence

Students progress through a structured learning journey that mirrors the medical device lifecycle, from needs identification to prototype refinement. This experiential approach integrates engineering, regulatory affairs, and ethics, promoting transdisciplinary competence. Medical device regulation merges engineering principles, legal standards, and healthcare needs, offering a holistic understanding of real-world development. Advanced courses in digital biomedical signal analysis, medical imaging, and AI applications foster interdisciplinary synergy, combining engineering, computer science, and medicine to advance healthcare solutions. Hands-on experiences, including implant safety assessment, computational biomechanics, and clinical exposure to diagnostic and therapeutic devices, deepen transdisciplinary learning by applying principles across diverse fields. Regulatory and policy education introduces key standards like ISO 13485, ISO 14971, IEC 60601, health insurance portability and accountability act (HIPAA), and general data protection regulation (GDPR), illustrating the intersection of regulatory affairs with engineering and healthcare.

2.5.4 Lessons Learned and Best Practices in Transdisciplinary Integration

Early exposure to the medical device lifecycle enhances systems thinking and student competence. The biodesign framework, supported by hands-on projects, integrates engineering skills while encouraging ethical problem-solving. Balancing analog and digital skills ensures comprehensive training in instrumentation and AI-driven health technologies. Integrating AI, digital health, and data science within ethical and regulatory frameworks prepares students to address evolving healthcare challenges. Industry and healthcare partnerships enrich learning, equipping graduates to innovate responsibly. This integrated approach prioritizes sustainability, patient-centered care, and regulatory competence, fostering biomedical engineers who contribute to an inclusive and equitable healthcare ecosystem.

2.6 CONCLUSION

As biomedical engineering evolves, education must adapt to prepare graduates for global health challenges. This requires an emphasis on multidisciplinarity, interdisciplinarity, and transdisciplinarity, alongside purposeful innovation. Biomedical engineering education must foster collaboration across biology, chemistry, engineering, medicine, and data science, equipping students with the technical skills, critical thinking, communication, and ethical decision-making necessary to address complex health issues. Collaboration with professionals in medicine, public health, and policy ensures holistic solutions to emerging challenges such as infectious diseases, aging populations, and health disparities.

Disciplinary expertise in various BME divisions, including biomaterials, biomechanics, bioinstrumentation, biomedical imaging, tissue engineering, bioinformatics, biosensors, and many others, provides a solid foundation, ensuring graduates are industry-ready while cultivating problem-solving skills. The adoption of curricular frameworks such as the Medical Device Lifecycle enhances this foundation by promoting cross-disciplinary integration, human-centered design, and real-world problem-solving. As a result, while specializing in their fields, graduates are also prepared to collaborate across disciplines, particularly in emerging technologies such as AI, personalized medicine, and digital health. Aligning educational practices with industry needs ensures that biomedical engineers will drive innovation, becoming leaders in healthcare technologies.

Furthermore, disciplinary depth is crucial for transformative innovations in prosthetics, diagnostics, therapeutic devices, and other advanced healthcare solutions. Biomedical engineers must adapt to evolving health challenges, offering sustainable, "out-of-the-box" solutions throughout their careers. As new technologies emerge, engineers will play a key role in integrating them into healthcare systems, navigating interoperability and clinical complexities. A sustained focus on disciplinarity will position biomedical engineering as a key driver of global health advancements, leaving a lasting impact on healthcare and society.

REFERENCES

Abu-Faraj, Ziad O. 2008. "Bioengineering/Biomedical Engineering Education and Career Development: Literature Review, Definitions, and Constructive Recommendations." *International Journal of Engineering Education* 24 (5): 990–1011.

Abu-Faraj, Ziad O. 2011. "Project Alexander the Great: An Analytical Comprehensive Study on the Global Spread of Bioengineering/Biomedical Engineering Education." In *Biomedical Engineering: Trends in Materials Science*, edited by A. N. Laskovski, 549–64. Rijeka: IntechOpen. https://doi.org/10.5772/13501.

Abu-Faraj, Ziad O. 2012a. "Bioengineering/Biomedical Engineering Education." In *Handbook of Research on Biomedical Engineering Education and Advanced Bioengineering Learning: Interdisciplinary Concepts*, 1–59. Hershey, PA: IGI Global. https://doi.org/10.4018/978-1-4666-0122-2.ch001.

Abu-Faraj, Ziad O., ed. 2012b. *Handbook of Research on Biomedical Engineering Education and Advanced Bioengineering Learning: Interdisciplinary Concepts.* 2 vols. Hershey, PA: IGI Global. https://doi.org/10.4018/978-1-4666-0122-2.

Abu-Faraj, Ziad O. 2025. "Accreditation in Biomedical Engineering Education." In *Perspectives in Biomedical Engineering Education*, edited by S. Dokos, B. C. C. Chan, and L. Kark. New York: Routledge, Taylor & Francis Group.

Banks, James. 2024. "Reversing the Innovation Pathway Could Be the Key to Cost-Efficient Health Care." *IEEE Pulse* 15 (1): 20–3. https://doi.org/10.1109/MPULS.2024.3370008.

Baturalp, T. B., S. Bozkurt, and C. Baldock. 2024. "The Future of Biomedical Engineering Education Is Transdisciplinary." *Australasian Physical & Engineering Sciences in Medicine* 47 (3): 779–82. https://doi.org/10.1007/s13246-024-01442-9.

The Business Research Company. 2025. *Bioengineering Technology Global Market Report 2025.* https://www.thebusinessresearchcompany.com/report/bioengineering-technology-global-market-report.

Choi, Bernard C. K., and Allan W. P. Pak. 2006. "Multidisciplinarity, Interdisciplinarity and Transdisciplinarity in Health Research, Services, Education and Policy: Definitions, Objectives, and Evidence of Effectiveness." *Clinical and Investigative Medicine* 29 (6): 351–64.

Fasco, Peter S., Shafik Asiimwe, George Ssekabira, and John A. Tushabe. 2024. "Enhancing Student Engagement and Learning Outcomes: Effective Strategies in Institutional Pedagogy." *Education Sciences* 5 (4): 758–67.

Feng, Xiang, Sami Ylirisku, Elina Kähkönen, Hannele Niemi, and Katja Hölttä-Otto. 2023. "Multidisciplinary Education Through Faculty Members' Conceptualisations of and Experiences in Engineering Education." *European Journal of Engineering Education* 48 (4): 707–23. https://doi.org/10.1080/03043797.2023.2185126.

Grand View Research. 2023. *Bioengineering Technology Market Size, Share and Trends Analysis Report by Product, by Application, by Region, and Segment Forecasts, 2024–2030*. https://www.grandviewresearch.com/industry-analysis/bioengineering-technology-market.

Harmon, Leon D. 1975. "Biomedical Engineering Education: How to Do What, with Which, and to Whom." *IEEE Transactions on Biomedical Engineering* 22 (2): 89–94. https://doi.org/10.1109/TBME.1975.324424.

Harris, Thomas R., John D. Bransford, and Sean P. Brophy. 2002. "Roles for Learning Sciences and Learning Technologies in Biomedical Engineering Education: A Review of Recent Advances." *Annual Review of Biomedical Engineering* 4 (1): 29–48. https://doi.org/10.1146/annurev.bioeng.4.091701.125502.

Hassan, Umar, Tania Zahra, and Sunil Bajpai. 2019. "Biomedical Engineering Education in India." *Biomedical Engineering Letters* 9 (4): 51–8. http://www.degruyter.com.

Interagency Working Group on Convergence. 2022. *Convergence Education: A Guide to Transdisciplinary STEM Learning and Teaching*. Washington, DC: National Science and Technology Council.

Kikuchi, Masashi. 2007. "Status and Future Prospects of Biomedical Engineering: A Japanese Perspective." *Biomedical Imaging and Intervention Journal* 3 (3): e37. https://doi.org/10.2349/biij.3.3.e37.

Klein, Julie Thompson. 2005. "Interdisciplinary Teamwork: The Dynamics of Collaboration and Integration." In *Interdisciplinary Collaboration: An Emerging Cognitive Science*, edited by S. J. Derry, C. D. Schunn and M. A. Gernsbacher, 1–28. Mahwah, NJ: Psychology Press. https://doi.org/10.4324/9781410613073.

Kolasa, Katarzyna. 2023. *The Digital Transformation of the Healthcare System: Healthcare 5.0*. New York: Routledge. https://doi.org/10.1080/13696998.2023.2295157.

Krishnan, Shankar. 2013. "Promoting Interdisciplinary Project-Based Learning to Build the Skill Sets for Research and Development of Medical Devices in Academia." In *Proceedings of the 2013 Annual International Conference of the IEEE Engineering in Medicine and Biology Society (EMBC)*, 6610207. https://doi.org/10.1109/EMBC.2013.6610207.

LaFrance, Danielle L., Michael J. Weiss, Elham Kazemi, John Gerenser, and James Dobres. 2019. "Multidisciplinary Teaming: Enhancing Collaboration Through Increased Understanding." *Journal of Autism and Developmental Disorders* 12 (3): 709–26. https://doi.org/10.1007/s40617-019-00331-y.

Lawlor, E. Francis, Matthew W. Kreuter, Amy K. Sebert-Kuhlmann, and Timothy D. McBride. 2015. "Methodological Innovations in Public Health Education: Transdisciplinary Problem Solving." *American Journal of Public Health* 105 (Suppl 1): S99–S103. https://doi.org/10.2105/AJPH.2014.302462.

Linsenmeier, Robert A., and David W. Gatchell. 2006. "Core Elements of an Undergraduate Biomedical Engineering Curriculum: State of the Art and Recommendations." In

Proceedings of the 2006 International Conference on Engineering Education (ICEE). https://www.ineer.org/Events/ICEE2006/papers/3179.pdf.

Linsenmeier, Robert A., and Ann Saterbak. 2020. "Fifty Years of Biomedical Engineering Undergraduate Education." *Annals of Biomedical Engineering* 48 (6): 1590–615. https://doi.org/10.1007/s10439-020-02494-0.

Martínez-Ávila, Martha, Roberto M. García-García, Sandra Guajardo-Flores, and Daniel Guajardo-Flores. 2023. "Soft Skills Development in Bioengineering Students Through Problem-Based Learning: An Analysis of Educational Impact." In *Proceedings of the 2023 Latin American and Caribbean Consortium of Engineering Institutions Conference (LACCEI).* https://doi.org/10.18687/LACCEI2023.1.1.1576.

Montesinos, Luis, David Ernesto Salinas-Navarro, and Alejandro Santos-Diaz. 2023. "Transdisciplinary Experiential Learning in Biomedical Engineering Education for Healthcare Systems Improvement." *BMC Medical Education* 23: 207. https://doi.org/10.1186/s12909-023-04171-x.

Nagel, Joachim H., Dick W. Slaaf, and John Barbenel. 2007. "Medical and Biological Engineering and Science in the European Higher Education Area." *Medical Engineering & Physics* 26 (3): 18–25.

Prestigiacomo, Rita, Chun Chuen Chan, and Lauren Kark. 2024. "A Biomedical Engineering Curriculum Development: A Qualitative Study Engaging Four Stakeholders." *European Journal of Education* 59 (2): e12632. https://doi.org/10.1111/ejed.12632.

Quon, Samuel, and Simon Low. 2024. "Bridging the Gap in Biomedical Engineering Education by Integrating Local Context." *Research in Medical Education* 13 (18): 1–3. https://doi.org/10.34172/rdme.33264.

Rodríguez Dueñas, William R., and Adriana M. Ríos Rincón. 2018. "Interdisciplinary Work as a Pedagogical Innovation for Biomedical Engineering and Health Science Students." *Journal of Engineering Education* 107 (2): 331–44.

Rooney, Shannon I., Christine E. King, Lauren Christian, Mukta Kavdia, Jacob C. Kays, and Sarah F. Shady. 2025. "Identifying and Overcoming Barriers to Classroom Engagement in Biomedical Engineering Education." *Biomedical Engineering Education.* https://doi.org/10.1007/s43683-025-00176-8.

Saltzman, W. Mark. 2015. *Biomedical Engineering: Bridging Medicine and Technology.* Cambridge: Cambridge University Press.

Singh, Anita, Daniel Ferry, and Simon Mills. 2018. "Improving Biomedical Engineering Education Through Continuity in Adaptive, Experiential, and Interdisciplinary Learning Environments." *Journal of Biomechanical Engineering* 140 (8): 081009. https://doi.org/10.1115/1.4040359.

Smith, C. A. 2024. "Promoting Cross-Functional Collaboration in L&D Leadership." *Join The Collective.* https://www.jointhecollective.com/article/promoting-cross-functional-collaboration-in-ld-leadership

Soares, Daniel, Ana Franco, Miguel Rocha, and Pedro Dias. 2024. "Do Birds of a Feather Flock Together? Lessons from an Interdisciplinary and Interinstitutional Community-Development Approach to Faculty Development." *International Journal for Academic Development* 29 (2): 205–18. https://doi.org/10.1080/1360144X.2024.2355527.

Tripp, Brian, and Erin E. Shortlidge. 2019. "A Framework to Guide Undergraduate Education in Interdisciplinary Science." *CBE—Life Sciences Education* 18 (2): ar22. https://doi.org/10.1187/cbe.18-11-0226.

UC Davis College of Engineering. 2022. *An Immersive Biomedical Engineering Experience for Undergrads Is Now the Whole Package*, August 31. https://engineering.ucdavis.edu/news/immersive-biomedical-engineering-experience-undergrads-now-whole-package.

University of Michigan. n.d. *Undergraduate Program: Biomedical Engineering.* https://bme.umich.edu/undergraduate/.

U.S. Bureau of Labor Statistics. 2024. *Occupational Outlook Handbook: Bioengineers and Biomedical Engineers.* https://www.bls.gov/ooh/architecture-and-engineering/biomedical-engineers.htm.

Weng, Xianbin, Weidong Niu, and Yubo Fan. 2009. "Educational Development of Biomedical Engineering in China." In *IFMBE Proceedings: World Congress on Medical Physics and Biomedical Engineering*, 978–83. https://doi.org/10.1007/978-3-642-03893-8_29.

White, James L., and Robert Plonsey. 1982. "Does Undergraduate Biomedical Engineering Education Produce Real Engineers?" *IEEE Transactions on Biomedical Engineering* 29 (5): 374–8. https://doi.org/10.1109/TBME.1982.324908.

3 Challenges in Biomedical Engineering Education

Brian P. Helmke and Renata F. Ramos

3.1 DESIGNING EDUCATIONAL PROGRAMS THAT PREPARE STUDENTS TO SUCCEED IN A RAPIDLY CHANGING FIELD

Biomedical engineering (BME) is a rapidly evolving field, driven by scientific discovery and technological innovation. The unique origins of BME programs, emerging from traditional engineering disciplines and expanding in response to medical and biological challenges, have resulted in a complex educational landscape. Designing effective educational programs requires not only the integration of core technical and professional competencies aligned with stakeholder needs but also the implementation of adaptive strategies that enable timely curricular iterations in response to developments in the field.

This chapter delineates the key challenges faced by BME educational programs and examines approaches and frameworks to support the alignment of curriculum with the evolving demands of the field.

3.2 CHALLENGE 1: DESIGNING A BME CURRICULUM THAT ALIGNS LEARNING OUTCOMES AND CAREER PATHS

3.2.1 Historical Perspective on Biomedical Engineering Education

Early biomedical engineering graduate programs were founded in the 1960s, as a result of academic researchers from "traditional" engineering disciplines (e.g., mechanical, electrical, and chemical) working to apply engineering principles to design solutions to medical problems. Undergraduate programs originated from departments with existing graduate programs in the subsequent decades. By 1980, 37 institutions offered undergraduate degrees in BME, enrolling nearly 3,000 students (Potvin et al. 1981; Robert A. Linsenmeier and Saterbak 2020). The creation of BME programs was accelerated in the 1990s due to efforts by the Whitaker Foundation, leading to over 80 undergraduate programs and nearly 14,000 students by 2005.

Over the years, BME programs have shifted from a "bridging the gap" model, equipping engineering students with the tools to understand and solve biological and medical problems, to a more integrative approach emphasizing problem-solving at the interface of engineering and the life sciences (Katona 2006).

The rapid expansion of BME programs, their origins from traditional engineering disciplines, and the inherently interdisciplinary nature of the field have contributed

DOI: 10.1201/9781003520313-3

to broad and varied curricula, with the profile of a BME graduate differing significantly from one program to another.

3.2.2 Identifying Core Technical Competencies in BME

Multiple efforts have sought to identify and define core technical competencies within BME curricula. One of the most comprehensive studies was done in 2004 by the Vanderbilt, Northwestern, Texas, Harvard/MIT Engineering Research Center (VaNTH ERC), aimed at determining the general topics encompassing the common or "core" curriculum across BME programs. The VaNTH ERC compiled information from 40 ABET-accredited programs and provided recommendations on the curricular requirements that defined BME undergraduate programs, based on the courses that were required by most of the existing programs at that time (Gatchell and Linsenmeier 2014; R.A. Linsenmeier 2003). The composition of the core curriculum was revisited during the Fourth BME Education Summit in 2019, reaching a similar conclusion (White et al. 2020).

However, while these studies have successfully outlined the core technical topics that characterize BME education, they fall short of defining the specific scope, depth, and competencies embedded within these courses. Consequently, the specific knowledge and skills BME graduates possess are still unclear to external stakeholders.

Furthermore, the BME field continues to evolve as new research directions and technologies emerge, prompting academic programs to expand the range of specialized topics in the curriculum. To address the agility of the field, many programs have incorporated areas of specializations, tracks, or technical electives in the curriculum to provide students with curricular flexibility based on the desired career outcomes (Amos and Dupont 2018). One group recently proposed a fundamental reconfiguration of the traditional BME curriculum, referred to as BME 2.0 (Miller et al. 2023), replacing the core courses identified in the VaNTH ERC study with a curricular model that reflects ongoing biotechnology research discoveries and developing technologies.

The breadth of career outcomes, combined with the accelerating pace of technological innovations, accentuates the challenge of defining the profile of a BME graduate. While articulating a shared set of core competencies could improve student preparation and employability, overly prescriptive curricula may limit the responsiveness needed to integrate emerging knowledge and skills. A more sustainable approach may lie in integrating core technical skills with professional competencies and in designing agile curricula capable of incorporating timely stakeholder input and adapting to the evolving demands of the field.

3.2.3 Complementary Competencies (Professional Skills) in BME Education

BME educational programs prepare students to address complex, multidisciplinary problems in a rapidly changing environment. While proficiency in discipline-specific technical areas remains essential, graduates must develop a range of complementary competencies to succeed beyond the classroom (Rivera et al. 2020).

These complementary competencies include professional skills such as communication, teamwork, life-long learning, ethical conduct, leadership, resilience, adaptability, and non-discipline-specific technical skills such as critical thinking and problem-solving. A growing body of literature has emphasized the importance of these essential skills to prepare engineering graduates to function competently and productively in their professional careers (Hirudayaraj et al. 2021; de Campos, de Resende, and Fagundes 2020; Dumitru and Halpern 2023; Maghiar and Brown 2022).

Recognition of the value of professional skills in engineering disciplines was formally established in 1996 in the United States when the ABET Board of Directors adopted a new set of standards, called Engineering Criteria 2000. The new ABET criteria retained traditional technical accreditation standards while explicitly incorporating professional competencies. These professional skills included teamwork, communication, lifelong learning, ethics, professionalism, and the broader impact of engineering solutions (Newstetter and Benkeser 2004; Volkwein et al. 2004; National Academy of Engineering 2018).

Within BME specifically, researchers have looked into the skills and competencies necessary for graduates to succeed in the workforce. A national survey distributed to 150 industry stakeholders identified problem-solving, communication, design, and teamwork as the most critical skills. In this study, both MedTech and BioTech industry respondents ranked professional skills above disciplinary skills. These findings were reaffirmed in the 2024 BME Educational Survey, in which industry participants identified communication, teamwork, critical thinking, and problem-solving as the most critical skills for BME graduates in industry. Collectively, these studies demonstrate that discipline-specific knowledge alone is insufficient to meet the expectations of engineering employees. Engineering and BME curricula must intentionally integrate complementary competencies to prepare graduates for the demands and complexity of the professional environment (Lam et al. 2025; White et al. 2020; Baura 2015).

3.2.4 Integration of Core Disciplinary and Complementary Professional Skills

There is a broad consensus that technical skills should remain central to the engineering curriculum and that professional competencies are essential for engineering graduates' success in the workplace. However, debate persists regarding the right balance and most effective strategies for integrating these domains. A 2020 review by Winiberg et al. examined existing literature and introduced a theoretical model grounded in a social realist framework to inform pedagogical strategies in engineering education. The study emphasized the value of an embedded model, one in which professional skills are not taught in isolation but are interwoven with core disciplinary content. This integration requires clearly defined student learning outcomes that include both technical and professional competencies, and aligning the curriculum design, instructional methods, and assessment strategies to support the integrated student learning outcomes (Winberg et al. 2020).

While not exclusive to BME, the integration of technical and professional skills presents distinct challenges for BME programs that underscore the need for a backward design approach to curricular design:

- Breadth and Multidisciplinarity of BME. The inherently multidisciplinary nature of BME introduces a wide-ranging curriculum that complicates the identification of core disciplinary content, while simultaneously reinforcing the need for graduates to develop strong complementary competencies such as teamwork, communication, and critical thinking. Technical expertise and professional skills cannot be addressed in isolation; effective BME programs must intentionally integrate both through pedagogical strategies that foster conceptual understanding and practical application across the curriculum.
- Diversity of Career Outcomes of BME Graduates and Core Competencies. Unlike many traditional engineering disciplines, BME graduates pursue diverse professional outcomes, including roles in industry, graduate research, and health professions. This diversity challenges programs to define a coherent set of "core" technical and professional competencies. Programs must, therefore, be intentional about developing an understanding of the career outcomes and design programs that establish core foundations, while incorporating flexibility that enables students to tailor their educational experience to align with varied professional goals.
- Need to Adapt to an Agile BME Field. As the field continues to evolve with technological and scientific advancements, educational programs must prepare students for long-term success by cultivating lifelong learning skills such as critical thinking, intellectual curiosity, adaptability, and self-directed learning. These skills become indispensable for navigating a dynamic professional environment and supporting sustained professional growth.

3.2.5 Pedagogical Approaches in BME Education

While no comprehensive study has quantified the extent to which active learning techniques are incorporated in BME curricula at different institutions, the growing body of BME education research suggests that many programs are incorporating innovative pedagogical strategies throughout the curriculum. A range of instructional approaches is used in BME, with those that integrate technical content and professional skills, such as PBL, engineering design, laboratories, and problem-solving studios, among the most commonly discussed (Sovilj, Lackovic, and Magjarevic 2012; LaPlaca, Newstetter, and Yoganathan 2001; Tompkins 2001; Le Doux and Waller 2016).

A survey of 50 programs presented at the 2019 BME Education Summit found that approximately 30% of required undergraduate courses incorporated PBL. Of those, about 65% involved the creation of a physical artifact or prototype (Billiar et al. 2022). The increasing employment and evaluation of innovative pedagogical strategies in BME education is further reflected in the launch of the journal *Biomedical*

Engineering Education (BIEE) in 2021, underscoring the growing emphasis on educational scholarship within the field.

Despite the advancements in BME education research, most programs have not taken an intentional and cohesive approach to integrating innovative pedagogical strategies at the curricular level. While many instructors employ active learning in their individual courses, such efforts are frequently isolated and not embedded within a coordinated, curriculum-wide strategy. As a result, disciplinary courses are often taught using traditional lecture-based methods, with more student-centered experiences largely confined to specific offerings such as project-based courses, laboratories, or senior capstone projects—many of which are led by teaching-focused faculty.

Co-curricular and experiential learning opportunities such as internships, clinical immersion programs, and undergraduate research have also been leveraged to reinforce classroom instruction and provide opportunities to practice the application of learned knowledge and skills. These experiences offer valuable exposure to real-world challenges; however, they remain inconsistently integrated into curricula and are often difficult to scale equitably across diverse student populations (Jamison et al. 2020, 2023).

Only a limited number of BME programs have adopted curricular models that systematically embed active learning throughout the curriculum. Even fewer employ pedagogical strategies intentionally to scaffold technical and professional competencies progressively across all academic years and courses. As the field continues to evolve, there is an increasing need for curricular designs that integrate instructional strategies and experiences longitudinally to support the achievement of desired technical and professional student learning outcomes for BME graduates (Huang-Saad, Stegemann, and Shea 2020).

3.2.6 Alignment of Curriculum and Career Outcomes

One of the earlier studies examining career outcomes surveyed 464 individuals who earned a bachelor's degree in BME. Among the respondents, 34% pursued careers in industry (with approximately half working in BME-related industries), 25% entered careers in medicine (primarily attending medical school), and 28% pursued graduate studies (with half enrolling in BME programs) (Linsenmeier and Saterbak 2020; Potvin et al. 1981). A subsequent study conducted in 2006 by the American Institute of Medical and Biological Engineering collected data from 1,352 students across multiple institutions. The results showed that 41% of students entered industry, 16% enrolled in medical school, and 35% pursued graduate education, with career outcomes varying by institution, location, and program emphasis. Although the distribution of these outcomes fluctuates slightly over time, it is commonly accepted that the predominant career paths for BME graduates are industry, graduate school, and medical school (Hart 2015).

However, defining career outcomes in broad terms, such as "graduate school" or "industry," limits the ability to determine the specific learning outcomes that will support the professional success of BME graduates. For example, the requirements to pursue a PhD in BME vary significantly depending on the research focus.

Furthermore, many graduating BME students pursue advanced degrees outside the BME field altogether, and only 64% of BME doctoral students have a bachelor's degree in the same field (National Science Foundation 2023). Similarly, while "industry" is often used to describe careers in the Biotechnology and Medical Device sectors, BME graduates pursue a wide range of career options in industry, including manufacturing, pharmaceuticals, and quality engineering, among others (Bureau of Labor Statistics 2025; Suresh et al. 2024).

Preparing BME students for professional practice requires designing learning outcomes that align with the expectations of these varying career paths. A recent study sought to identify the skills most valued by stakeholders across various sectors that recruit BME graduates. Researchers interviewed 63 stakeholders—48 from industry (medical device, biotechnology, and pharmaceutical), ten from academia, three from the medical field, and two from the legal field—to identify the critical skills prioritized by each sector. The interview data were classified into four main categories: professional skills, technical skills, knowledge, and experiences. Findings from this study revealed a misalignment in the skills and experiences valued by academic and industry stakeholders. The authors emphasized the importance of designing a core BME curriculum that intentionally integrates professional skills and experiences with technical skills and knowledge. While this study is limited by its sample size and lacks a multi-institutional context, it presents a valuable framework for discussing the value of aligning curricular content to stakeholder needs. These findings underscore the need for academic programs to continuously assess and revise curricular content in response to evolving professional expectations, thereby designing more agile and responsive educational models (Rivera et al. 2020).

While this section describes curricular challenges in terms of content, pedagogical strategies, and stakeholder input, the process of curricular reform should not be limited to curricular elements alone. Meaningful change requires both top-down, policy-driven initiatives and bottom-up efforts grounded in implementation strategies and supported by committed change agents (Kandiko Howson and Kingsbury 2023).

3.3 CHALLENGE 2: CREATING NEW PROGRAMS THAT CAN ADAPT TO THE RAPIDLY EVOLVING BME DISCIPLINE

3.3.1 Continuous Improvement Strategies

As outlined earlier, past adaptations of curricular and pedagogical approaches have relied on large-scale efforts such as the VaNTH ERC study and educational summit conferences. These efforts occurred at single points in time, required a large effort to bring the BME community together for discussion, and made recommendations for significant revisions that were difficult to implement. In contrast, advances in healthcare technology and the emergence of new engineering challenges in BME occur rapidly, especially with the advent of digital technologies (Industry 4.0) such as the IoT and AI. In engineering practice, strategies for continuous improvement aim to increase efficiency and productivity through ongoing, gradual process changes supported by documentation and validation (Singh and Singh 2013; Vinodh et al. 2020).

For example, innovating product designs while simultaneously meeting regulatory standards in the medical device industry may involve continuous quality improvement strategies such as quality management standards, total quality management (TQM), or Six Sigma. Continuous productivity improvement strategies may include just-in-time (JIT) manufacturing, lean thinking to minimize waste, or implementing the Theory of Constraints to optimize throughput (Brown et al. 2008). The disparity between improvement strategies in BME education and in BME-related industries suggests a gap that will impact the ability of BME education programs to prepare students for the workplace. Thus, a strategy for continuous improvement in educational programs that adapt to the rapidly evolving BME field represents a challenge for BME education.

3.3.2 Change Management in Education

Historically, the curriculum was defined as a collection of knowledge or a method of organizing disciplinary content (Walkington 2010). A more contemporary approach includes in the curriculum definition a broad array of learner experiences inside and outside the classroom that promote self-discovery (Law 2022; Kumar and Rewari 2022). As a result, curriculum designers must consider dynamic and complex interactions among technological, social, political, and economic issues that impact learners and the learning environment. For example, to succeed in Industry 4.0, BME students might require technical skills in areas such as AI, machine learning, data science, robotics, and remote sensing in patients. They also require professional skills such as creative problem-solving, adaptive thinking, emotional and social intelligence, and communication. Students' lived experiences also influence technical and professional development as they progress through a curriculum. Since all these factors change rapidly, educational institutions need strategies to respond to and manage curricular change to prepare students for the professional workforce.

One theoretical approach to change management involves describing the curriculum as a complex system (Law 2022). Complexity theory describes the relationship between humans and the environment, represented in this case by the teaching and learning or workplace environment. The social, political, and technological aspects of the workplace (i.e., the external environment) determine the proficiencies needed by learners for successful careers. Educators respond by adjusting components of the curriculum to align with the needs of the workplace. This response requires input from multiple stakeholders, including employers, alumni, educators, parents, and students (Kumar and Rewari 2022). For example, BME programs often form external advisory boards with representatives from industry, government, alumni, and academia to inform program policy choices related in part to curriculum and assessment. Curricular changes provide students with new experiences and skills that they bring to the workplace, often leading to technological innovation. The interdisciplinary contributions of BMEs have resulted in advances in nanomedicine, immune therapies for cancer, and remote patient monitoring systems, for example. Thus, complexity theory in education describes both individuals' impacts on the workplace and their adaptation to changing workplace needs.

A theoretical framework for change strategies in undergraduate STEM education builds from conceptual and empirical literature (Henderson, Beach, and Finkelstein 2011). Education change occurs along two dimensions: from individuals to environments and structures and from prescribed outcomes to emergent outcomes. Along these dimensions, four categories of change exist: (1) disseminating curriculum and pedagogy; (2) developing reflective teachers; (3) enacting policy; and (4) developing shared vision. Change agents include disciplinary-based STEM education researchers, faculty development researchers, and higher education researchers, representing communities that are mutually independent but with complementary expertise.

Disseminating curriculum and pedagogy relies on individual change agents as experts to transfer particular instructional strategies or conceptions of teaching and learning to individuals with less expertise, leading to prescribed outcomes. Examples of this category include workshops or seminars intended to share "best practices" to achieve specific learning outcomes. Developing reflective teachers focuses on individuals and emergent outcomes by encouraging instructors to reflect on their experiences and expertise to develop new teaching practices and conceptions. Examples include faculty learning communities and other peer support strategies. Enacting policy emphasizes change agents developing environments where instructors engage in specific teaching practices, resulting in prescribed outcomes. For example, a post-tenure review process with a goal of improving teaching represents an environmental factor to incentivize faculty development activities. Finally, developing a shared vision involves instructors and other stakeholders in a department or program developing a collective vision and designing a teaching and learning environment consistent with this vision. Based on their analysis, Henderson et al. (Henderson, Beach, and Finkelstein 2011) determined that successful strategies align with the beliefs of the individuals involved, involve long-term efforts over a semester or more, and are compatible with the complex education system in the department or program. Interestingly, disseminating best practices and enforcing top-down mandates were the least successful change strategies.

A model for successful educational change in engineering relies on four common features: context, strategies, drivers, and mechanisms for sustaining change (Graham 2012). "Context" is a shared purpose among a community ranging from faculty to administrators, often driven by an imperative for change, such as externally imposed reforms or an established culture of innovation. "Strategies" for successful change are interconnected, wide-ranging, and ambitious, seeking to create a unique or premium educational approach that sets a benchmark for engineering education. "Drivers" of change exist at all levels of a program, including school leaders, department heads, and faculty. Finally, "mechanisms for sustaining change" exist in resilient programs that involve a wide pool of faculty delivering changed courses, a well-disseminated long-term assessment of the impact of the change, and an ongoing process of reinvention to remain in a leadership position as a program.

Combining strategies for successful change with mechanisms for sustaining change leads to a conceptual representation from the individual courses to the system or environment level (Kolmos, Hadgraft, and Holgaard 2016). Modifying individual courses without changing the structure of the curriculum represents an "add-on" strategy of change. An "integration" strategy involves working with a wider group of faculty, and perhaps department heads to map and coordinate learning outcomes across multiple courses. This level meets the needs of accreditation agencies focused on outcomes for program graduates. A "re-building" strategy occurs at the institutional level, creating shared vision and values to address the needs of a wide variety of stakeholders. Desired outcomes for students emerge from coordinating courses across disciplines, for example.

When implementing change processes across these levels, one must consider both courses in the curriculum and organizational culture. At the individual (add-on) level, instructor beliefs and concepts will influence the changes made to teaching and learning in individual courses. At systemic levels (integration and rebuilding), sharing of ideas, concepts, and beliefs among faculty or across the institution is important. Thus, change processes will necessarily involve both individual instructors' impact on student learning and organizational approaches to supporting faculty and students in the teaching and learning environment. These change processes require leaders at all three levels, since top-down mandates are not expected to be successful (Henderson, Beach, and Finkelstein 2011). Add-on strategies by individual instructors in response to external requirements represent a bottom-up approach associated with academic freedom (Kolmos, Hadgraft, and Holgaard 2016). Integration strategies at the program level rely on a strategic coordinator, such as a curriculum chair, to motivate groups of faculty, and rebuilding strategies evolve from a shared vision and values. These latter two systems approaches involve both bottom-up and top-down involvement to implement change.

How does an organization implement these theoretical and conceptual models to effect change in a curriculum? The process extends beyond organizing content to involve stakeholders such as students, teachers, institutions, employers, and governments. Principles guiding the process derive from the models above, emphasizing a wide array of participants and perspectives, integrating bottom-up individual efforts with top-down collective vision, and embracing change as a journey rather than a fixed blueprint (Walkington 2010). Each stage in the process of establishing need and context for change, disseminating and refining curriculum vision, designing and developing the curriculum, and implementing change involves cycles of feedback and learning. Successful change agents continually evaluate decision-making processes through reflective practices, leading to cycles within a cycle of change. This approach establishes a continuous process of assessment and revision that mimics continuous improvement processes in engineering practice. Most importantly, faculty and administrator buy-in through active engagement leads to the creation of agile programs capable of quickly adapting to changes in technology and environment in a dynamic workplace.

3.3.3 Creating Agile Programs

The goal of creating an agile program is to respond in a timely manner to changes in the workplace. Some have postulated that major changes in industry, the discipline, and students occur about every ten years, necessitating curriculum updates more often to keep pace (Fowler et al. 2016). Recent advances in BME include new healthcare technologies such as cellular and molecular treatments and wearable patient sensing and intervention devices. In addition, a recent model identified gaps in awareness of BME career paths that decrease students' expectancy for success after graduation (Suresh et al. 2024). An agile program facilitates more rapid realignment of teaching, SOs, and workplace expectations.

Agility at the program level involves contributions from instructional designers and faculty developers, representing a fourth strategy for implementing curriculum change in the conceptual model of Kolmos et al. (2016). Faculty developers may serve as faculty collaborators through consulting and feedback about individual courses (add-on strategy), or they may serve as change agents at the systemic level by advocating for change to departmental leaders (integration) or institutional administration (rebuilding). As faculty developers and teaching and learning centers shift their focus from individual courses to learning environments, they support organizational change at the interface between bottom-up and top-down approaches. For example, after identifying curricular gaps by mapping course objectives to educational program goals, a medical education program was able to implement a process for curriculum revision based on a Theory of Change model that involved a program leader, school administrators, and faculty instructors (Worden and Bray 2025). The change process engaged stakeholders intentionally and transparently, which enhanced buy-in and supported strategic thinking.

BME departments have collaborated with faculty developers to establish curriculum change processes and engage widespread faculty support (Patrick et al. 2022; Barker et al. 2024). In these examples, the processes began with the collection of data from a variety of sources, including student surveys, course materials, instructor feedback, alumni and industry stakeholders, and accrediting agencies. Mapping course learning outcomes to curriculum outcomes represented a core activity, and input from other stakeholders helped to identify gaps and redundancies in the existing curriculum. These processes then informed curriculum change in alignment with student career paths, accreditation requirements, and the department's strategic plan (Patrick et al. 2022). Periodic data acquisition, such as from annual student exit surveys and external advisory board meetings, informs an ongoing process of assessment and adjustment, representing a continuous improvement model in BME curriculum design.

3.4 CHALLENGE 3: EDUCATING BME STUDENTS TO ADAPT TO A GLOBAL WORKFORCE

The US framework for BME education has substantially influenced curriculum development in other countries. The development of BME programs in Asia and Europe coincides with the proliferation of the BME field in the US Early BME programs were established in several countries in Asia in the 1970s, and the first undergraduate programs in Europe were launched in the 1990s (Dermitzakis et al. 2021; Lin et al. 2016). Non-US BME programs have evolved within the context of their socioeconomic and cultural environment; however, commonalities in the curriculum strongly suggest that early US work, such as the VaNTH ERC, has been instrumental in defining BME curriculum across the world (Linsenmeier 2003; Lithgow 2001; Abu-Faraj 2008). For example, a comparative analysis of universities from Europe and Australia contrasts their curriculum with that of US universities and uses the context to justify discrepancies (Lithgow 2001). Similarly, some universities in Asia and Africa have launched new programs adapted from US BME curricula to better align with the specific social, cultural, and technological needs of the region (Abu-Faraj 2008; Ahluwalia et al. 2015). In a global economy, an emerging challenge is to create BME education systems within regional contextual differences so that BME students are capable of adaptation to a global workforce.

As of 2010, 40 of 77 countries in Europe had BME undergraduate programs, and most were created after 2000 (Magjarevic et al. 2010). The European focus on equipping engineering students for the workplace emphasizes employability based on technical and professional skills (Spinks, Silburn, and Birchall 2006; International Engineering Alliance 2021) and sustainability goals (Lantada 2022; Gardelle 2025). Importantly, government agencies such as the Royal Academy of Engineering and accrediting bodies such as the European Network for Accreditation of Engineering Education recognize that systemic efforts are required in addition to individual sharing of best practices in classroom pedagogy (Graham 2012; Henderson, Beach, and Finkelstein 2011).

Several European projects to bridge academia and industry in BME education have focused on connecting research, technology development, and building students' skills and competencies (Magjarevic et al. 2010). The Medical Engineering Listed Education and Training Information Project was founded in 2000 as an initiative of the International Federation for Medical and Biological Engineering (IFMBE) to establish a web-based resource for information on training, education, and research activities related to BME education in Europe. The project identified 50 universities offering 26 undergraduate and 30 postgraduate BME programs. Programs assessed their curricula using methods such as quality assessment schemes, student surveys, employer feedback on graduate employability, and external evaluators. Only four years later, the Chart (Chartography of Medical and Biological Engineering in Europe) Project identified over 200 European institutions offering BME programs at bachelor, master, and/or PhD level. Although most were BME specializations within other engineering disciplines, integrated BME programs leading to a BME diploma were beginning to appear. In 2004–2005, the IFMBE and the European Alliance for Medical and Biological Engineering and Science organized the BIOMEDEA project to establish guidelines for quality assurance and accreditation of educational programs as well as certification of biomedical and clinical engineers. Finally, the European Commission created the Tempus funding scheme to support multi-institution partnerships to develop and disseminate new curricula and pedagogies and to promote quality assurance strategies. By 2010, 299 BME bachelor's, master's, and PhD programs were documented at 148 universities in 40 European countries (Bliznakov and Pallikarakis 2012). These projects demonstrate the rapid expansion of BME education in Europe, leading to an increased number of BMEs available for the workforce.

In Asia, a survey of institutions in ten countries revealed curricula that are designed about 30% based on basic knowledge, such as mathematics and physiology, and about 40% based on specialized knowledge in areas including medical instrumentation, biomaterials, bio-information, and biomechanics. Most BME programs require internship experiences in hospitals or biomedical engineering practice. Approximately half of BME graduates work in biomedical-related fields. The most common career paths for BMEs are as service or sales engineers, primarily in medical device companies, and as clinical engineers, especially in Japan, Taiwan, Singapore, Malaysia, and China. The growth of BME education and professional practice in these countries has societal impacts. The availability of BME education programs, which support BME research efforts, correlates with higher healthcare quality in Southeast Asian nations (Fermin and Tan 2021). Outcomes like these are leading to efforts to establish new BME programs in the Philippines (Fermin and Tan 2021), and India is supporting engineering education reform to create an "efficient skilling ecosystem" that will bridge the academia-industry gap in disciplines such as BME (Kumar and Rewari 2022).

Engineering education in Australia reflects a need to address multiple stakeholders in industry, academia, and government (Walkington 2010). Assessment and accreditation standards include both technical competencies, including sustainability and other societal impact considerations, and professional and personal attributes, including ethics, communication, and creativity (Engineers Australia 2019). In BME, traditional curricula contained a limited number of courses related to traditional engineering career opportunities (Lithgow 2001). This design is built on historical growth in medical physics and clinical engineering in this region. More recently, the need for dialogue among educational institutions and stakeholders to create a comprehensive BME curriculum has been demonstrated (Prestigiacomo, Chan, and Kark 2024). This BME curriculum would include both interdisciplinary technical proficiencies and a broad set of interprofessional skills, including interdisciplinary teamwork, team and project management, creativity and innovation, communication, entrepreneurship, leadership, and empathy toward patients and clinical users. Input from industry partners and recent graduates highlighted the need for technical skills related to regulatory standards, data analysis, software engineering, and manufacturing. These ideas aligned with professional practice in the workplace. Input from current BME students and academic staff highlighted aspects of professional practice, experiential learning, and societal impact. Examples included industry internships, a broad choice of BME electives, and history/social science courses related to sociotechnical topics. These suggestions related to the stakeholders' formative experiences in academia. Although this study was performed in Australia, the results demonstrate the need for input from multiple stakeholders when designing or revising BME curricula.

A primary goal of education systems in Africa is to develop engineers with expert skills through individualized programs that cater to the specific social, cultural, and technological needs of the region. Historically, very few African institutions offered BME courses. Existing courses were heavily based on Western curricula and emphasized niche subjects like micro-electro-mechanical devices or cell engineering. One strategy to broaden the availability of BME education resources involved implementing an open-source approach through workshops and online repositories (Ahluwalia et al. 2015). The approach leveraged expertise from local stakeholders in participating countries, encouraging ownership of student training and continuity of the innovation process. In Nigeria, BME professional practice has grown from maintaining and repairing medical equipment to also include problem-solving in the biological and medical fields (Oyejide et al. 2025). In 2016, the University of Ilorin (Unilorin) became the first university in Nigeria to admit students directly into a degree-awarding BME undergraduate program. More universities now offer BME or BME-related degree programs, but curriculum design is often limited by resources, faculty expertise, and institutional priorities. Education leaders in Nigeria and other African countries recognize the importance of continuing to grow BME education to support the improvement of healthcare system quality and accessibility in their countries (Raxworthy, Ssekitoleko, and Makobore 2022). Recommendations include developing BME curricula that support economical and viable health technologies appropriate for the local context. As technical capability and capacity improve, curricula should prepare BME students to contribute to defining a regulatory environment that allows for efficient and safe translation of technology to clinical applications.

Historically, comprehensive BME education programs in the Middle East and North Africa (MENA) region only existed at three universities in Israel (Ben Gurion University, Tel Aviv University, and the Technion). The Jordan University of Science and Technology (JUST) and the American University College of Science and Technology (AUST) in Lebanon established comprehensive BME programs in 1998 and 2002, respectively (Abu-Faraj 2006; Abdulhay et al. 2017). Both curricula were designed with the objective of accreditation by ABET, the primary accreditation body in the United States. The program at JUST was assessed comprehensively using both student performance metrics and surveys of students, faculty, and employers (Abdulhay et al. 2017). Empirical analysis of the curriculum at AUST and several other institutions in the MENA region revealed a need for supporting collaborations among academic programs, medical centers, and industry (Abu-Faraj 2014). In Turkey, Başkent University established the first biomedical engineering department offering an undergraduate degree in 2000 (Ün 2022). Since then, BME curriculum designs in Turkey have tended to mimic existing science and engineering programs due to faculty availability and government approval processes, leading to less diversity of topic areas than in US programs. In addition, the supply of BME students appears to exceed the industry need, suggesting academic programs need to solicit stakeholder input in ways other countries and regions have done. Overall, the diverse perspectives on curriculum development strategies and stakeholder requirements among countries create variable outcomes for students seeking careers in BME.

As a field, BME started in Latin America in the 1970s in Argentina, Brazil, and Mexico. Most of the early programs were established by researchers trained in the United States to develop a workforce capable of understanding electronic devices in healthcare settings (Ríos Rincón et al. 2010; Fandiño 2017; Cuautle et al. 2020). While curricular structure was similar to US programs, the focus was not on the design or development of techniques and equipment but rather on training high-level professionals to install, maintain, and use biomedical systems and equipment. In recent years, the number of programs has grown significantly, from a few offerings in the 1970s to more than 90 programs in 2017, most of them in Mexico and Colombia. Despite the growth observed in the number of programs and countries offering BME programs, the educational content has not evolved with recent technological and research advances, and programs have remained focused on training engineers to manage and maintain the technical infrastructure of healthcare systems (J. Azpiroz-Leehan et al. 2016). Recent studies that looked into career opportunities for BME graduates in Mexico show that while current programs accurately prepare students for the workforce, most job offerings are for low-paying sales, service, and hospital maintenance positions. There is a growing need to shift educational models from a maintenance-oriented curriculum to a project-based, experiential learning model emphasizing translational research topics and professional skills development. This new approach would present an area of opportunity to educate engineers who are competent in the design and development of medical devices and can innovate to impact the quality of the local healthcare system (Joaquín Azpiroz-Leehan et al. 2020, 2015; Gallo et al. 2024).

In developing countries around the world, addressing sustainability in BME education often means addressing public health needs and challenges, which depend on the local context in the country or region (Douglas 2011). As a result, BME programs are encouraged to focus on collaborating with local communities through governments, non-governmental organizations, healthcare providers, and industry. In some cases, partnerships between institutions in developed and developing countries enable the transfer of skills while addressing local constraints in engineering design and solution spaces. Care must be taken to prioritize local perspectives and social justice to reach equitable engineering solutions. A "descriptive meaning" of engineering globalization, applying engineering principles to problems across international and cultural boundaries (Newberry 2004), may not be sufficient. In developed countries, the tendency in BME education is to add requirements such as foreign language proficiency or international studies topics using an add-on strategy (Kolmos, Hadgraft, and Holgaard 2016). Similarly, requiring study abroad does not typically reduce the compulsory technical course content in the curriculum. A "normative meaning" of engineering globalization involves cultural exchange to achieve a shared meaning of reality, but it also risks inequities associated with which group's preferences or interests are promoted through globalization. BME faculty might propose systemic approaches to prepare graduates with skills, competencies, and international experiences for a global workplace. Newberry (2004) argues for a "transformative meaning" of engineering globalization in which the mission of engineering education emphasizes students' critical thinking, analysis, and synthesis skills while including cultural, ethical, environmental, sustainability, and global justice considerations. Resistance to this idea often centers around the objection to a rebuilding strategy (Kolmos, Hadgraft, and Holgaard 2016) that replaces some advanced technical content in the curriculum with depth in professional and affective competencies. Many BME curricula are already well-positioned, since they are inherently interdisciplinary and responsive to multiple stakeholders in industry, healthcare, and regulatory agencies.

BME education worldwide includes diverse origins and perspectives influenced by international standards of engineering practice and local contexts in individual regions and countries. These local contexts provide both challenges and opportunities for BMEs to impact healthcare. As a result, the challenge for agile BME education systems is to train students who can participate in the global workforce to impact healthcare locally.

3.5 CONCLUSION

The discipline of BME education has grown rapidly since its origin in the 1960s. As new engineering challenges emerge and biomedical sciences and healthcare strategies advance, BME curricula attempting to achieve technical depth in multiple traditional engineering disciplines appear out of date. Modern BME curricula design learning outcomes that align with the expectations of available career paths in a range of industries and professional settings. A dynamic, interdisciplinary workplace requires agile BME programs that adapt quickly while maintaining core values in both engineering content and professional competencies. Adaptability of BME programs involves continuous improvement through change management strategies that include perspectives from multiple stakeholders. In a global economy, BME students expect to impact healthcare in localities in all parts of the world. BME programs need to adapt the scope and breadth of curriculum content to balance technical skills with cultural responsiveness, ethics, and social justice. BME curricula that satisfy a transformative definition of engineering globalization will prepare students both for successful careers and for advancing contributions to human health worldwide.

REFERENCES

Abdulhay, Enas, Ruba Khnouf, Shireen Haddad, and Areen Al-Bashir. 2017. "Improvement of Medical Content in the Curriculum of Biomedical Engineering Based on Assessment of Students' Outcomes." *BMC Medical Education* 17 (129). https://doi.org/10.1186/s12909-017-0968-2.

Abu-Faraj, Ziad O. 2006. "A Premier Comprehensive Curriculum in Biomedical Engineering within the Middle East and Northern African Region." In *2005 IEEE Engineering in Medicine and Biology Conference*. https://doi.org/10.1109/IEMBS.2005.1616418.

Abu-Faraj, Ziad O. 2008. "Bioengineering/Biomedical Engineering Education and Career Development: Literature Review, Definitions, and Constructive Recommendations." *International Journal of Engineering Education* 24 (5): 990–1011.

Abu-Faraj, Ziad O. 2014. "Biomedical Engineering Education in the Middle East and North Africa." In *2nd Middle East Conference on Biomedical Engineering*, 317–20. https://doi.org/10.1109/MECBME.2014.6783268.

Ahluwalia, Arti, Daniel Atwine, Carmelo De Maria, Charles Ibingira, Emmanuel Kipkorir, Fasil Kiros, June Madete, et al. 2015. "Open Biomedical Engineering Education in Africa." In *2015 37th Annual International Conference of the IEEE Engineering in Medicine and Biology Society (EMBC)*, 3687–90. https://doi.org/10.1109/EMBC.2015.7319193.

Amos, Jennifer R., and Gabriella R. Dupont. 2018. "Work in Progress: Are We on Track with Tracks?" In *2018 ASEE Annual Conference & Exposition*. https://peer.asee.org/board-3-work-in-progress-are-we-on-track-with-tracks.

Azpiroz-Leehan, Joaquín, Fabiola Martínez-Licona, E. Gerardo Urbina-Medal, Miguel Cadena-Méndez, and Emilio Sacristán-Rock. 2015. "Critical Assessment and Outlook for the 50 Biomedical Engineering Undergraduate Programs in Mexico." In *2015 Annual International Conference of the IEEE Engineering in Medicine and Biology Society (EMBC)*, 3973–6. https://doi.org/10.1109/EMBC.2015.7319264.

Azpiroz-Leehan, Joaquín, Fabiola Martínez-Licona, E. Gerardo Urbina-Medal, Miguel Cadena-Méndez, and Emilio Sacristán-Rock. 2016. "Biomedical Engineering in Latin America: A Survey of 90 Undergraduate Programs." *IFMBE Proceedings* 60. https://doi.org/10.1007/978-981-10-4086-3_27.

Azpiroz-Leehan, Joaquín, Emilio Sacristán-Rock, Gerardo Urbina-Medal, and Fabiola M. Martínez-Licona. 2020. "Updating the Biomedical Engineering Curriculum in Latin America: Moving from Management and Maintenance to Design and Development of Medical Devices." In *2020 Annual International Conference of the IEEE Engineering in Medicine and Biology Society (EMBC)*, 6028–31. https://doi.org/10.1109/EMBC44109.2020.9175362.

Barker, Shannon, Brian P. Helmke, Lynn Mandeltort, Jessica Taggart, and Timothy E. Allen. 2024. "Work in Progress: A Collaborative, Principle-Focused Curriculum Design Process for a BME Undergraduate Program." In *2024 ASEE Annual Conference & Exposition*. https://peer.asee.org/board-7-work-in-progress-a-collaborative-principle-focused-curriculum-design-process-for-a-bme-undergraduate-program.

Baura, Gail D. 2015. "Educating for Industry: A Call to Action for Bio-Biomedical Engineering Professors and Students." *IEEE Pulse* 6 (2): 5–9.

Billiar, Kristen, Donald P. Gaver, Kenneth Barbee, Anita Singh, John D. DesJardins, Beth Pruitt, Joe Tranquillo, et al. 2022. "Learning Environments and Evidence-Based Practices in Bioengineering and Biomedical Engineering." *Biomedical Engineering Education* 2 (1): 1–16. https://doi.org/10.1007/s43683-021-00062-z.

Bliznakov, Zhivko, and Nicolas Pallikarakis. 2012. "Overview of Biomedical Engineering Education Programs in Europe: The Results of the CRH-BME Project Survey." In *5th European Conference of the International Federation for Medical and Biological Engineering*, edited by Ákos Jobbágy, 1414–17. Berlin: Springer. https://doi.org/10.1007/978-3-642-23508-5_365.

Brown, Alan, Julie Eatock, Dorian Dixon, Brian J. Meenan, and John Anderson. 2008. "Quality and Continuous Improvement in Medical Device Manufacturing." *The TQM Journal* 20 (6): 541–55. https://doi.org/10.1108/17542730810909329.

Bureau of Labor Statistics. 2025. *Bioengineers and Biomedical Engineers*. Accessed June 5, 2025. https://www.bls.gov/ooh/architecture-and-engineering/biomedical-engineers.htm.

Campos, Débora Barni de, Luis Mauricio Martins de Resende, and Alexandre Borges Fagundes. 2020. *The Importance of Soft Skills for Engineering*. https://www.researchgate.net/publication/343908179_The_Importance_of_Soft_Skills_for_the_Engineering.

Cuautle, José de Jesús Agustín Flores, Citlalli Jessica Trujillo Romero, Rigoberto Martínez Méndez, Blanca Estela González Sánchez, and Ingrid Lizette Sánchez Carmona. 2020. "Desarrollo y tendencias de la ingeniería biomédica en México." *ReCIBE. Revista Electrónica de Computación, Informática, Biomédica y Electrónica* 9 (1): 1–11.

Dermitzakis, Aris, Christos Alexandropoulos, Maria Fermani, and Nicolas Pallikarakis. 2021. "Biomedical Engineering Education in Europe: A 30 Years Review." In *8th European Medical and Biological Engineering Conference*, edited by Tomaz Jarm, Aleksandra Cvetkoska, Samo Mahnič-Kalamiza, and Damijan Miklavcic, 208–17. Cham: Springer International Publishing. https://doi.org/10.1007/978-3-030-64610-3_24.

Douglas, Tania S. 2011. "Biomedical Engineering Education in Developing Countries: Research Synthesis." In *2011 Annual International Conference of the IEEE Engineering in Medicine and Biology Society (EMBC)*, 3628–30. https://doi.org/10.1109/IEMBS.2011.6090609.

Dumitru, Daniela, and Diane F. Halpern. 2023. "Critical Thinking: Creating Job-Proof Skills for the Future of Work." *Journal of Intelligence* 11 (10): 194. https://doi.org/10.3390/jintelligence11100194.

Engineers Australia. 2019. *Stage 1 Competency Standard Professional Engineer*. https://www.engineersaustralia.org.au/publications/stage-1-competency-standard-professional-engineers.

Fandiño, Clarena Cruz. 2017. "La ingeniería biomédica: Aplicación e impacto de la tecnología en salud." *#ashtag* 11: 23–36. https://doi.org/10.52143/2346139X.530.

Fermin, Jamie Ledesma, and Myles Joshua Toledo Tan. 2021. "The Need for the Establishment of Biomedical Engineering as an Academic and Professional Discipline in the Philippines—A Quantitative Argument." *IEEE Access* 9: 3097–111. https://doi.org/10.1109/ACCESS.2020.3046655.

Fowler, Debra A., Chelsea A. H. Bakenhus, Merwyn M. Kothmann, Maria L. Macik, Nate Poling, and Sherri MacWillie. 2016. "Redesigning Natural Resources Curricula: A Redesign Process Model at Texas A&M University." *Natural Sciences Education* 45 (1): 1–10. https://doi.org/10.4195/nse2015.09.0019.

Gallo, Lucila M. Figueroa, María F. Lencina, Facundo A. Lucianna, Carmelo Felice, and Rossana Madrid. 2024. "Degree Integration Projects in Biomedical Engineering: Design of a Didactic Sequence to Promote Learning." In *Advances in Bioengineering and Clinical Engineering*. https://doi.org/10.1007/978-3-031-61973-1_33.

Gardelle, L. 2025. "Sustainability in Engineering Education in Europe Over the Last 15 Years: Visions and Tendencies among Educators as Revealed by a Literature Review." *European Journal of Engineering Education*. https://doi.org/10.1080/03043797.2025.2474044.

Gatchell, David, and Robert Linsenmeier. 2014. "Similarities and Differences in Undergraduate Biomedical Engineering Curricula in the United States." In *2014 ASEE Annual Conference & Exposition Proceedings*, 24.1082.1–14. Indianapolis, IN: ASEE Conferences. https://doi.org/10.18260/1-2-23015.

Graham, Ruth. 2012. *Achieving Excellence in Engineering Education: The Ingredients of Successful Change*. London: Royal Academy of Engineering.

International Engineering Alliance. 2021. *Graduate Attributes and Professional Competencies*. https://www.internationalengineeringalliance.org/.

Hart, Richard T. 2015. "Biomedical Engineering Accredited Undergraduate Programs: Four Decades of Growth." *Annals of Biomedical Engineering* 43 (8): 1713–15. https://doi.org/10.1007/s10439-015-1319-2.

Henderson, Charles, Andrea Beach, and Noah Finkelstein. 2011. "Facilitating Change in Undergraduate STEM Instructional Practices: An Analytic Review of the Literature." *Journal of Research in Science Teaching* 48 (8): 952–84. https://doi.org/10.1002/tea.20439.

Hirudayaraj, Malar, Rose Baker, Francie Baker, and Mike Eastman. 2021. "Soft Skills for Entry-Level Engineers: What Employers Want." *Education Sciences* 11 (10): 641. https://doi.org/10.3390/educsci11100641.

Huang-Saad, Aileen, Jan Stegemann, and Lonnie Shea. 2020. "Developing a Model for Integrating Professional Practice and Evidence-Based Teaching Practices into BME Curriculum." *Annals of Biomedical Engineering* 48 (2): 881–92. https://doi.org/10.1007/s10439-019-02427-6.

Jamison, Cassandra Sue Ellen, Aileen Huang-Saad, Shanna R. Daly, and Lisa R. Lattuca. 2020. "The Value of Co-Curricular Experiences: Perspectives of Third-Year Biomedical Engineering Students." In *2020 ASEE Annual Conference & Exposition*. https://peer.asee.org/the-value-of-co-curricular-experiences-perspectives-of-third-year-biomedical-engineering-students.

Jamison, Cassandra Sue Ellen, Lisa R. Lattuca, Shanna R. Daly, and Aileen Huang-Saad. 2023. "Biomedical Engineering Students' Perceived Learning Through Co-Curriculars." *Studies in Engineering Education* 4 (1). https://doi.org/10.21061/see.94.

Kandiko Howson, Camille, and Martyn Kingsbury. 2023. "Curriculum Change as Transformational Learning." *Teaching in Higher Education* 28 (8): 1847–66. https://doi.org/10.1080/13562517.2021.1940923.

Katona, Peter G. 2006. "Biomedical Engineering and the Whitaker Foundation: A Thirty-Year Partnership." *Annals of Biomedical Engineering* 34 (6): 904–16. https://doi.org/10.1007/s10439-006-9087-7.

Kolmos, Anette, Roger G. Hadgraft, and Jette Egelund Holgaard. 2016. "Response Strategies for Curriculum Change in Engineering." *International Journal of Technology and Design Education* 26 (3): 391–411. https://doi.org/10.1007/s10798-015-9319-y.

Kumar, Vikas, and Mohit Rewari. 2022. "A Responsible Approach to Higher Education Curriculum Design." *International Journal of Educational Reform* 31 (4): 422–41. https://doi.org/10.1177/10567879221110509.

Lam, Gabrielle, Isgard Hueck, Christian Rivera, and Patricia Widder. 2025. "A Future-Focused Lens to Equipping Biomedical Engineering Graduates for an Evolving Field." *Biomedical Engineering Education*. https://doi.org/10.1007/s43683-025-00186-6.

Lantada, Antonio D. 2022. "Toward a More Ethical and Sustainable Biomedical Engineering Education." *IEEE Pulse* 13 (3): 26–9.

LaPlaca, Michelle C., Wendy C. Newstetter, and Ajit P. Yoganathan. 2001. "Problem-Based Learning in Biomedical Engineering Curricula." In *31st Annual Frontiers in Education Conference. Impact on Engineering and Science Education. Conference Proceedings*, vol. 2, F3E–16. https://doi.org/10.1109/FIE.2001.963748.

Law, Mei Yuan. 2022. "A Review of Curriculum Change and Innovation for Higher Education." *Journal of Education and Training Studies* 10 (2): 16–23. https://doi.org/10.11114/jets.v10i2.5448.

Le Doux, Joseph M., and Alisha A. Waller. 2016. *The Problem Solving Studio: An Apprenticeship Environment for Aspiring Engineers*. https://www.researchgate.net/publication/312095211_The_problem_solving_studio_An_apprenticeship_environment_for_aspiring_engineers.

Lin, Kang-Ping, Mei-Fen Chen, Cheng-Lung Tsai, and Kao Tsai. 2016. "Status of Biomedical Engineering Education in the Asia Pacific." In *XIV Mediterranean Conference on Medical and Biological Engineering and Computing 2016*, edited by Efthyvoulos Kyriacou, Stelios Christofides and Constantinos S. Pattichis, 1331–4. Cham: Springer International Publishing. https://doi.org/10.1007/978-3-319-32703-7_256.

Linsenmeier, Robert A. 2003. "What Makes a Biomedical Engineer?" *IEEE Engineering in Medicine and Biology Magazine* 22 (4): 32–8. https://doi.org/10.1109/MEMB.2003.1237489.

Linsenmeier, Robert A., and Ann Saterbak. 2020. "Fifty Years of Biomedical Engineering Undergraduate Education." *Annals of Biomedical Engineering* 48 (6): 1590–615. https://doi.org/10.1007/s10439-020-02494-0.

Lithgow, Brian J. 2001. "Biomedical Engineering Curriculum: A Comparison Between the USA, Europe, and Australia." In *2001 Conference Proceedings of the 23rd Annual International Conference of the IEEE Engineering in Medicine and Biology Society*, vol. 4, 4016–19. https://doi.org/10.1109/IEMBS.2001.1019726.

Maghiar, Mihai, and Casey Brown. 2022. "A Qualitative Multi-Disciplinary Analysis of Employers' Technology Competency Perceptions for Graduates' Readiness to the Workforce." *Cogent Education* 9 (1): 2147777. https://doi.org/10.1080/2331186X.2022.2147777.

Magjarevic, Ratko, Igor Lackovic, Zhivko Bliznakov, and Nicolas Pallikarakis. 2010. "Challenges of the Biomedical Engineering Education in Europe." In *2010 Annual International Conference of the IEEE Engineering in Medicine and Biology*, 2959–62. https://doi.org/10.1109/IEMBS.2010.5626263.

Miller, Michael I., Andrew O. Brightman, Frederick H. Epstein, K. Jane Grande-Allen, Jordan J. Green, Eileen Haase, Cato T. Laurencin, et al. 2023. "BME 2.0: Engineering the Future of Medicine." *BME Frontiers* 4: 0001. https://doi.org/10.34133/bmef.0001.

National Academy of Engineering. 2018. *Understanding the Educational and Career Pathways of Engineers*. Washington, DC: National Academies Press. https://doi.org/10.17226/25284.

National Science Foundation. 2023. *Survey of Earned Doctorates*. https://ncses.nsf.gov/surveys/earned-doctorates/2023#data.

Newberry, Byron. 2004. "Engineering Globalization: Oxymoron or Opportunity?" *IEEE Technology and Society Magazine*: 29–35. https://doi.org/10.1109/ISTAS.2004.1314322.

Newstetter, Wendy, and Paul Benkeser. "Integrating Soft Skills in a BME Curriculum." Paper presented at the 2004 *Annual Conference, Salt Lake City*, Utah, June 20–23, 2004. https://doi.org/10.18260/1-2--13281.

Oyejide, Ayodele James, Oluwatosin David Abodunrin, Ebenezer Oluwatosin Atoyebi, Bola Oni, Joy Ene Idoko, Ayoade Adetunji Adeyemi, Goodnews Akindele, and Sadiq Adewale Adedayo. 2025. "Landscape of Biomedical Engineering and Technology in Nigeria: A Perspective." *Biomedical Engineering Education*, May. https://doi.org/10.1007/s43683-025-00187-5.

Patrick, Charles W., James Machek, Reza Avazmohammadi, Daniel L. Alge, Charles W. Peak, and Michael McShane. 2022. "Process for Faculty-Driven, Data-Informed Curriculum Continuity Review in Biomedical Engineering." *Biomedical Engineering Education* 2 (2): 265–80. https://doi.org/10.1007/s43683-021-00063-y.

Potvin, Alfred R., Francis M. Long, John G. Webster, and Richard J. Jendrucko. 1981. "Biomedical Engineering Education: Enrollment, Courses, Degrees, and Employment." *IEEE Transactions on Biomedical Engineering* BME-28 (1): 22–8. https://doi.org/10.1109/TBME.1981.324841.

Prestigiacomo, Rita, Chun Chuen Chan, and Lauren Kark. 2024. "A Biomedical Engineering Curriculum Development: A Qualitative Study Engaging Four Stakeholders." *European Journal of Education* 59 (2): e12632. https://doi.org/10.1111/ejed.12632.

Raxworthy, Matthew, Robert Ssekitoleko, and Philip N. Makobore. 2022. *Biomedical Engineering as a Driver for Healthcare Improvements in East Africa*. https://eprints.whiterose.ac.uk/196342/7/BME-Driver_Report_Final_Digital.pdf.

Ríos Rincón, Adriana María, Antonio Miguel Cruz, Luis Eduardo Rodríguez Cheu, and Javier Chaparro. 2010. "La ingeniería biomédica en Colombia: Una perspectiva desde la formación del pregrado." *Revista Ingeniería Biomédica* 4 (7): 23–34.

Rivera, Christian Poblete, Aileen Huang-Saad, Cassandra Sue Ellen Jamison, and Annie Wang. 2020. "Preparing Early-Career Biomedical Undergraduates Through Investigations of Stakeholder Needs: A Qualitative Analysis." In *2020 ASEE Annual Conference & Exposition*. https://peer.asee.org/preparing-early-career-biomedical-undergraduates-through-investigations-of-stakeholder-needs-a-qualitative-analysis.

Singh, Jagdeep, and Harwinder Singh. 2013. "Continuous Improvement Strategies: An Overview." *SSRN Scholarly Paper*. Rochester, NY: Social Science Research Network. https://papers.ssrn.com/abstract=2255815.

Sovilj, Snezana, Igor Lackovic, and Ratko Magjarevic. 2012. "The Role of Laboratories and Projects in Biomedical Engineering Education." In *5th European Conference of the International Federation for Medical and Biological Engineering*, edited by Ákos Jobbágy, 1422–5. Berlin: Springer. https://doi.org/10.1007/978-3-642-23508-5_367.

Spinks, Nigel, Nick Silburn, and David Birchall. 2006. *Educating Engineers for the 21st Century: The Industry View*. London: Royal Academy of Engineering.

Suresh, Deepthi E., Julie P. Martin, Annamarie Lunkes, and Paul A. Jensen. 2024. "Modeling Career Paths in Biomedical Quality Engineering." *Biomedical Engineering Education* 4 (2): 339–59. https://doi.org/10.1007/s43683-024-00150-w.

Tompkins, Willis. 2001. "Using Design as the Backbone of a BME Curriculum." In *2001 ASEE Annual Conference & Exposition*, 6.1104.1–9. https://peer.asee.org/using-design-as-the-backbone-of-a-bme-curriculum.

Ün, M. Kerem. 2022. "Editorial: A Historical Perspective to Biomedical Engineering and Biomedical Engineering Education in Turkey." *International Journal of Advances in Biomedical Engineering* 1 (1): 1–8.

Vinodh, S., Jiju Antony, Rohit Agrawal, and Jacqueline Ann Douglas. 2020. "Integration of Continuous Improvement Strategies with Industry 4.0: A Systematic Review and Agenda for Further Research." *The TQM Journal* 33 (2): 441–72. https://doi.org/10.1108/TQM-07-2020-0157.

Volkwein, J. Fredericks, Lisa R. Lattuca, Patrick T. Terenzini, Linda C. Strauss, and Javzan Sukhbaatar. 2004. *Engineering Change: A Study of the Impact of EC2000*. Baltimore: ABET.

Walkington, Jackie. 2010. "A Process for Curriculum Change in Engineering Education." *European Journal of Engineering Education* 27 (2): 133–48.

White, John A., Donald P. Gaver, Robert J. Butera, Bernard Choi, Mary J. Dunlop, K. Jane Grande-Allen, Anna Grosberg, et al. 2020. "Core Competencies for Undergraduates in Bioengineering and Biomedical Engineering: Findings, Consequences, and Recommendations." *Annals of Biomedical Engineering* 48 (3): 905–12. https://doi.org/10.1007/s10439-020-02468-2.

Winberg, Christine, Mike Bramhall, David Greenfield, Patrick Johnson, Peter Rowlett, Oliver Lewis, Jeff Waldock, and Karin Wolff. 2020. "Developing Employability in Engineering Education: A Systematic Review of the Literature." *European Journal of Engineering Education* 45 (2): 165–80. https://doi.org/10.1080/03043797.2018.1534086.

Worden, Mary Kate, and Megan J. Bray. 2025. "A Theory of Change Approach to Curricular Revision: Filling a Curricular Gap Identified through Curriculum Mapping." *BMC Medical Education* 25 (1): 533. https://doi.org/10.1186/s12909-025-07100-2.

4 Accreditation in Biomedical Engineering Education

Ziad O. Abu-Faraj

4.1 INTRODUCTION: ACCREDITATION AS A PILLAR OF QUALITY IN BIOMEDICAL ENGINEERING

In a world shaped by rapid technological advances and modern healthcare demands, biomedical engineering (BME) education emerges as a critical frontier where biological science, engineering, and medicine converge. Accreditation ensures that academic programs meet rigorous quality standards while remaining aligned with industry and societal needs. Foundational studies (Nagel 2001; Enderle et al. 2003; Abu-Faraj 2011, 2012) highlight accreditation's role in fostering innovation through standardized yet flexible curricula. By integrating engineering principles with biomedical sciences, accreditation enables graduates to address interdisciplinary healthcare challenges, sustaining the global demand for high-quality BME programs.

Accreditation extends beyond academics, preparing graduates for the complexities of healthcare. Hart (2015) and Linsenmeier and Saterbak (2020) documented the global expansion of BME programs, reflecting the field's evolution. As of January 2025, 142 ABET-accredited Biomedical Engineering programs offering Bachelor of Science (BS) and Bachelor of Engineering (BE) degrees exist across 11 countries, along with 32 accredited Bioengineering programs in the United States (ABET 2025). This growth underscores the importance of equipping students with industry-relevant skills, clinical experience, and research expertise. By fostering continuous improvement, accreditation ensures that graduates are prepared for current challenges and future healthcare transformations.

This chapter explores accreditation's role in shaping BME education, examining general and program-specific criteria that govern student performance, faculty qualifications, and curriculum design while aligning programs with industry needs. It discusses the mapping of PEOs to SOs to ensure competency attainment, alongside continuous improvement processes, institutional support, faculty development, and facilities. Ultimately, accreditation drives BME education forward, ensuring that programs evolve to meet healthcare demands and prepare graduates for leadership in medical technology and innovation.

DOI: 10.1201/9781003520313-4

4.1.1 Accreditation: Ensuring Quality and Industry Relevance

Accreditation validates academic rigor while aligning BME programs with evolving healthcare and technological needs. In an era of rapid medical advancements, programs must remain dynamic, adaptable, and forward-thinking. Moreover, accreditation ensures that curricula balance technical knowledge with practical clinical applications, bridging academic learning with industry expectations. Beyond academic assurance, it also aligns BME programs with strategic needs in medicine and engineering. As healthcare systems integrate advanced technologies, the demand for skilled biomedical engineers increases. Consequently, accreditation provides a framework for curriculum refinement and institutional alignment with global healthcare priorities, fostering continuous improvement. Table 4.1 highlights international accreditation bodies, reflecting a global commitment to quality BME education. Furthermore, Enderle et al. (2003) emphasize systematic planning in ABET accreditation, guiding institutions through evolving standards. By supporting educational objectives and program outcomes, accreditation ensures graduates acquire the knowledge and skills to drive healthcare innovation.

4.1.2 Accreditation's Role in Adapting to Industry and Educational Advancements

BME education must evolve alongside technological advancements, healthcare needs, and interdisciplinary knowledge integration. Programs must establish strong

TABLE 4.1
Leading international accreditation bodies and their commissions for biomedical engineering programs

Accreditation Body	Corresponding Commission/Unit	Region
ABET (Accreditation Board for Engineering and Technology, Inc.)	Engineering Accreditation Commission (EAC)	United States
EUR-ACE (European Accreditation of Engineering Programs)	European Network for Accreditation of Engineering Education (ENAEE)	Europe
Washington Accord	International Engineering Alliance (IEA)	Global
Canadian Engineering Accreditation Board (CEAB)	CEAB under Engineers Canada	Canada
Engineering Council UK (ECUK)	ECUK Professional Engineering Institutions (PEIs)	United Kingdom
Asia Pacific Accreditation and Certification Commission (APACC)	APACC Standards	Asia-Pacific
Engineers Australia (EA)	EA Accreditation for Engineering and Technology	Australia
China Engineering Education Accreditation Association (CEEAA)	CEEAA Standards	China
National Board of Accreditation (NBA)	Engineering Accreditation Committee (EAC)	India
Consejo de Acreditación de la Enseñanza de la Ingeniería (CACEI)	Ingeniería y Tecnología (Engineering and Technology)	Mexico

engineering foundations while incorporating emerging fields such as AI, medical robotics, and personalized medicine, alongside ethical considerations and healthcare policies. Accreditation ensures rigorous academic standards while enabling adaptation to industry shifts. Through advisory boards and industry input, accreditation frameworks align curricula with evolving healthcare trends, fostering continuous improvement.

To remain relevant, program leadership must champion innovation and stakeholder engagement. Collaboration with accrediting bodies, industry partners, and faculty ensures that curricula integrate interdisciplinary approaches, emerging technologies, and experiential learning opportunities such as clinical immersion and co-op programs. Feedback from alumni, industry advisory boards (IABs), and employers refines PEOs and SOs, ensuring that programs not only meet accreditation standards but also anticipate future healthcare trends.

Frank et al. (2020) highlight accreditation's role in maintaining curricular alignment with technological advancements. Accreditation supports continuous evaluation, enabling programs to incorporate innovations such as wearable health technologies, 3D bioprinting, and gene editing. Thus, accreditation sustains BME education's quality while ensuring its evolution to meet the dynamic needs of healthcare and society.

4.2 ACCREDITATION CRITERIA: FOUNDATIONS FOR PROGRAM COMPLIANCE

Accreditation standards ensure consistency and excellence across academic programs, defining expectations at various degree levels. General criteria establish fundamental requirements, including student performance, PEOs, SOs, continuous improvement, faculty qualifications, curriculum, facilities, and institutional support. These criteria ensure rigorous academic and operational standards, while program-specific criteria address the unique needs of specialized fields like biomedical engineering, ensuring that programs meet the unique needs of their respective disciplines. Accreditation frameworks balance broad academic rigor with specialized expertise, enabling alignment with institutional missions and evolving industry demands. Adopting the ABET model, this section explores how accreditation criteria serve as pillars for quality assurance and continuous improvement.

4.2.1 General Criteria: Establishing a Broad Foundation

General criteria provide a standardized framework for accredited engineering programs, addressing key elements such as student performance, curriculum breadth and depth, continuous improvement, faculty qualifications, institutional support, and facilities. Programs must align with these criteria to demonstrate commitment to industry standards and graduate preparedness. The ABET Criteria for Accrediting Engineering Programs, 2025–2026, ensure rigorous academic standards while fostering responsiveness to technological advancements (ABET 2024a). Continuous improvement through data-driven assessment and evaluation reinforces the dynamic nature of engineering education. Table 4.2 summarizes these guidelines, establishing a foundation for quality, sustainability, and innovation.

TABLE 4.2
Key components of ABET general criteria for accrediting engineering programs

General Criterion	Description
Students	Admissions, progress, and outcomes
PEOs	Long-term accomplishments expected of graduates
SOs	Knowledge, skills, and abilities students must attain by graduation
Continuous improvement	Mechanisms for assessment and refinement
Curriculum	Ensuring breadth and depth of knowledge
Faculty	Qualifications and professional development
Facilities	Adequate resources for effective learning
Institutional support	Sustained commitment to program success

4.2.2 Program Criteria: Discipline-Specific Requirements

The Bioengineering and Biomedical Engineering Program Criteria ensure alignment with the interdisciplinary demands of the field. According to ABET's Criteria for Accrediting Engineering Programs, 2025–2026, accredited programs must offer a curriculum combining both breadth and depth in engineering and scientific principles. The curriculum must cover foundational courses in engineering principles, biology, human physiology, chemistry, calculus-based physics, mathematics (through differential equations), and statistics, preparing students to address bio/biomedical engineering challenges. Practical experience is essential, requiring students to analyze and design biomedical systems, devices, and processes while conducting measurements on living systems and interpreting data. These criteria ensure that graduates develop both technical expertise and an understanding of the interaction between biological systems and engineering solutions. Faculty qualifications and professional development remain critical in maintaining academic rigor and fostering innovation. Table 4.3 outlines the key components shaping SOs and professional preparedness (ABET 2024a).

4.2.3 Integrating General and Program-Specific Criteria in Curriculum Design

Effective curriculum development integrates general and program-specific accreditation criteria, ensuring that students gain technical competencies, interdisciplinary knowledge, and problem-solving skills to address challenges in healthcare and medical technology. Mapping general criteria, such as faculty qualifications and SOs, to program-specific requirements in biological sciences, physiology, and data measurement in living systems ensures academic rigor and industry relevance. Moreover, aligning curricula with international accreditation frameworks such as the Bologna Process, Washington Accord, and EUR-ACE Framework Standards fosters continuous improvement through structured learning outcomes, credit allocation, and

TABLE 4.3
ABET EAC program criteria for bioengineering, biomedical, and similarly named engineering programs

Component	Description
Curriculum	The structure of the curriculum must provide both breadth and depth across the range of engineering and science topics consistent with the PEOs and SOs.
Application of principles	The curriculum must include experience in applying principles of engineering, biology, human physiology, chemistry, calculus-based physics, mathematics (through differential equations), and statistics.
Problem-solving in biomedical engineering	Students must gain the ability to solve bio/biomedical engineering problems, including those associated with the interaction between living and non-living systems.
Design, analysis, and realization	Programs must emphasize analyzing, modeling, designing, and realizing bio/biomedical engineering devices, systems, components, or processes.
Data measurement and interpretation	The curriculum must also include making measurements on and interpreting data from living systems.

assessment. As noted by Boev, Gruenwald, and Heitmann (2014), this alignment enhances program quality and ensures compliance with global standards. For biomedical engineering programs, such structured approaches reinforce competencies essential for future careers while promoting sustained program enhancement.

4.3 ESTABLISHING PROGRAM FOUNDATIONS: STUDENTS, PEOS, AND SOS

A BME program's foundation lies in preparing students for professional success while aligning with institutional goals and societal needs. This foundation is built on fostering student progress, defining PEOs, and establishing measurable SOs. Together, these elements ensure academic and professional excellence. According to ABET's Criteria for Accrediting Engineering Programs, 2025–2026, accredited programs must offer a curriculum combining both breadth and depth in engineering and scientific principles. Students are central to this framework, with their success supported through rigorous evaluation and alignment with programmatic and institutional expectations. PEOs bridge academic goals with constituencies' expectations, while SOs define the competencies required to meet professional challenges. This section explores these foundational components, their alignment with institutional priorities, and the mechanisms ensuring continuous improvement (ABET 2024a).

4.3.1 Empowering Student Success: The Core of Academic Excellence

Student success is the cornerstone of academic excellence, emphasizing intellectual growth, critical thinking, and professional preparedness. Accreditation ensures rigorous academic standards while fostering transparency, accountability, and continuous improvement (APL nextED 2024). External peer evaluation upholds educational quality, reinforcing student achievement (Kumar et al. 2020). Accreditation criteria require assessing student performance and progress to support academic and career readiness (ABET 2024a). Programs must implement clear policies on admissions, credit transfers, and graduation requirements, ensuring fairness and integrity. In BME, these measures equip students with technical expertise and interdisciplinary awareness, preparing them for ethical and professional challenges in healthcare and technology. By embedding these principles, BME programs cultivate engineers who drive innovation and address global challenges.

4.3.2 Engaging Program Constituencies in PEO Development and Review

Engaging program constituencies is fundamental to establishing and maintaining effective PEOs. Program constituencies are groups or individuals with a vested interest in program outcomes and the ability to provide valuable insights aligning with the institution's mission and societal needs. These include faculty, students, alumni, the IAB, employers, and other stakeholders. Their involvement ensures that PEOs reflect diverse academic and professional expectations. Programs must document periodic reviews through constituency participation, reinforcing alignment with institutional goals and enhancing PEO credibility (ABET 2024a).

ABET defines PEOs as broad statements outlining graduate accomplishments within a few years post-graduation. Their development requires systematic input and alignment with institutional goals. Continuous feedback from healthcare professionals, employers, and regulatory bodies strengthens program relevance, ensuring graduates address ethical, technological, and societal challenges. This engagement fosters innovation and enhances program integrity. Enderle et al. (2003) underscore the role of constituency involvement in sustaining program quality, reinforcing the need for structured review processes.

4.3.3 Alignment of PEOs With Institutional Mission, Vision, and Constituency Needs

A BME program's mission and vision define its strategic direction, shaping long-term objectives. The mission articulates core purposes and societal impact, while the vision outlines future aspirations. These statements must align with institutional goals to foster innovation, leadership, and societal contributions. Constituency engagement ensures that PEOs remain relevant and industry-responsive. The IAB provides external perspectives on curriculum and industry trends, reinforcing academic rigor.

Aligning a BME program's mission with constituency needs requires sustained collaboration. Constituencies refine program objectives, curriculum, and assessment strategies, with documented input ensuring accountability. Failing to engage constituencies risks undermining program integrity and accreditation standing. As Teitel (1994) notes, advisory committees bridge educational programs with their broader environment, making constituency engagement essential for academic and industry relevance.

4.3.4 Mapping PEOs to SOs to Ensure Competency Attainment

Systematically mapping PEOs to SOs ensures that graduates develop essential competencies. PEOs define long-term accomplishments, while SOs specify knowledge, skills, and abilities demonstrated at graduation. This mapping enables curriculum evaluation and continuous improvement. ABET (2024a) outlines SOs (1–7) as a framework for competency assessment. While programs may define their own SOs, they must align them with ABET's framework to meet accreditation standards. Consequently, many adopt ABET's outcomes verbatim, ensuring consistency in competency attainment, as reflected in Table 4.4.

A structured mapping mechanism links each PEO to corresponding SOs, demonstrating how graduates achieve long-term objectives. Programs commonly use a comprehensive table associating PEOs with SOs, supported by a narrative explaining the rationale behind the mapping. Transparency in this process strengthens accreditation compliance and curriculum refinement. Osman et al. (2018) highlight structured mapping as a key component in sustaining program quality and ensuring accreditation alignment.

4.3.5 Integrating Feedback Loops for Relevance and Effectiveness

A structured feedback loop ensures that PEOs remain relevant and effective. Input from program constituencies guides program assessment and revision. Annual meetings provide a forum for reviewing PEO alignment with industry trends, with meeting minutes serving as documentation for decision-making. This cyclical process allows program leadership to reassess and realign PEOs with academic and professional goals. Moreover, by continuously engaging external stakeholders, BME

TABLE 4.4
ABET (2024a) SOs (1–7) for engineering programs

SO #	Student Outcome
SO1	An ability to identify, formulate, and solve complex engineering problems by applying principles of engineering, science, and mathematics
SO2	An ability to apply engineering design to produce solutions that meet specified needs with consideration of public health, safety, and welfare, as well as global, cultural, social, environmental, and economic factors
SO3	An ability to communicate effectively with a range of audiences
SO4	An ability to recognize ethical and professional responsibilities in engineering situations and make informed judgments, which must consider the impact of engineering solutions in global, economic, environmental, and societal contexts
SO5	An ability to function effectively on a team whose members together provide leadership, create a collaborative and inclusive environment, establish goals, plan tasks, and meet objectives
SO6	An ability to develop and conduct appropriate experimentation, analyze and interpret data, and use engineering judgment to draw conclusions
SO7	An ability to acquire and apply new knowledge as needed, using appropriate learning strategies

programs maintain agility in responding to advancements in biomedical engineering. The feedback loop fosters ongoing dialogue, strengthening academic excellence and accreditation compliance. This iterative approach ensures graduates acquire the competencies required for success while reinforcing the program's commitment to continuous improvement.

4.4 ENSURING CONTINUOUS IMPROVEMENT: PROCESSES FOR PROGRAM ASSESSMENT AND EVALUATION

Continuous improvement in academic programs relies on structured assessment and evaluation to enhance student learning and program effectiveness, ensuring alignment with evolving educational and industry standards. This ongoing process mirrors the plan-do-check-act (PDCA) framework (Deming 1986), integrating assessment, evaluation, and refinement cycles. Accreditation requires programs to regularly assess SOs and evaluate effectiveness (ABET 2024a), ensuring data-driven decisions for curriculum development and program enhancement. Assessment systematically collects data through direct and indirect measures—such as exams, projects, and surveys—while evaluation interprets these results to identify gaps and guide improvements. A structured feedback loop, supported by PDCA, ensures timely refinements based on both internal and external inputs, fostering academic excellence and adaptability.

4.4.1 Documented Assessment and Evaluation Processes

Effective continuous improvement requires well-documented assessment and evaluation processes, using flowcharts, tables, and narratives to ensure transparency and sustainability. Flowcharts illustrate the cyclical nature of assessment, while spreadsheets track performance trends over time, aiding in data-driven decision-making. Assessment involves systematically collecting data to measure SOs through both direct and indirect measures. Direct assessment includes tangible evidence such as exams and projects, while indirect assessment captures students' perceptions via surveys or interviews.

Evaluation, in contrast, interprets the collected data to assess how well the program meets its goals and identifies areas for improvement. In addition, accreditation guidelines emphasize sustainable and accurate assessment practices. Regular assessment ensures valid measurement of SOs, preventing reliance on superficial metrics. A balanced approach—incorporating both direct and indirect measures—avoids biases that could obscure critical insights. Evaluation results must be comprehensive, considering all relevant data to support informed curricular decisions. By maintaining rigorous documentation and transparent processes, programs ensure alignment with accreditation requirements, driving continuous refinement in response to educational and industry advancements.

4.4.2 Leveraging Assessment Results for Continuous Improvement

Assessment results must be systematically analyzed and translated into actionable improvements. Faculty retreats and curriculum committee reviews provide structured mechanisms to integrate findings into decision-making, refining instructional strategies and program outcomes. For instance, if students struggle with quantitative reasoning (aligning with SO1), integrating PBL modules can address deficiencies, while inconsistencies in technical communication skills (aligning with SO3) may necessitate writing-intensive assignments or oral presentation workshops.

A quantitative approach, such as percentile rankings, helps interpret assessment data by categorizing students into performance levels: "*Exceeded Expectations*," "*Met Expectations*," "*Proceeding Towards Expectations*," and "*Did Not Meet Expectations*." This enables faculty to implement targeted academic interventions for students at all performance levels. It is important to note that this approach is not prescriptive but suggestive, offering flexibility to adapt to the unique needs and context of the program. Other approaches exist for analyzing and interpreting assessment data, each providing different insights based on methodology and objectives. Embedding structured assessment reviews within the continuous improvement cycle ensures evidence-based changes that align with program goals. By refining instructional strategies based on assessment trends, program leadership ensures a responsive academic environment that meets both educational and professional expectations.

4.4.3 Involvement of Program Constituencies and Feedback Loops to Drive Responsive Changes

Responsive changes are data-driven modifications made within a program to enhance its educational effectiveness, based on systematic assessment and feedback from the program's various constituencies. These changes ensure that adjustments in curriculum, instructional strategies, or resource allocation align with performance trends and evolving industry expectations, fostering a dynamic learning environment. A structured approach involves leveraging feedback loops to analyze performance data. For instance, SO1 can be assessed through four key performance indicators (KPIs): Problem Identification, Problem Formulation, Solution Development, and Solution Implementation. These KPIs can be measured within a course like *Advanced Engineering Analysis* using a frequency distribution and a four-tier scale (Poor, Fair, Good, and Excellent), with the satisfactory threshold set at 70% of students achieving a quality point average above 3.0 on a 4.0 scale. A web diagram can visualize assessment trends, plotting current and past cycle values to show changes in performance. If certain KPIs show no progress or a decline, a review of instructional methods is necessary. For example, if "*Solution Development*" underperforms, incorporating more PBL or adjusting course content may improve results. The effectiveness of prior interventions should be critically reviewed, ensuring that modifications are based on actual impacts, not just historical data. This iterative cycle fosters continuous improvement, allowing the program to refine its approach over time. Engagement from the program's various constituencies—faculty, students, and industry partners—is essential in keeping the program responsive, data-informed, and aligned with academic and professional expectations.

4.5 ADVANCING STANDARDS: ALIGNMENT OF CURRICULUM, FACULTY, FACILITIES, AND INSTITUTIONAL SUPPORT

Advancing BME education requires aligning curriculum, faculty, facilities, and institutional support with accreditation standards to ensure academic rigor and continuous improvement. ABET's Engineering Accreditation Commission (2024a) provides a structured framework for assessing these elements, ensuring responsiveness to technological and healthcare advancements. A well-designed curriculum integrates mathematics, basic sciences, and engineering with specialized biomedical coursework to develop problem-solving skills, ethical awareness, and interdisciplinary collaboration. Faculty expertise and sufficiency are crucial for delivering this curriculum, requiring a qualified academic body engaged in teaching, research, and professional practice. State-of-the-art laboratories, computational resources, adequate library services, and clinical training spaces foster experiential learning and technical proficiency, while institutional support sustains faculty development, infrastructure, and student engagement. Effective program leadership ensures compliance with accreditation criteria while fostering innovation, diversity, and excellence. The following sections will explore curriculum development, assessment and evaluation, accreditation policies, and mechanisms for faculty development and facility enhancement.

4.5.1 Processes for Curriculum Development, Assessment, and Evaluation Aligned With Accreditation Standards

To prepare students for professional practice, BME programs must align their curriculum with educational standards that support SOs and PEOs. Accreditation emphasizes key subject areas, including a minimum of 30 semester credit hours in mathematics and basic sciences—such as chemistry, physics, biology, and other natural sciences—and at least 45 semester credit hours, covering engineering and computer sciences, as well as engineering design, which is integral to the profession. This section of the curriculum must integrate modern engineering tools and methodologies, reflecting the ever-evolving landscape of biomedical engineering. The iterative design process requires students to identify problems, develop solutions, and consider constraints such as accessibility, cost, regulatory requirements, ergonomics, and sustainability. Through this process, students learn to apply mathematical, scientific, and engineering knowledge to real-world challenges. A culminating major engineering design experience ensures that they synthesize coursework, incorporate engineering standards, and solve complex problems, preparing them for professional practice (ABET 2024a).

The curriculum must also address societal, ethical, legal, and professional responsibilities, preparing students to engage with interdisciplinary issues in healthcare and policy. To remain relevant, curriculum development requires continuous collaboration with faculty, industry, and alumni. Regular reviews help incorporate emerging technologies and methodologies, ensuring alignment with evolving professional demands (ABET 2024a). The assessment of SOs must be systematic and sustainable, with representative sampling to identify areas for improvement. Efficient data collection through learning management systems (LMSs) supports evidence-based decision-making, enhancing curricular updates, faculty development, and resource allocation. This iterative process fosters continuous improvement while maintaining accreditation compliance (ABET 2024a).

Educational innovations have significantly influenced biomedical engineering (BME) curricula. The VaNTH-ERC, supported by the National Science Foundation, developed reusable learning materials based on the How People Learn framework, which emphasizes inquiry and critical thinking. Challenge-Based Instruction further aligned student learning with industry needs (Brophy 2003). The Whitaker Foundation (U.S. National Science Foundation 2008) fostered industry-academic collaboration, advocating for curricula that blend life sciences, advanced engineering tools, and quantitative modeling to address medically relevant challenges. ABET's accreditation framework ensures that programs uphold academic rigor while adapting to real-world applications, driving the continued advancement of biomedical engineering education (Abu-Faraj 2012).

4.5.2 Faculty Development, Facilities, and Institutional Support for Meeting Accreditation Criteria

Faculty development, high-quality facilities, and institutional support are all integral to maintaining accreditation and academic excellence in BME. Programs must ensure faculty possess expertise across curricular areas and engage in teaching, research, and professional practice, with qualifications such as advanced degrees, teaching effectiveness, and scholarly contributions being crucial. Strong ties with industry ensure that curricula meet workforce demands, while faculty governance and involvement in program assessment foster continuous improvement (ABET 2024a). High-quality facilities, including classrooms, laboratories, and computing resources, are essential for achieving program outcomes, requiring them to be well-maintained, accessible, and aligned with instructional needs. Adequate library services and information infrastructure further support instruction and research, with students provided appropriate guidance in the use of tools, equipment, and laboratories. Equipment must be systematically maintained, repaired, and upgraded to ensure functionality and alignment with evolving program requirements. Effective coordination ensures efficient use of multidisciplinary resources, supporting both learning and accreditation compliance (ABET 2024a). Institutional support, encompassing financial resources, staffing, and leadership, is crucial for program sustainability, with faculty retention and development dependent on professional growth opportunities, competitive compensation, and a supportive academic environment. Institutional leadership must also promote collaboration among faculty, students, and administrators, fostering student success and preventing resource limitations (ABET 2024a). Prioritizing faculty development, state-of-the-art facilities, and institutional support allows BME programs to maintain accreditation and adapt to evolving academic and industry needs.

4.5.3 Role of Accreditation Policies in Ensuring Compliance With Program and Institutional Goals

Accreditation policies align BME programs with institutional goals, ensuring compliance with quality standards. Program leadership must be familiar with these policies to uphold transparency and accountability in accreditation (ABET 2024b). Compliance involves accurately representing accreditation status, avoiding misleading claims about its duration, and ensuring that the status is clearly communicated. Accreditation statements, PEOs, and SOs must be publicly posted to demonstrate a commitment to continuous improvement. The program name must adhere to accreditation agency requirements, and all documentation must be in English for unbiased evaluation. Accreditation ensures that curricular pathways meet academic standards and that the review process is supported by appropriate resources, including access to individuals, facilities that are adequate and safe for their intended purposes, and supporting materials adequate for the visiting team to perform its review. Continuous monitoring and refinement of program objectives, aligned with institutional goals, support growth, quality education, and institutional accountability. Effective communication during the review process fosters a positive outcome for both the program and the accreditation team.

4.6 ACCREDITATION AS A DRIVER OF EXCELLENCE

Accreditation drives excellence in biomedical engineering education by establishing rigorous benchmarks that ensure program quality, relevance, and continuous improvement. It aligns educational objectives with industry standards, fostering engagement among faculty, students, and institutional leadership to maintain academic rigor and professional readiness. Faculty development ensures that educators stay at the forefront of interdisciplinary integration, innovation, and research excellence, while accreditation mandates robust infrastructure, including well-equipped laboratories, modern computing resources, adequate library services, and strategic partnerships. This integration of engineering and biological sciences, alongside the role of postgraduate programs, is essential for addressing challenges in the field. The emerging challenges and opportunities in biomedical engineering accreditation underscore its impact on educational quality and professional preparation.

4.6.1 Integrating Engineering and Biological Disciplines in Biomedical Education

Integrating engineering and biological disciplines is vital in shaping a biomedical engineering curriculum that meets the evolving demands of healthcare and biotechnology. Unlike traditional engineering fields, biomedical engineering merges engineering problem-solving with biological and physiological processes of living systems. This interdisciplinary approach enhances students' ability to design medical devices, develop bioinformatics tools, and create solutions that improve patient outcomes. A challenge in this integration is ensuring that engineering principles, such as mechanics and materials science, are applied to biological problems while considering biological systems' dynamic and nonlinear nature.

Pedagogical strategies must promote synthesis across disciplines, using PBL, collaborative research, and hands-on laboratory experiences. These methods foster a mindset that embraces both analytical rigor and biological complexity, preparing students to navigate challenges at the interface of engineering and life sciences, where innovation faces regulatory, ethical, and translational hurdles (Abu-Faraj and Rihana 2025). Continuous curriculum refinement, faculty expertise, and strong industry-academia partnerships are essential for preparing students to lead advancements in medical technology, tissue engineering, and bioinstrumentation, while maintaining engineering excellence.

4.6.2 Entry Criteria for Graduate Programs in Biomedical Engineering and Allied Health Disciplines

Excellence in BME education begins with accredited undergraduate programs that equip graduates for industry roles and graduate studies in diverse fields, including medicine, law, business, and regulatory affairs. Graduate BME programs build on this foundation, offering specialization opportunities in areas such as medical device design, biomechanics, and biomedical imaging. For example, graduates specializing in biomechanics contribute to improving clinical decision-making and patient mobility in orthopedic corrective procedures for children with cerebral palsy. Accredited BME programs also serve as a gateway to multiple career paths, including medicine, law, and entrepreneurship, enabling graduates to leverage engineering expertise in healthcare, policy, and business. While inclusivity in graduate programs enriches the field, it is vital to maintain rigorous admission standards and offer preparatory support to ensure success (Abu-Faraj and Rihana 2025). Structured admission policies aligned with industry standards and accreditation guidelines are necessary to address challenges in diverse graduate admissions.

4.6.3 Infrastructure and Resources Supporting Program Compliance

An accredited BME program must elevate its infrastructure to foster an exceptional learning and research environment. This includes specialized facilities, advanced computing resources, collaborative workspaces, and a robust library system. Excellence in infrastructure is not just about resource availability but also about how effectively these assets are integrated into the academic experience. Enderle et al. (2003) emphasize that leading programs surpass accreditation requirements by incorporating real-world applications and industry-aligned experiences. By fostering a technologically advanced learning ecosystem, BME programs can position themselves as global leaders in education, continuously improving through accreditation processes.

4.6.4 Bridging the Gap Between Academia and Industry

The gap between academia and industry arises from differences in curricula, research focuses, and technological advancements. Accreditation ensures that curricula remain adaptable to technological trends and aligned with industry needs, closing gaps in applied training and industry collaboration. Programs can foster industry-academic connections through advisory boards, internships, and faculty involvement in industry research, ensuring that students gain both theoretical and practical expertise. Bikard and Marx (2020) emphasize the role of geographic hubs in facilitating the transfer of academic research into real-world innovations. Even without proximity to hubs, BME programs can bridge the gap by fostering global partnerships and local industry connections, ensuring that graduates are prepared for emerging challenges.

4.6.5 Future Challenges and Opportunities in Biomedical Engineering Accreditation

The future of BME accreditation intersects with global challenges such as aging populations, urbanization, environmental degradation, and health disparities. Accreditation must evolve beyond traditional standards to address societal needs, such as sustainable solutions, disaster response technologies, and age-inclusive innovations. Issues such as resource scarcity and climate change require interdisciplinary approaches integrating environmental science, ethics, and law. Accreditation should ensure adaptability, preparing students to anticipate and innovate in response to emerging challenges, including legal considerations. As BME programs align with real-world demands, accreditation offers an opportunity to position BME as a globally responsible and forward-thinking discipline. This evolution requires curricula that are technically rigorous, ethically grounded, and socially responsible, ensuring that BME graduates are prepared for leadership in an interconnected world. Accreditation can guide BME programs in shaping a sustainable, healthy, and equitable future.

4.7 CONCLUSION

Biomedical engineering education is a dynamic and evolving process of continuous improvement, where academic rigor and practical relevance converge to prepare students for the changing landscape of healthcare, technology, and society. Accreditation serves as both a guide and a catalyst, ensuring that programs align with industry needs, foster interdisciplinary collaboration, and integrate foundational principles with technological advancements. Accredited programs emphasize theoretical knowledge alongside experiential learning, equipping graduates with the expertise and confidence to innovate in a competitive global environment. Beyond academics, accreditation cultivates ethical responsibility and social impact, empowering students to contribute meaningfully to the biomedical field and broader society. While the accreditation process is not prescriptive, it provides a structured yet adaptive framework that enables institutions to shape programs according to their unique missions while maintaining high educational standards.

The lasting impact of an accredited Biomedical Engineering program is reflected in the experiences of its graduates. Beyond academic achievements, students express a profound sense of belonging, as noted during one program visit: "*We feel we are in the comfort of our home!*" This sentiment embodies the nurturing environment fostered by accreditation—one that provides not only technical knowledge but also personal growth and a strong academic community. Accreditation ensures that students are guided through their educational journey with confidence, fostering resilience and a commitment to innovation. More than a credential, it is a transformative experience that shapes skilled professionals and adaptive leaders dedicated to advancing the biomedical engineering field and making meaningful contributions to global healthcare.

REFERENCES

ABET. 2024a. *ABET Engineering Accreditation Commission: Criteria for Accrediting Engineering Programs. Effective for Reviews During the 2025–2026 Accreditation Cycle. Incorporates All Changes Approved by the ABET Board of Delegates Engineering Area Delegation as of October 25, 2024.* https://www.abet.org/accreditation/accreditation-criteria/criteria-for-accrediting-engineering-programs-2025-2026/#1.

ABET. 2024b. *Accreditation Policies and Procedures Manual 2024–2025.* https://www.abet.org/accreditation/accreditation-criteria/accreditation-policy-and-procedure-manual-appm-2024-2025/.

ABET. 2025. *Find Programs.* Accessed January 24, 2025. https://amspub.abet.org/aps/name-search?searchType=program.

Abu-Faraj, Ziad O. 2011. "Project Alexander the Great: An Analytical Comprehensive Study on the Global Spread of Bioengineering/Biomedical Engineering Education." In *Biomedical Engineering: Trends in Materials Science*, edited by A. N. Laskovski, 549–64. Rijeka: IntechOpen. https://doi.org/10.5772/13501.

Abu-Faraj, Ziad O., ed. 2012. *Handbook of Research on Biomedical Engineering Education and Advanced Bioengineering Learning: Interdisciplinary Concepts.* Hershey, PA: IGI Global. https://doi.org/10.4018/978-1-4666-0122-2.ch001.

Abu-Faraj, Ziad O., and Salim A. Rihana. 2025. "Integrating Disciplinarity in Biomedical Engineering Education." In *Perspectives in Biomedical Engineering Education*, edited by S. Dokos, B. C. C. Chan, and L. Kark, xx–xx. New York: Routledge, Taylor & Francis Group.

APL nextED. 2024. *Unlocking the Power of Accreditation: A Pathway to Academic Excellence.* https://aplnexted.com/accreditation-power/.

Bikard, Michaël, and Matt Marx. 2020. "Bridging Academia and Industry: How Geographic Hubs Connect University Science and Corporate Technology." *Management Science* 66 (8): 3295–798. https://doi.org/10.1287/mnsc.2019.3385.

Boev, Oleg V., Norman Gruenwald, and Gerhard Heitmann. 2014. *Engineering Curriculum Design Aligned with Accreditation Standards.* Wismar: Hochschule Wismar, University of Applied Sciences Technology, Business and Design. ISBN 978-3-639-66368-6.

Brophy, Sean P. 2003. "Constructing Shareable Learning Materials in Bioengineering Education." *IEEE Engineering in Medicine and Biology Magazine* 22 (4): 39–46.

Deming, W. Edwards. 1986. *Out of the Crisis.* Cambridge, MA: Center for Advanced Engineering Study, Massachusetts Institute of Technology.

Enderle, John, Gerald Gassert, Sheila Blanchard, Paul King, David Beasley, Philip Hale Jr., and David Aldridge. 2003. "The ABCs of Preparing for ABET." *IEEE Engineering in Medicine and Biology Magazine* 22 (4): 122–32. https://doi.org/10.1109/MEMB.2003.1237513.

Frank, Jason R., Scott Taber, Marta van Zanten, Fedde Scheele, and Dominique Blouin. 2020. "The Role of Accreditation in 21st Century Health Professions Education: Report of an International Consensus Group." *BMC Medical Education* 20 (Suppl 1): 305. https://doi.org/10.1186/s12909-020-02121-5.

Hart, Richard T. 2015. "Biomedical Engineering Accredited Undergraduate Programs: Four Decades of Growth." *Annals of Biomedical Engineering* 43 (8): 1713–15. https://doi.org/10.1007/s10439-015-1319-2.

Kumar, Pradeep, Bharti Shukla, and Devendra Passey. 2020. "Impact of Accreditation on Quality and Excellence of Higher Education Institutions." *Revista Investigación Operacional* 41 (2): 151–67.

Linsenmeier, Robert A., and Ann Saterbak. 2020. “Fifty Years of Biomedical Engineering Undergraduate Education.” *Annals of Biomedical Engineering* 48 (6): 1590–615. https://doi.org/10.1007/s10439-020-02491-7.

Nagel, Joachim H. 2001. “Accreditation of Biomedical Engineering Programs in Europe: Challenge and Opportunity.” In *2001 Conference Proceedings of the 23rd Annual International Conference of the IEEE Engineering in Medicine and Biology Society*, vol. 1, 1–4. https://doi.org/10.1109/IEMBS.2001.1019556.

Osman, Abdu, Azman Yahya, and Mohamed B. Kamal. 2018. “A Benchmark Collection for Mapping Program Educational Objectives to ABET Student Outcomes: Accreditation.” In *5th International Symposium on Data Mining Applications*, edited by M. Alenezi and B. Qureshi, 46–60. Advances in Intelligent Systems and Computing, vol. 753. Cham: Springer. https://doi.org/10.1007/978-3-319-78753-4_5.

Teitel, Lee. 1994. *The Advisory Committee Advantage: Creating an Effective Strategy for Programmatic Improvement (ASHE-ERIC Higher Education Report No. 1).* Washington, DC: ERIC Clearinghouse on Higher Education.

U.S. National Science Foundation. 2008. *The Whitaker Foundation Biomedical Engineering Education Summit Meetings.* https://www.nsf.gov/awardsearch/showAward?AWD_ID=0757969.

5 Pedagogical Perspectives on Teaching Prototyping in Biomedical Engineering Education

Matthew Wettergreen

5.1 INTRODUCTION

In 2004, the biomedical engineering (BME) capstone course at Rice University was one semester long, and student teams were all assigned the same project. This project culminated in a detailed written report outlining a proposed medical device design solution and the necessary verification and validation tests, but no physical prototypes were built. Recognizing that biomedical engineers needed to create functional, testable devices to be credible and competitive, course director Dr. Maria Oden initiated a curriculum redesign. This transformation ultimately led to the creation of the Oshman Engineering Design Kitchen (OEDK), a dedicated space for collaborative prototyping and a model for hands-on BME education.

Ten years later, hands-on outcomes are clear: first-year students, not just final-year students, were developing real solutions to real problems. One team designed a device to help astronauts drink coffee aboard the International Space Station. Another built a robotic reaching arm for a teenager who used a wheelchair. Another prototyped a solution for the Houston Zoo's giraffe population. These achievements were made possible by hands-on prototyping. Some of these students were in the BME program and among the first graduates to participate in the act of transforming abstract ideas into functional approximations of a final solution in the OEDK. At Rice and elsewhere, prototyping has become a vital pedagogical tool to bridge the gap between concept and implementation.

Prototyping is the process of creating physical or digital artifacts to solve a problem. A prototype is a physical or digital representation of the solution. A prototype can be a napkin sketch, a rough foam model, or a functional electromechanical device. In the engineering design process, prototyping holds an important role in helping teams and individuals convert their solution options from an idea into a physical reality. Prototypes are not complete, and sometimes not even functional. The word's root in Greek derives from "primitive" or "primitive form." The concept of "first" is imbued in the word, and most prototypes have characteristics of the first

DOI: 10.1201/9781003520313-5

versions of what will ultimately become manufactured products that you can purchase online or at stores (need confirmation of this from Socrates).

Prototyping is an effective pedagogical method in BME education. Hands-on activities that require building, iterating, and testing are among the most effective ways to promote engagement and knowledge retention in engineering students (Smith et al. 2005). Studies have shown that students working on physical prototypes report greater confidence, satisfaction, and long-term retention of skills (Bethke et al. 2024; Higbee and Miller 2019). This effect is impactful in BME education, where the need for user-centered design and real-world application is high. Introducing physical prototyping early in the curriculum supports active learning and gives students a more integrated understanding of engineering design, technical tools, and clinical needs. Rather than addressing theoretical problems, students are challenged to produce, test, and refine tangible solutions, preparing them for professional practice.

Prototyping has always been about exploring ideas through physical realization, but its applications and methods have evolved significantly. Historically, prototyping emerged from hands-on engineering disciplines such as mechanical and aerospace engineering, where physical models were used to test and improve designs. National Aeronautics and Space Administration (NASA), for example, promoted a "design-by-prototype" approach, prioritizing physical builds as a means of iterative problem-solving and innovation (Mulenburg and Gundo 2002). By the early 2000s, digital tools such as computer-aided design (CAD), computer-aided engineering, and 3D printing allowed more advanced prototyping in engineering education, particularly in BME education. As prototyping methods evolved, so did their educational relevance. Structured integration of prototyping into engineering curricula became increasingly common, reflecting a need to align student training with professional design practices. This shift helped to develop engineering judgment and emphasized the importance of iterative, real-world problem-solving (Detand, Bastiaens, and Grimonprez 2010). Many technologies now exist that support prototyping for engineering students, including hybrid methods, which allow imaging technologies to convert physical models into digital formats for enhanced exploration and documentation (Kohtala et al. 2018).

Prototypes exist across a number of scales and complexities—they may be constructed from simple materials (like yarn or tape), or they may be fully functional and created with all the tools of a makerspace. A prototype can be a simple napkin sketch or a complex machine with moving parts. Some prototypes are functional, while some are merely representational. In many cases, prototypes exist as an artifact or a temporary state of design—this allows prototypes to be ugly, lack function, be at the wrong scale, or be constructed from the wrong materials.

While every stage of the design process has its advocates, it would not be surprising if prototyping emerged as a favorite for many designers. Prototyping is the FUN step; designers get to make things with their hands, or digitally design things that are then made by machines. Prototypes are something to be proud of and share with others; they are a snapshot of a designer's current solution and their talent to create a physical or digital representation of that solution. The steps leading up to prototyping build an understanding of the problem, but do not commit to a solution. Prototyping is one of the first steps where the designer commits to a solution, or a range of solutions, and that is demonstrated through the properties of the prototype. This prototype is the designer's first stab at something creative and new. Prototyping is the *most* visible by-product of the entire design process, and it is what everyone wants to see and touch.

Prototyping can bridge theoretical learning and real-world problem-solving. The use of prototyping in BME education can span the entire undergraduate curriculum, evolving in complexity and purpose over time. In early courses like first-year cornerstone design, students can be introduced to prototyping through simple, low-fidelity materials. These experiences build foundational teamwork, creativity, and communication skills, and an orientation toward design process knowledge. As students advance into sophomore and junior-level courses, they can use more specialized tools (e.g., CAD software, electronics, laser cutters, and 3D printers) and tackle increasingly complex problems. These intermediate experiences can develop medium-fidelity prototypes, which combine appropriate materials with partial functionality. By their final year, a capstone project should require a team to design, build, and test a fully refined prototype for real-world clients. All of these projects can integrate technical knowledge, design methodology, and communication skills into a comprehensive design process. Employers value this progression: students who have engaged in prototyping across the curriculum graduate with more substantial portfolios, greater technical confidence, and a more precise understanding of engineering practice.

ABET accreditation criteria have helped drive the incorporation of prototyping into and across the BME curriculum. Specifically, outcomes 3.2 and 3.6 have been used to underscore the value of physical prototyping as an integral part of engineering education and program success. Outcome 2 emphasizes the ability to "apply engineering design to produce solutions that meet specified needs with consideration of public health, safety, and welfare." Outcome 6 stresses the ability to "develop and conduct appropriate experimentation, analyze and interpret data, and use engineering judgment to draw conclusions" ("Criteria for Accrediting Engineering Programs, 2025–2026" 2024).

Prototypes offer many advantages when applied to the steps of problem-solving. Each prototype is a chance to test a concept, or an assumption, visually represent brainstormed ideas, compare to a teammate's solution, help decide which feature to include, or communicate complex concepts to a client (Wettergreen et al. 2020). At the onset of the design process, prototypes convert ideas that only exist in the head of the designer into tangible representations and realizations. This physical representation helps communicate with stakeholders. Later prototypes help to verify hypotheses and test assumptions about a problem/solution; the medium of a prototype allows meaningful conversations with users, customers, and clients over the project's life. Another distinct benefit of prototyping is that it allows the designer or the team to explore many design alternatives quickly, producing as many prototypes as there are ideas about the solution. While producing multiple prototypes may seem resource-intensive, it is, in fact, a highly cost-effective way to de-risk design decisions. Because early prototypes can be made from inexpensive materials (e.g., cardboard, tape, and foam), they offer low-stakes environments for learning, testing, and innovation.

This chapter covers the three main dimensions of prototyping: low-, medium-, and high-fidelity prototypes. Low-fidelity prototypes are early, unrefined versions of a design solution, often produced from simple, low-cost materials, and lacking many of the characteristics of a fully realized solution. A medium-fidelity prototype includes a number of features that resemble a final, idealized solution. This prototype is constructed from parts that hold their shape more readily or are made of more appropriate materials. A high-fidelity prototype includes most, if not all, of the features of an idealized design solution, meets all of the intended design criteria, and is fabricated from appropriate materials. Each of these levels has a different set of materials and tools to produce them, and as prototypes evolve, the production tools also evolve. As instructors, the types of prototypes students in BME education should be expected to produce should be dependent upon instruction time, available tools, and student educational level.

This chapter further provides a framework for BME educators to integrate prototyping meaningfully into the BME undergraduate curricula. We introduce three levels of prototype fidelity—low, medium, and high—and explain how expectations for student work can be calibrated based on available tools, instructional time, and academic level.

Throughout the chapter, we emphasize that successful prototyping education depends not only on materials and tools but also on well-structured support systems, both visible (like makerspaces) and invisible (such as mentorship networks). We offer concrete pedagogical strategies to help instructors scaffold tool instruction, manage project scope, and foster hands-on learning in resource-constrained settings or locations set up as ad hoc prototyping areas (Wettergreen et al. 2023). Above all, prototyping is an avenue that allows students to take creative risks, learn from failure, and build functional, impactful solutions to real problems. This chapter aims to help BME educators develop learning experiences for students that make this possible, regardless of their own technical expertise in prototyping.

5.2 DIMENSIONS OF PROTOTYPING IN BME EDUCATION

5.2.1 Prototypes Exist at Different Fidelity Levels

Prototypes are the result of the process of *prototyping,* and they are created at specific levels of complexity called *fidelity (or resolution).* Three major organizing levels of prototype fidelity exist that broadly characterize the technical sophistication or representative complexity of the solution: low fidelity, medium fidelity, and high fidelity. Fidelity impacts both how a prototype communicates ideas and how it functions in testing. Technical sophistication is defined as the academic or technical level of knowledge required to execute a desired design block or feature (e.g., Python-technical sophistication that is non-basic), and complexity is defined as the depth of information imbued in a prototype. A table that discusses and overviews the differences between these three levels of prototypes can be found in Table 5.1, breaking down the differences between these prototypes, the time it takes to produce them, and the materials that can be included in their construction.

TABLE 5.1
The difference between low-, medium-, and high-fidelity prototypes

	Low Fidelity	Medium Fidelity	High Fidelity
Purpose	Early prototypes produced rapidly; explore ideas, communicate concepts, and seek basic functionality	Middle iterative prototypes; somewhat demonstrate function and test specific design features, have some refined features	Late refined prototypes; high functionality, high sophistication through iteration, closely resemble a manufactured object
Materials	Any readily available or low-cost material: paper, cardboard, foam, wood, velcro, PVC, and pipe cleaners	More appropriate or processed materials: wood, plastics, hardware, simple electronics, and 3D printed pieces	Refined or custom materials selected for project specificity: ordered parts, machined/molded parts, custom 3D prints, and functional electronics
Tools	Basic: cardboard, office or craft supplies, sketching, 3D pen, basic hand tools, and TinkerCAD	Intermediate: laser cutter, SolidWorks, 3D printer, Arduino, basic composite materials	Advanced: custom 3D prints, CNC machines, mill/lathe, plasma/water jet cutter, and molding/casting equipment
Time investment	Low effort; minutes to hours	Moderate time and effort; days to weeks	Significant planning and build time; weeks to months
Design constraints to consider	Few constraints; focus is on communicating concepts and actions	Some design constraints considered: materials, partial function, and usability are considered and tested	All major constraints are addressed: manufacturability, safety, aesthetics, cost, and full functionality. These guide the design and inform final testing and refinement

5.2.1.1 Low-Fidelity Prototypes

Low-fidelity prototypes are early prototypes produced rapidly that are often non-functional, representational, or serve simply as physical objects to communicate the designer's ideas. These prototypes are completed quickly to test ideas that the designer or the team has about a particular solution. There is no requirement that this prototype works nor that it be created at the correct scale or be aesthetically pleasing. These prototypes are not generally intended to work, though low-fidelity and low-cost prototyping are synonymous with producing functional solutions in many parts of the world. Low-fidelity prototypes can be constructed quickly and rapidly in a short period of time, without the need for careful scheduling or planning. Low-fidelity prototypes, which do not intend to demonstrate function, cannot be tested based on how well they achieve their intended design solution. A person or a design team can create many versions of low-fidelity prototypes to explore alternatives. Low-fidelity prototypes can be produced with readily available materials, such as sketching materials, office supplies, craft supplies, cardboard, and Arduino-based electronics for proof-of-concept testing, or readily available materials that can be quickly shaped and formed.

5.2.1.2 Medium-Fidelity Prototypes

Medium-fidelity prototypes are evolved versions of low-fidelity prototypes, containing many refined features. The goal of a medium-fidelity prototype is to achieve some of the design objectives of the intended solution; in this prototype, some of the design blocks may begin to demonstrate function closer to the designer's intention. Some of the materials included in these prototypes have been selected based on need, rather than what was readily available. Some materials may be more rigid, hold their shape, or be more challenging to shape and form than low-fidelity versions. Medium-fidelity prototypes are created with more care, sustained effort, and by applying tools and skill proficiency. The crafting and refinement of medium-fidelity prototypes requires a measurable amount of time and must be accounted for in project planning. Because these prototypes have been refined to achieve design objectives, they can be used for verification and functional testing. Areas of difficulty in creating medium-fidelity prototypes relate to students and student teams failing to be able to use materials, tools, and processes to achieve functional outcomes of their prototypes. Medium-fidelity prototypes may be constructed from materials that need to be ordered, and tools that would be found in a makerspace or maker-focused classroom: 3D printing, laser cutting, Arduino integrated projects, electronics with breadboards, and basic use of composite materials (silicones and urethanes).

5.2.1.3 High-Fidelity Prototypes

High-fidelity prototypes are refined, functional prototypes that can closely resemble a manufactured object. This prototype aims to demonstrate all of the design goals of an intended or idealized solution. The key to the high-fidelity prototype is that not only does the solution look refined, but it also *is* refined, matching most of the intended functionality of the solution that will be tested on the user. The design blocks or criteria have been iterated over successive prototypes.

Tests have been conducted on previous prototypes, which have resulted in the high-fidelity prototypes' achievement of design outcomes. High-fidelity prototypes require the usage of and proficiency in specific machines and tools: CNC machining, injection molding, integrated mechano-electrical systems, microfluidics, and how to achieve consistent functionality in these tools. They are constructed of appropriate materials that match the mechanical and materials properties of the desired solution, and these materials are rarely readily available; often, they are custom-fabricated or ordered specifically for the prototype's need. Due to the difficulty of refining these prototypes, the fabrication of these prototypes can take long periods of time to create, months, or even longer. High-fidelity prototypes are the physical embodiment of all the effort that a team has invested in their design project. This physical (or digital or electronic-based) solution may look simple, but it is imbued with the complexity, ingenuity, and effort of the design process and the design team.

5.3 DESIGN GOALS VARY WITH FIDELITY LEVEL

In the process of iteration, students need to have particular goals for their prototypes that map to their design criteria (objectives or constraints). However, students may struggle to achieve specific design criteria as a function of fidelity or as a result of the prototype goal. Table 5.2 reflects how the design goals of a prototype change depending on the fidelity.

Expanding beyond fidelity, prototypes can also be described across other dimensions. Here we describe these other dimensions and then feature examples of these prototypes in Chapter 3.1. While fidelity of prototypes refers to a prototype's level of refinement toward functionality, there is another method to categorize prototypes, and that is by their goal. The five main types of prototypes that a team or individual might produce are Representational, Mockup/Visual, Proof-of-Concept, Ergonomic, and Functional prototypes.

TABLE 5.2
How design criteria vary based on the fidelity of the prototype

Design Criteria	Level of Importance			Justification
	Low	**Medium**	**High**	
Ease of use	Less important	Top priority	Top priority	Ease of use is emphasized in medium- and high-fidelity prototypes because healthcare devices must often be operated quickly and intuitively. User-friendly designs improve accessibility and reduce the risk of user error.
Ease of maintenance	Not important	Minimal	Top priority	Ease of maintenance is important in high-fidelity prototypes where long-term use and reliability are considered. In healthcare settings, devices must be easily repaired to ensure patient safety.
User experience quality	Not important	Important	Top priority	As prototypes evolve, user experience becomes critical to ensure comfort, usability, and effectiveness in real scenarios.
Aesthetics	Not important	Important	Top priority	Aesthetics are not a significant focus during early prototyping, where function is prioritized. However, aesthetics gain importance in medium- and high-fidelity prototypes as visual appeal can influence user perception, especially in healthcare designs.
Safety	Not important	Not important	Top priority	Safety is crucial in high-fidelity prototypes so that devices may be tested for real-world use. Safety is not important in low- and medium-fidelity stages because the prototypes are not used in real settings and pose minimal risk.

(Continued)

TABLE 5.2 (Continued)
How design criteria vary based on the fidelity of the prototype

Design Criteria	Level of Importance: Low	Medium	High	Justification
Cost	Not important	Not important	Top priority	In the prototyping process in all BME undergraduate education, cost as a design criterion rarely functions effectively as a minimizing criterion. Students buy and use materials based on what is available and in their budget.
Communicates function	Top priority	Less important	Less important	Early prototypes quickly convey how a device will work, even while lacking functionality. A strong visual or physical representation helps teammates, mentors, and users understand the concept.
Transparency of action	Top priority	Less important	Less important	At low-fidelity scales, clearly showing how the mechanism works is essential to communicating ideas. As prototypes advance, internal components may be hidden or refined, making transparency less important.
Functionality of action	Not important to important	Top priority	Top priority	Early prototypes sometimes sacrifice full functionality to explore other concepts. However, demonstrating the intended action is critical for medium and high fidelity.

5.3.1 Representational Prototypes—"Symbolizing Design and Features"

These early prototypes represent the pieces and parts of a prototype using analogical materials or physical representations of what the designer ultimately envisions will serve as the function of an object. The scale of these prototypes does not matter, nor does it matter what materials make up their composition. These prototypes are predominantly focused on communicating multiple ideas or concepts about function. They are frequently completed quickly and discarded after the idea has been adopted or discussed. Prototypes in this category may have concepts that are copied over into future prototypes.

5.3.2 Mockup or Visual Prototypes—"Looks Like"

These prototypes are created to communicate features that describe (visually) what a final device will look like. This includes aspects such as what size it might be, what colors a user dashboard might have, or what the user interface might present. Mockups of this type offer no functionality but might be the approximate size of the final solution; they are only created to answer questions about how the device will look and be interacted with. Prototypes of this sort frequently have features directly adopted into higher-fidelity prototypes.

5.3.3 Proof-of-Concept Prototypes—"Works Like"

Proof-of-concept prototypes answer the question "How will this prototype work?" They often demonstrate some aspects of the desired function of the solution to help the design team understand whether their intended idea will actually work. Prototypes of this nature might be created with the wrong materials but at the correct scale; intended features of the solution may be missing, but one critical function may be demonstrated (Bushnell et al. 2013). The core functionality of this prototype is often used to make critical next-step solution decisions; the results of these decisions are almost always present as core functionality in later prototypes.

5.3.4 Ergonomic Prototype—"Feels Like"

An ergonomic prototype is similar to a mockup or visual prototype in that the prototype's goal is to represent information to a user without providing a functional solution. However, ergonomic prototypes might explore how the hand wraps around a solution or how the body fits inside a harness system. Ergonomic prototypes are typically at the correct scale of the final solution because they are designed to exist as an interface that will test assumptions of the user interacting with the device. This prototype is highly functional, and its features and functions are adopted in later prototypes.

5.3.5 Functional Prototypes—"Looks Like, Feels Like, Works Like"

Functional prototypes combine validated assumptions and accrued knowledge of a design project into one prototype. These prototypes are not only at the correct scale but also integrated, including multiple features and functions intended for the final solution. Functional prototypes may undergo many revisions and iterations before being delivered to the client. Early functional prototypes may look messy, but they have integrated functions. Late-stage functional prototypes are likely to have gone through many revisions and now resemble the final object in functionality, human factors, materials, finish, and design objectives. This final level of refinement and completion is highly challenging to achieve; it is not often accomplished by design teams outside of long-term curricular engagements. In the process of iteration, students need to have particular goals.

5.4 TEACHING PROTOTYPING ACROSS THE BME CURRICULUM

Strong BME programs incorporate prototyping not only in capstone projects but as a core pedagogical strategy woven throughout the undergraduate curriculum (Higbee and Miller 2019). Hands-on design experiences, scaffolded from early exposure to advanced integration, help students develop the technical, creative, and collaborative skills essential for biomedical innovation.

Introducing prototyping early, particularly in first-year design courses, gives students a chance to build confidence, learn the design process experientially, and develop comfort with basic tools and materials. As students progress, their work becomes more sophisticated and increasingly tied to the biological and clinical contexts central to BME. This gradual evolution prepares students for the complexity and accountability of senior-year capstone design. To visualize this progression, Table 5.3 outlines how prototyping instruction and expectations can evolve from the first year to the final year, aligning fidelity level, tools, curricular content, and technical preparation.

The progression in Table 5.3 intentionally scaffolds prototyping across the BME curriculum, with design activities increasing in fidelity, function, and integration with core BME content. This progression has been adapted in part from the Engineering Design Minor at the OEDK, where prototyping is central to all of the education, and a curriculum was developed as elective courses for all of the engineers at Rice. This curriculum has been capitalized heavily by the BME students.

Early experiences like first-year design have demonstrated powerful downstream effects: students who take introductory design courses were shown to be stronger problem solvers, more confident with tools, and better collaborators during capstone. These findings are echoed in longitudinal studies and informal assessments from faculty and industry mentors alike (Wettergreen et al. 2020; Bethke et al. 2024).

By the middle years, students should understand not just how to build prototypes but also how to build the right refined prototypes for biomedical contexts—models that respect clinical standards of care, consider material constraints, and incorporate technical sophistication. Senior year should challenge students to integrate these lessons in a high-stakes setting, producing functional devices with real users and stakeholders in mind.

5.5 VISIBLE AND INVISIBLE SUPPORT STRUCTURES FOR BME PROTOTYPING EDUCATION

5.5.1 Makerspaces as Visible Infrastructure to Support BME Students

A global interest in designing and building physical objects has resulted in the academic makerspace, design studio, or fab lab (call it what you will) as a hub for hands-on activities. Due to the versatility of where these spaces can live, they can be found in various spaces on university campuses and communities inside of libraries, as standalone buildings, or in urban innovation centers. In higher education, makerspaces unify previously dispersed resources—machine shops, electronics labs, and wet labs—into a cohesive, collaborative environment. The educational philosophy behind makerspaces emphasizes learning by doing, where students solve open-ended problems through iteration and experimentation. Reports such as the NAE's Grand Challenges and the United Nations' Sustainable Development Goals (SDGs) have supported integrating PjBL models in makerspaces.

A critical insight about makerspaces is that they should be driven by educational goals. As Wilczynski et al. observe, successful makerspaces align their programming with curricular needs, focusing on engineers' development before producing

TABLE 5.3
Scaffolding of prototyping in the BME curriculum

Academic Year	Prototyping Focus	Educational Activities	Learning Outcomes	Scaffolding Goals
Years 1–2 (Foundational Exposure)	- Emphasis on low-fidelity prototyping - Introduction to basic tools, materials, and makerspace access - Use of Arduino, breadboards, simple CAD, and 3D printing	- Hands-on labs - Hackathons - Design sprints - Cornerstone design course (e.g., ENGI 120: Introduction to Engineering Design)	- Understand the design process - Gain confidence with tools - Develop teamwork and communication skills - Set design criteria, evaluate alternatives (Bethke et al. 2024; Brandel, Chang, and Wettergreen 2022)	- Establish a prototyping mindset - Practice iteration and decision-making - Prepare for tool integration in 200- and 300-level courses
Years 2–3 (Intermediate Design Courses)	- Introduction to medium fidelity prototyping - Use of CAD, 3D printing, molding, basic electronics, and composite materials	- Team-based projects in design-focused electives - Bioinstrumentation, biomechanics, and biomaterials courses - "Canned" projects to introduce specialty tools	- Apply the design process to discipline-specific problems - Improve prototyping functionality - Work with clinical or contextual constraints (IJEE)	- Link tool choice to project needs - Scaffold skills for functional integration - Build comfort with complexity in preparation for a capstone project
Year 4 (Capstone Design and Advanced Courses)	- Focus on medium-to-high-fidelity prototypes - Integrated systems: sensors, CAD-CAM, clinical usability - Emphasis on manufacturability and testability	- Industry- or hospital-partnered projects - User-centered design and clinical immersion - Full-year design course with staged reviews	- Demonstrate the entire design process - Validate prototypes through testing and user feedback - Communicate with stakeholders professionally (Saterbak and Wettergreen 2022; "Criteria for Accrediting Engineering Programs, 2025–2026" 2024)	- Deliver functional, testable devices - Understand prototype-to-product transition - Develop professional readiness for industry or graduate study

engineering artifacts. Makerspaces are most impactful when integrated into coursework, where prototyping serves as a vehicle for learning, rather than an end in itself (Wilczynski and Adrezin 2016). Similarly, in Wettergreen et al., we highlight that the three priorities of a makerspace are, in order, (1) people, (2) programming, and (3) tools. This visible support structure exists to support BME students in their prototyping efforts (Wettergreen et al. 2020).

5.5.2 Key Physical Tools for the BME Student

The prototyping tools in a makerspace span a wide range of technical complexity and sophistication, from basic hand tools to advanced digital fabrication equipment.

Common tools used in BME prototyping include the following:

- *3D printers* for simple shapes and rapid iteration of complex geometries
- *Laser cutters* for precision machining of wood or acrylic components
- *Biofabrication tools*, such as bioprinters, for controlled deposition of biomaterials
- *Electronics* for creating sensor-based systems or repeatable methods of action
- *Microcontrollers and Microprocessors* (e.g., Arduino and Raspberry Pi) for creating interactive or automated systems

Many resources exist to describe or teach the use of these tools. However, few sources focus on how to use these tools well, with skill, efficiency, and intentionality. Educators should help students distinguish between tool *operation* and tool *technique*, guiding students toward finesse and high-quality application of the tool, not simply novelty. For an overview of the types of advanced manufacturing tools that are available in most makerspaces, and how to achieve high-quality outputs from the application of these tools, check out the following suggested resources:

- Making It: Manufacturing Techniques for Product Design by Chris Lefteri (Lefteri 2019)
- Manufacturing Processes for Design Professionals by Rob Thompson (Thompson 2007)
- The 3D Printing Handbook: Technologies, Design, and Applications by Ben Redwood, Filemon Schoffer, and Brian Garret (Redwood et al. 2017)
- Practical Electronics for Inventors by Paul Sherz and Simon Monk (Scherz and Monk 2016)
- Making Things Move by Dustyn Roberts (Roberts 2010)
- Getting Started with Arduino by Massimo Banzi and Michael Shiloh (Banzi and Shiloh 2022)

5.5.3 Invisible Support Structures

Student prototyping is significantly enhanced when they are supported by what is called a Web of Mentors—a diverse network of faculty, peers, industry professionals, and clinicians. In fact, at the OEDK, we have seen this structure as a key mediator of success by applying a high-touch support system for students in multiple areas: process, technical, communication, and professional skills. This mentorship structure can take many forms, but ideally provides support across several domains: technical guidance, project management, communication, and professional development. At the OEDK, we classify mentorship in three ways: academic, peer, and industrial mentoring, and have developed our Web of Mentors model based on existing pedagogy and best professional practices (Vygotsky 1978; National Center for Faculty Development & Diversity 2025).

Academic mentoring involves using faculty or course instructors who meet regularly with students in the program and provide key insights and advice. This type of support orients students to the design processes related to the course and provides deep content area details for students. These faculty and course members can direct students to unknown resources and give them feedback related to problems they will experience in the timeline of their class project. These faculty can listen to their concerns and uncertainty while providing deep content expertise and direct access to resources. An example would be to point students to governing equations for a particular project.

The second type of mentoring is peer-based mentoring. These individuals provide empathy, encouragement, and tactical advice based on shared experiences and vocabulary. This peer mentorship can often come in the form of a teaching assistant (TA) or a prototyping lab assistant and exists in an ongoing mentorship relationship or JIT. This type of mentor could also be a peer writing mentor who reviews technical documents and provides expertise. An example of this type of support might be: "We also struggled with testing—we ran over 100 iterations."

A third type of mentoring would come from technical or professional sources, such as industry professionals, alums, or other BME engineers. These individuals provide relevancy, real-world expectations, and feedback to any type of education or project that teams are working on. This mentorship helps students connect with industry practices. Mentorship of this sort can be JIT as needed or during design reviews. An example of the type of feedback that would be received in this arena would be: "In industry, we'd machine this part to meet ISO tolerances."

5.6 PEDAGOGICAL BENEFITS OF THE PHYSICAL PRESENCE OF A MAKERSPACE

Makerspaces can be engines for collaborative learning. Many effective makerspaces leverage these opportunities due to their open layout, which allows all users to see each other working and interact directly. This open structure of these spaces fosters peer-to-peer interaction, multidisciplinary teamwork, and spontaneous knowledge exchange. Engagement in real-world projects within makerspaces supports multiple outcomes for students, for project partners, and for universities.

Students benefit from being present in a makerspace in several ways. First, by spending time in the makerspace, they can acquire skills. Second, by working alongside their peers, they can experience professional growth. Finally, one of the benefits of makerspaces is that they provide exposure to real-world problems.

Universities benefit from makerspaces in ways that improve their programs' overall education and prestige. Students who graduate from makerspaces often reflect positive feelings toward those makerspaces (Wettergreen et al. 2025). The curriculum from these makerspaces is often updated to reflect the current tools and best practices of teaching these tools, since many of these tools have emerged in the past 20 years. Finally, the projects that come out of these makerspaces, especially in BME or collaborative capstone, are fundamentally dramatic and worth sharing with the community.

Partners and communities are perhaps the most positively affected by makerspaces. These partners have access to emerging talent, students who have worked in the makerspaces and can demonstrate foundational engineering talents and professional skills that are valuable to employers. Partners and communities receive increased visibility on campuses as they have their real-world projects run by students. Finally, partners benefit from fresh innovation that student teams can provide. Such partnerships also ground academic projects in reality, giving students a preview of the professional landscape and the constraints of real-world engineering practice.

5.7 CHALLENGES: COST, ACCESS, AND SAFETY REGULATIONS IN BIOMEDICAL PROTOTYPING

Despite their benefits, makerspaces present challenges, particularly in BME contexts. These include high operational costs, regulatory and human subjects testing hurdles, and access equity. Fully staffed makerspaces with various tools demand a commensurate financial investment, which is difficult to justify for one department (BME or any department!). As a limited solution, small makerspaces in a classroom can be launched with hundreds of dollars in low-fidelity prototyping supplies and simple machines to accelerate prototyping, such as hand tools and 3D printers.

Specific to BME education, overcoming regulatory and human subjects testing in a makerspace can be challenging. Biomedical projects often raise biosafety or patient-interaction concerns. The challenges of user testing or human testing are often exacerbated in a public makerspace, which is not a hospital or testing environment. Finally, not all students in BME have equal access to tools or space, which means that students are graduating worldwide with a wide range of skills and outcomes related to the application of medical devices and prototyping inside makerspace environments. Strategies such as low-fidelity prototyping, portable toolkits, or decentralized instructional models can help mitigate these issues while still offering meaningful hands-on learning.

5.8 PROTOTYPING CAN HAPPEN ANYWHERE: ADAPTING TO LIMITED-RESOURCE SETTINGS

A pervasive global misconception in academic settings is that prototyping must occur in formal (and often expensive) makerspaces. In reality, *prototyping can happen anywhere*. In many parts of the world, people prototype solutions in the moment, using what is immediately available where they currently are, be it urban environments, rural settings, markets, or makeshift workshops.

This type of prototyping to solve immediate problems is common in agriculture and livestock management. These industries are often large plots of land with many types of structures and competing types of programming running concurrently. Common to farming is the reality that something is always breaking, and most things are just barely working to begin with. Many problems that arise are immediate and critical to the function of the farm, such as if animal fencing breaks, the irrigation system springs a leak, or machines will not run. In these cases, problems need to be solved immediately, and the focus is not on whether it looks good, but whether the solution works (Pario Perra 2010).

Many BME programs engage students in design for low-resource or global health settings; a subset of these programs takes students to these settings, where access to sophisticated tools may be limited. Teaching prototyping in these contexts requires adaptability and creativity: students must repurpose materials, simulate functionality with simple analogs, and build directly using locally available supplies. Instructors can structure activities around frugal innovation, challenge students to prototype without digital fabrication, and use constraints as teaching tools. Emphasizing these real-world limitations prepares students for diverse professional environments and reinforces that effective biomedical solutions are not always built in ideal conditions.

This scarcity and solution-oriented mindset is valuable in BME education, especially in high-resource settings. When a clinical device fails in the field or an irrigation system leaks, the priority is immediate, functional repair, not elegance or aesthetics. These rapid, situational problem-solving acts *are* prototyping and embody the essence of practical ingenuity. BME educators should help students unlearn the myth of the perfect workspace. Prototyping can happen: in classrooms with prototyping carts, anywhere with cardboard and tape, or in field settings, using found materials (Wettergreen et al. 2025).

5.9 PEDAGOGICAL STRATEGIES FOR EFFECTIVE PROTOTYPING EDUCATION

A number of pedagogical strategies can be employed to support effective prototyping in BME education. These strategies are applicable not only at the senior capstone level but throughout all stages of the undergraduate curriculum. Foundational to this approach is an emphasis on *practical ingenuity*, encouraging students to begin with resourceful, low-cost methods rather than relying immediately on advanced tools or technologies.

Importantly, BME educators themselves do not need to be experts in prototyping to facilitate successful SOs. With the right strategies in place, students can learn and thrive in prototyping efforts regardless of whether a formal makerspace exists on campus or whether the educator is trained on this prototyping equipment. Educators can instead focus on fostering a mindset of exploration, iteration, and resourcefulness that empowers students to build confidently with the available tools and materials.

5.9.1 Celebrate Practical Ingenuity and Start With Low-Fidelity Prototyping

At the OEDK, we have refined many strategies that prioritize hands-on learning and creativity in developing functional prototypes over the past 15 years. One foundational

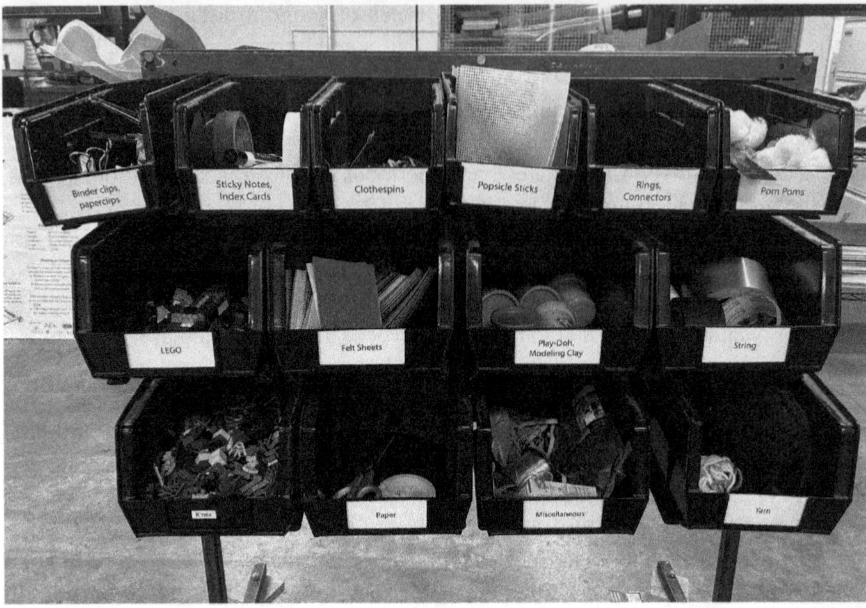
Binder clips, paperclips
Sticky Notes, Index Cards
Clothespins
Popsicle Sticks
Rings, Connectors
Pom Poms
LEGO
Felt Sheets
Play-Doh, Modeling Clay
String

FIGURE 5.1 Low-fidelity prototyping cart stocked with simple, affordable materials, allowing quick, accessible design

principle is to celebrate *practical ingenuity*—the idea that everything can be a raw material, and that prototyping success stems from how creatively materials are used, not how advanced they are.

One effective practice is using low-fidelity prototyping carts stocked with simple, affordable materials. These enable students to begin building immediately, lowering the barrier to entry. Figure 5.1 shows our low-fidelity prototyping cart, which includes many simple and readily available materials. These materials may vary by geographical location, but variants are readily available worldwide.

We also implement the *30-minute prototype* exercise, where each team member builds a prototype, any prototype, in 30 minutes. The prototype can be large or small, communicate a function, or exercise a design block, but it must be finished at the end of the period. Teams then review each prototype, consolidate the strongest elements, and refine the idea into a single direction. This quick-start method emphasizes momentum over perfection and helps develop team consensus through action.

5.9.2 Lay a Foundation for Tool Use Excellence

Building early tool confidence is essential for all students. This tool's confidence is crucial as first-year students arrive at college with a range of skills. Unfortunately, this delta can exacerbate a lack of confidence when peers compare each other.

At the OEDK, we train students through skill-based Fabrication Workshops, or "Fabshops," two-hour hands-on skills-building workshops that teach safe and effective use of hand and power tools. While these workshops are offered across a spectrum of skills and tools, the foundational ones are on safe and effective use of hand and power tools. Later workshops are optional, but the hand and power tools workshops are mandatory for first-year students. Often led by the instructors of the first-year design course, students learn how to use basic hand and power tools while building from the plans for a basic birdhouse. These skills workshops can be taught inside a class or extracurricularly, but students in courses that require prototyping can be asked to attend extracurricular workshops to support their skills growth.

5.9.3 Use Real-World Challenges to Drive Engagement

When students recognize that a design challenge is rooted in a real-world need, they treat the project as real, increasing engagement significantly. At the OEDK, we integrate short design exercises centered on practical healthcare or industry challenges to contextualize prototyping activities. These assignments help students appreciate the stakes of design decisions and the role of prototyping in solving authentic problems. Examples of these projects are motivated by global challenges such as access to clean water or the development of a safer Bajaj, a three-wheeled motorized vehicle commonly used for transportation in many developing countries. The following are additional concepts that can support educators' ability to help students effectively prototype in their BME education.

5.10 STRESS THE USE OF LOW-FIDELITY PROTOTYPING AS A STARTING POINT

Regardless of academic level, we stress that each project should begin with low-fidelity prototyping and practical ingenuity as a starting point for all of their prototypes. This approach allows for rapid iteration, encourages creative problem-solving, and provides a low-risk way to test ideas. For students and educators who are still building technical expertise, low-fidelity prototyping offers an accessible entry point that does not require extensive tool training.

In Brandel et al., we have shown that starting with low-fidelity models gives students valuable "momentum," improving morale and increasing the quality of final outcomes. Our teaching philosophy, shaped by global fieldwork and conversations with craftspeople, prioritizes quick, functional construction using low-cost, widely available materials. Rather than begin with a budget, students are taught to begin with *making* (Brandel, Chang, and Wettergreen 2022).

Many low-fidelity prototyping tools have a low investment cost, which means that they can be picked up and used effectively and quickly. Figure 5.2 shows a sample of some of the low-fidelity prototypes that have been generated through two-hour prototypes or semester-long projects. These low-fidelity prototypes reflect design intention while also being low-cost and easy to produce and modify.

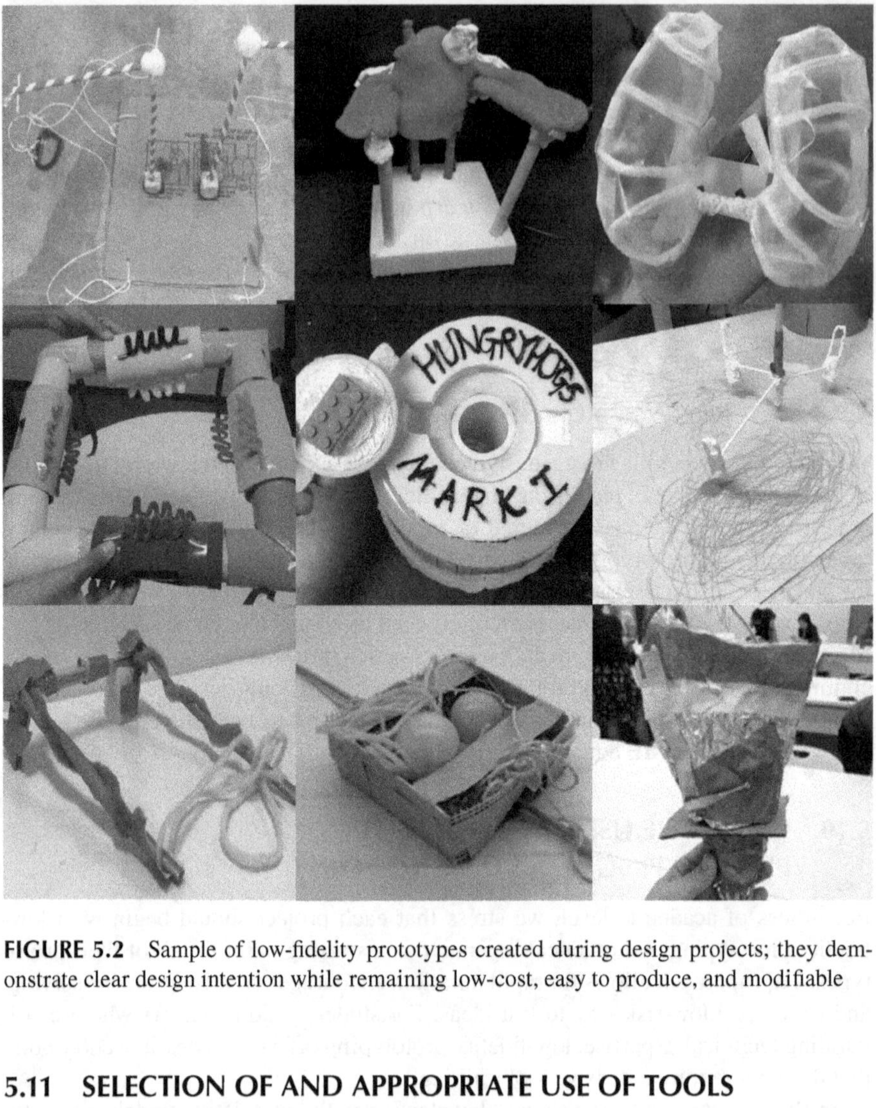

FIGURE 5.2 Sample of low-fidelity prototypes created during design projects; they demonstrate clear design intention while remaining low-cost, easy to produce, and modifiable

5.11 SELECTION OF AND APPROPRIATE USE OF TOOLS

Low-fidelity prototypes need not be condemned to being produced with simple materials and lacking function. Figure 5.3 shows several versions of an elbow mannequin assembled with rubber bands, wood, and plastic. This prototype has both low/medium fidelity aspects but was constructed with only hand and power tools, minimal material cost, and is fully functioning. Students need to be taught that the goal is to realize function quickly and simply, and that low-fidelity prototypes can help achieve that.

Because students are resistant to spending time using low-fidelity prototyping as a method for developing solutions, they are more likely to select more challenging tools or materials to use. Thus, a critical part of prototyping education is helping students make smart tool choices. We stress that students should not jump to

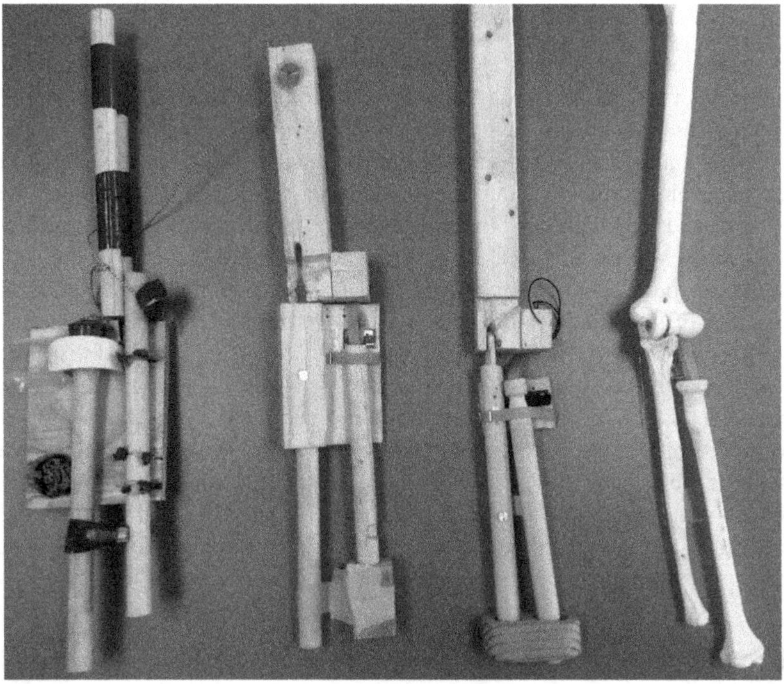

FIGURE 5.3 Functional elbow mannequin prototypes progressing from low to medium fidelity (left to right), built with simple materials to quickly test key functions

a higher-fidelity prototype or a more technologically complex fabrication method until they have answered key questions about their prototype, such as identifying design blocks, features, and general scale. Many students gravitate toward advanced tools (e.g., Computer Numerical Control (CNC) machines and Printed Circuit Board (PCB) design software) before they are ready, underestimating the learning curve and time investment. In such cases, educators should intervene. For example, at the OEDK, students often propose designing custom PCBs; we redirect them to faster, more flexible alternatives like breadboards or perf boards to accelerate testing and learning. Tool complexity should be introduced progressively. As noted in prior work (Brandel, Chang, and Wettergreen 2022), mastery of a few accessible tools often yields better learning outcomes than exposure to many. Table 5.2 reflects the types of prototyping tools available in makerspaces and their relative characteristics to help BME educators select appropriate tools for their classes.

Brandel et al. demonstrated that students perform better with easy-to-learn tools, independent of which tools are well supported by instruction from the course or the MBE instructor (Brandel, Chang, and Wettergreen 2022). Taking this into consideration, and the fact that student self-reporting overestimates tool knowledge, the resulting conclusion is that faculty need to require students to learn some prototyping techniques.

5.11.1 Scaffolding Tool Instruction and Project Scoping

Appropriate selection of tools also leads to the scaffolding of tool instruction and stratification of project scoping. In all of the BME projects and classes, across the curriculum, instructors need to have an understanding of the complexity of the project, intended outcomes, and the tools that students cannot only use, but *should* and *should not* use to develop solutions. Educators should match the complexity of tools to the students' level and the time available for instruction. For instance, first- and second-year students might work with CAD, 3D printing, and basic electronics, but should avoid projects that require advanced techniques such as CNC machining or silicone molding.

This progression can be enforced by setting "guardrails" on project selection during the scoping process. Faculty should curate projects based on available instruction time and student readiness. For example, first-year students might be steered away from geometrically complex parts that require subtractive manufacturing. At the same time, seniors might be encouraged to pursue projects that involve integrating mechano-electrical systems. Instructors must also "right-size" project goals to align with prototyping goals, factoring in the tools and skills students are expected to develop within the given timeframe. Figure 5.4 can assist professors in selecting specific prototyping methods dependent upon the project length and student level.

5.11.2 Stressing the Design–Make–Test Iterative Cycle

Prototypes, like good ideas, change and mature over time. Moving from a napkin sketch to a functional prototype takes time, as well as iteration and evolution of the pieces and parts. In many projects, prototypes take an evolutionary path toward completion, gaining functions, shedding parts, and morphing into the final design. Students at all levels should be encouraged to produce *many* prototypes, as evolving ideas. The design–make–test cycle fosters a mindset of improvement and resilience—students should be encouraged to build, test, cannibalize, and rebuild their prototypes as they move toward optimal solutions.

This design–build–test cycle can look different for each team, project, and class. A generalized schema is the following:

- First-year students should be challenged to focus on executing the design process well and demonstrate iterative prototypes, starting with low-fidelity prototypes. Their final prototype can reflect iteration based on trial-and-error alone, with simple testing and results informing iteration that is discussed, but not necessarily required.
- Senior-level iteration should incorporate multiple evolved prototypes using CAD, 3D printing, and electronics, with intermittent testing results and documentation as the driver for prototyping iteration. Final prototypes should be the result of this iteration and reflect refined CAD drawings, precision fabrication, and documentation as key deliverables.
- There is some flexibility between these two ends of the spectrum. Generally, second- through third-year students should be capable of experimenting with functional iterations of medium-fidelity prototypes, and these prototypes should be the product of multiple prototyping processes.

Category	Tool/Skill	Tool/Skill	Relative Difficulty (low/medium/high)	Time investment to learn	Part complexity	Part Customization	Variety of workable materials	Minimum time to apply technique	Part repeatability	2D vs. 3D	Quality of Final Shape
Hand Operated Tools	Hand Tools (use of basic tools: hammer, screwdriver, pliers, wire crimper)	Hand Tools	★☆☆☆☆	★☆☆☆☆	★★☆☆☆	★★☆☆☆	★★★★★	★☆☆☆☆	★★☆☆☆	EITHER	★★☆☆☆
Hand Operated Tools	Physical Prototyping (putting things together, fixing or modifying machines around the house)	Physical Prototyping	★☆☆☆☆	★☆☆☆☆	★★☆☆☆	★★★☆☆	★★★★★	★☆☆☆☆	★★★☆☆	EITHER	★★★☆☆
Hand Operated Tools	Power Tools (use of power tools to cut, shape, or join material)	Power Tools	★★☆☆☆	★★☆☆☆	★★★☆☆	★★★☆☆	★★★★★	★☆☆☆☆	★★★☆☆	EITHER	★★☆☆☆
Hand Operated Tools	3D Pen Drawing - 3Doodler or others (making representations of objects, creating functional structures)	3D Pen Drawing	★☆☆☆☆	★☆☆☆☆	★★☆☆☆	★★★★★	★★★☆☆	★☆☆☆☆	★★☆☆☆	EITHER	★☆☆☆☆
Hand Operated Tools	Sanding/Painting/Finishing (how to sand/file/prepare a surface and then coat the surface with paint/stain/etc.)	Post-Processing	★☆☆☆☆	★☆☆☆☆	★☆☆☆☆	★★★★★	★★★★★	★☆☆☆☆	★★★☆☆	EITHER	★★★★☆
Eng. Visual Design	Drawing and Sketching by hand (making representations of objects with pen and paper)	Drawing/Sketching	★☆☆☆☆	★☆☆☆☆	★☆☆☆☆	★★★★★	★☆☆☆☆	★☆☆☆☆	★★☆☆☆	2D	★★☆☆☆
Eng. Visual Design	Computer Aided Design (TinkerCAD)	Computer Aided Design (TinkerCAD)	★☆☆☆☆	★☆☆☆☆	★★☆☆☆	★★★★★	★★★★★	★☆☆☆☆	★★★★★	3D	N/A
Eng. Visual Design	Computer Aided Design (SolidWorks or other industry standard)	Computer Aided Design (SolidWorks or other industry standard)	★★★★☆	★★★★☆	★★★☆☆	★★★★★	★★★★★	★★★☆☆	★★★★★	3D	N/A
Electronics	Electronics (ability to create circuits or use a microcontroller to make things responsive)	Electronics	★★★☆☆	★★★★☆	★★★★☆	★★★★☆	N/A	★★★☆☆	★★★★★	3D	★★★★☆
Advanced Manufacturing	Laser Cutter (operating a laser cutter to cut or etch planar objects)	Laser Cutter	★★★☆☆	★★★☆☆	★★★☆☆	★★★☆☆	★★☆☆☆	★★★☆☆	★★★★★	2D	★★★★☆
Advanced Manufacturing	3D Printing (DOWNLOAD parts / operate a 3D printer to produce objects)	3D Printer - downloaded parts	★★★☆☆	★☆☆☆☆	★★★☆☆	★☆☆☆☆	1 (PLA)	★★★☆☆	★★★★★	3D	★★☆☆☆
Advanced Manufacturing	3D Printing (DESIGN parts / operate a 3D printer to produce objects)	3D Printer - custom parts	★★★★☆	★★★★☆	★★★☆☆	★★★★★	★★★☆☆	★★★☆☆	★★★★★	3D	★★★☆☆
	Plasma Cutter (operating a plasma cutter to cut planar metal sheets)	Plasma Cutter	★★★☆☆	★★★☆☆	★★★★☆	★★★☆☆	★☆☆☆☆	★★★☆☆	★★★★★	2D	★★★★☆

FIGURE 5.4 Characteristics of various prototyping methods to assist BME educators in selecting tools for their classes (design of table inspired by material from Brandel et al. (Brandel, Chang, and Wettergreen 2022)

5.11.3 Balancing Teaching Prototyping Skills and Other Content to BME Students

Given the time constraints, BME educators must weigh how much emphasis to place on tool instruction versus prototyping skills and other course content (e.g., physiology, design process, and gene therapy). The following are three educational models BME educators can use to prioritize their learning objectives, further visualized in a pie graph format in Figure 5.5.

5.11.3.1 Prioritizing the Design Process or Content Knowledge

In this model, instructors seek to have teams make progress on real-world projects or primarily focus on helping students acquire conceptual knowledge. Students would apply the process knowledge or content knowledge to their specific project. This prioritization is the prevailing model of well-executed first-year and capstone design. A content-based course example would be a PBL-based course on Bioengineering Fundamentals. In both examples, collaboration, design, creative thinking, or content knowledge are stressed. Only a minimum amount of class time is allocated to the teaching of specific skills, with the emphasis on strong design execution or content acquisition. For first-year design, this skills instruction might be an introduction to the most accessible tools, like hand tools, power tools, or simple CAD programs like TinkerCAD. This approach builds strong design skills or content knowledge, but either limits technical prototyping excellence (such as in first-year design) or assumes foundational student skills (such as in capstone design). Many instances of this model may exist in one program's BME curriculum.

5.11.3.2 Prioritizing Prototyping

In this model, instructors prioritize a wide array of prototyping methods, tools, and machines to promote prototyping excellence. This broadens tool familiarity but

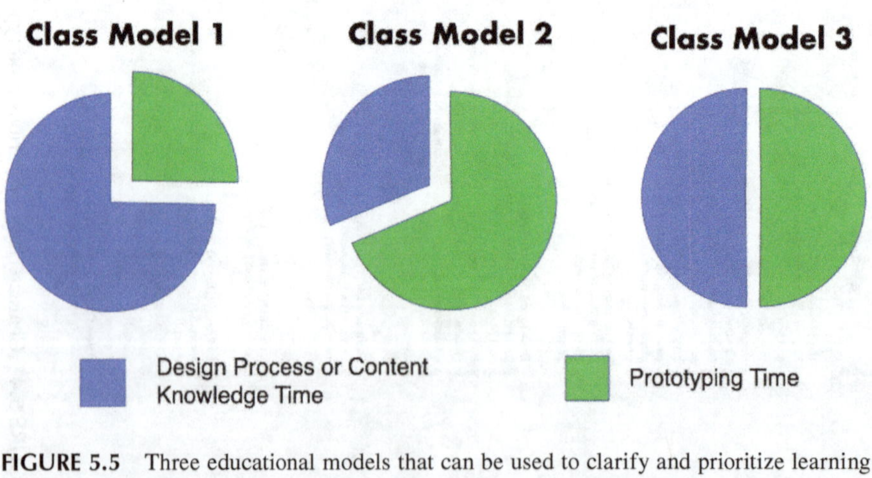

FIGURE 5.5 Three educational models that can be used to clarify and prioritize learning objectives in BME courses

leaves less time for content knowledge acquisition or design process-based instruction. This model is effective in the middle of the curriculum, teaching students who already have a foundation in design and some prototyping experience but need to develop proficiency in iteration, refinement, and prototyping evolution. There is a need for only one version of this course in any BME curriculum, focusing on the most valuable tools for BME students.

5.11.3.3 Balanced Approach

A third model aims for balance between the two, teaching just a few advanced tools (e.g., 3D printing and laser cutting) to a higher level of proficiency, while still covering the foundational design process or content knowledge. This model can be effective at higher academic levels, assuming foundational design and basic prototyping skills, while teaching only the prototyping skill that will be emphasized for a particular course. Examples of this approach include a system perspective on physiology where MATLAB is employed, or a Point of Care Diagnostics course where these specialized laboratory techniques are taught alongside POC content. Another example is where CAD and FEA are taught with the design-build-iterate cycle, requiring the 3D printing of evolutionary prototypes.

5.12 CONCLUSION AND FUTURE DIRECTIONS

This chapter provides BME educators with foundational concepts in prototyping and offers strategies for incorporating hands-on prototyping throughout the undergraduate biomedical engineering curriculum. It emphasizes how prototyping supports rapid iteration, problem-solving, and technical skill development at all levels of instruction. The subsequent Chapter 5 presents specific examples of prototypes, accompanied by visuals and analysis, to reinforce the pedagogical approaches discussed here.

We have highlighted how prototyping can be embedded throughout the curriculum, with expectations calibrated to the fidelity of prototypes and the instructional time available for teaching specific tools and techniques. It is unreasonable to expect students to produce refined, high-functioning prototypes without adequate training in fabrication methods, especially at lower (first- and second-year students) levels. However, this limitation can be transformed into a pedagogical strength. In early foundational courses, students can be introduced to fundamental prototyping methods that prioritize problem-solving, quick iteration, and a reliance on the design process. As students advance and gain experience with tools and materials, educators can progressively emphasize refinement, functionality, and performance based on real-world criteria. Several key pedagogical insights are condensed for BME educators:

5.12.1 BME Education Benefits From Hands-On Prototyping Across the Curriculum

Hands-on prototyping is an active form of learning that cultivates hand-eye coordination, physical material knowledge, tool usage, communication, and incorporates multiple perspectives. This dynamic mix of skills and practices increases engagement, which leads to enhanced knowledge acquisition and transfer (Smith et al. 2005).

5.12.2 Prototypes Exist Across a Continuum of Fidelity (or Resolution)

Prototypes may be classified as low, medium, or high fidelity, depending on their technical complexity and the degree to which they function. Students can produce prototypes at all these levels, but their ability to do so successfully depends on structured access to tools, materials, machines, and education. First-year students should be able to produce semi-functional low- or medium-fidelity prototypes in one semester. Seniors should be expected to produce fully functional medium-fidelity prototypes over a year, and those prototypes should include some features that are high fidelity.

5.12.3 Prototyping Should Always Begin With Low Fidelity

Regardless of educational level, available tools, or individual student skills, early design solutions should start with low-fidelity prototypes. Applying this method allows multiple prototypes to be completed rapidly and at a low cost, so it is advantageous to start here before moving on to a higher fidelity. Encouraging the practice of low-fidelity prototyping cultivates resourcefulness and creative problem-solving in students.

5.12.4 Tool Instruction Should Be Scaffolded Across the BME Curriculum

Students must be given the training and time to develop the skills necessary to produce refined prototypes. Instruction in tool usage should be introduced incrementally across the curriculum, with expectations for prototype refinement aligned with project outcomes. First-year students should be explicitly taught the tools they are expected to use. Upper-level students should be expected to produce work that reflects a commitment to self-directed study and practice using advanced tools.

5.12.5 BME Education Should Stress the Importance of Design Iteration

Similar to the need for tool instruction to be spread across the curriculum, space must be created for design iteration. In early courses, students should be required to demonstrate iteration from early sketched ideas, through low or medium-fidelity prototypes with design reviews that stress iteration and evolution of functionality. In later courses for upper-class students, design teams should submit to formal design reviews, including analysis of prototypes with an emphasis on iteration in fidelity, function, and testing.

5.12.6 Projects Must Be Matched to Students' Technical Skills

Expectations for project outcomes should be responsive to students' current technical readiness and then accommodate the amount of time available in a class for tool instruction, prototype iteration, and project complexity. Thus, BME educators should select projects that are appropriate in scope. Freshman projects should include between two and three critical functions and can be completed only using knowledge that will be taught to the students in the semester. Capstone projects may be more ambitious, building on known skills students have acquired through the curriculum, what will be taught to these students over the year, and an expectation that students will self-teach a limited number of skills and apply them in their prototype development.

5.12.7 Makerspaces Are Essential Infrastructure for Prototyping Education

The emergence of makerspaces has been one of the most impactful developments of the past 25 years in engineering education. BME is among the disciplines that have benefited the most. These spaces enable BME programs to meet hands-on learning goals aligned with ABET requirements while supporting a broad range of prototyping activities. Makerspaces can support semester-long courses (e.g., first-year design and final-year capstone) and short-form experiences like hackathons or skill-building workshops. The BME curriculum is enhanced and supported by makerspaces.

5.12.8 Prototyping Can Happen Anywhere

While some institutions are fortunate to host large, dedicated fabrication spaces, others rely on adaptable classrooms or mobile toolkits. Makerspaces can range from fully equipped facilities to temporary "pop-up" environments with basic tools and locally sourced materials. Educators should focus less on what is lacking and more on how to scaffold meaningful prototyping experiences with available resources: prototyping can happen anywhere.

5.12.9 Mentorship Networks Accelerate Student Development

Students can benefit from a "web of mentors" that includes faculty, peers, technical staff, clinicians, and industry partners. These mentors can help students overcome technical hurdles, access new tools, and refine their approaches. A strong mentorship network enables students to extend their capabilities beyond what would be possible in isolation.

While this chapter focuses on foundational strategies for incorporating prototyping into BME education, educators should also anticipate emerging trends shaping future curricula. For example, integrating computational modeling and AI-driven design tools, such as generative design platforms, offers new avenues for rapid iteration and personalization in prototyping. Additionally, advances in fields like bioprinting, soft robotics, and innovative materials are beginning to influence both instructional methods and the types of prototypes students can create. Achieving this level of curricular innovation requires sustained collaboration among academic institutions, industry partners, and clinical stakeholders. Many programs already embrace these partnerships to develop meaningful, translational design experiences. The subsequent chapter highlights specific tools and techniques supporting these real-world projects.

ACKNOWLEDGMENTS

This work was completed around the world at various universities, and in the United States at the OEDK, and spans many courses in the design curriculum over the previous 15 years. Thanks to Paige Rennie for copyediting, prototyping topic suggestions, and formatting changes. Thanks to Katherine Sammy for the reference formatting, research, document, figure, and table preparation. Photos from this chapter have been collected through traditional curricular instruction, where, at the beginning of the semester, students acknowledge their approval for future usage of these materials, based on the syllabus.

REFERENCES

ABET. 2024. *Criteria for Accrediting Engineering Programs, 2025–2026*. https://www.abet.org.

Banzi, Massimo, and Michael Shiloh. 2022. *Getting Started with Arduino*. San Francisco: Make Community.

Bethke, Eliot, Ali Ansari, Jennifer Amos, Joe Bradley, Ruth Ochia, and Holly Golecki. 2024. "Bridging Extracurricular Skill Needs in Bioengineering Capstone Design with Just-in-Time Workshops." Paper presented at *2024 ASEE Annual Conference & Exposition*. Portland, OR, June.

Brandel, Joshua, Andersen Chang, and Matthew Wettergreen. 2022. "The Impact of Appropriate Prototyping Tool Choices on Achieving Functionality for Novices." *International Journal of Engineering Education* 38 (6): 1730–46.

Bushnell, Tyler, Scott Steber, Annika Matta, Mark Cutkosky, and Larry Leifer. 2013. "Using a 'Dark Horse' Prototype to Manage Innovative Teams." In *Proceedings of the 3rd International Conference on Integration of Design, Engineering and Management for Innovation*, 8, edited by A. A. Fernandes, R. M. Natal Jorge, L. Patrício, A. Medeiros, Porto, Portugal, 4-6th September 2013. https://doi.org/10.13140/2.1.2361.7602

Detand, Jan, Ronald Bastiaens, and Bart Grimonprez. 2010. "The Role of Prototyping in Product Development." In *Proceedings of the 4th International PMI Conference*, Ghent, January. https://www.researchgate.net/publication/240045178_The_role_of_prototyping_in_product_development.

Higbee, Steven, and Sharon Miller. 2019. "Work in Progress: Vertical Integration of Engineering Design in an Undergraduate BME Curriculum." Paper presented at *2019 ASEE Annual Conference & Exposition*, Tampa, FL, June.

Kohtala, S. M. I., Jørgen Andreas Bogen Erichsen, Heikki Sjöman, and Martin Steinert. 2018. "Augmenting Physical Prototype Activities in Early-Stage Product Development." In *Proceedings of NordDesign 2018 (DS 91)*, August14 – 17, 2018, Linköping, Sweden. https://www.designsociety.org/publication/40955/augmenting_physical_prototype_activities_in_early-stage_product_development.

Lefteri, Chris, and Central Saint Martins College of Art and Design (London, England). 2019. *Making It: Manufacturing Techniques for Product Design*. London: Laurence King Publishing.

Mulenburg, Gerald, and Daniel Gundo. 2002. "Design by Prototype: Examples from the National Aeronautics and Space Administration." *NASA Ames Research Center*. 11th International Conference on the Management of Technology. Miami FL, March 10-14, 2002. https://ntrs.nasa.gov/api/citations/20040081092/downloads/20040081092.pdf

National Center for Faculty Development & Diversity. 2025. *NCFDD Mentor Map*. Accessed June 1, 2025. https://www.ncfdd.org/ncfddmentormap.

Pario Perra, Daniele. 2010. *Low Cost Design. Ediz. Italiana e Inglese*. Edited by Daniele Pario Perra. Milan: Silvana.

Redwood, Ben, Filemon Schöffer, and Brian Garret. 2017. *The 3D Printing Handbook: Technologies, Design and Applications*. Amsterdam: 3D Hubs B.V.

Roberts, Dustyn. 2010. *Making Things Move: DIY Mechanisms for Inventors, Hobbyists, and Artists*. New York: McGraw-Hill Education.

Saterbak, A., Wettergreen, M. 2022. Introduction to Engineering Design. Springer Cham, Switzerland: Springer AG. https://doi.org/10.1007/978-3-031-02093-3

Scherz, Paul, and Simon Monk. 2016. *Practical Electronics for Inventors*. 4th ed. New York: McGraw-Hill Education.

Smith, Karl A., Sheri D. Sheppard, David W. Johnson, and Roger T. Johnson. 2005. "Pedagogies of Engagement: Classroom-Based Practices." *Journal of Engineering Education* 94 (1): 87–101.

Thompson, Rob. 2007. *Manufacturing Processes for Design Professionals*. New York: W. W. Norton.

Vygotsky, Lev S. 1978. *Mind in Society: The Development of Higher Psychological Processes*. Vol. 86. Cambridge, MA: Harvard University Press.

Wettergreen, M. A, Walters, G., Mihas, P., and Maples, G. 2025. *Beyond Skills: Makerspace Participation Supports Well-Being*. IJAMM. https://doi.org/10.21428/70cb44c5.bb017743

Wettergreen, Matthew A., Ann Saterbak, Amy Kavalewitz, Alex Nunez-Thompson, Veronica Leautaud, Theresa Mkandawire, Matthew Petney, Carlos Dos Santos, and Maria Oden. 2020. "Makerspaces in Low-, Middle-, and High-Income Countries to Support Student Development of Engineering Design Skills." *International Journal of Engineering Education* 36 (4): 1234–51.

Wettergreen, Matthew A., Luis Felipe Dobles Junqueira, Shea Hagy, Emilio Da Cruz Brandao, and Amy Kavalewitz Dern. 2023. "From Place to Place: Harnessing Pop-up Makerspaces to Enable Hands-on Study Abroad Programs." *Contexts* 8 (13): 14.

Wilczynski, Vince, and Ronald Adrezin. 2016. "Higher Education Makerspaces and Engineering Education." In *Proceedings of the ASME 2016 International Mechanical Engineering Congress and Exposition*, November 11–17, 2016. V005T06A013. ASME. https://doi.org/10.1115/IMECE2016-68048

6 Teaching Innovation in Biomedical Engineering—The Need-Driven Biodesign Process of Innovating Health Technologies

Mark Seow Khoon Chong, Lyn Denend, and David B. Grayden

6.1 INTRODUCTION

6.1.1 Design and Innovation in Biomedical Engineering (BME) Programs

Biomedical engineers need more than just technical proficiency to thrive in the health and biomedical sectors. They must have an ability to understand the diverse (and sometimes divergent) interests of healthcare stakeholders in order to develop crucial insights that lead to creative problem-solving. Increasingly, biomedical engineering programs around the world are incorporating design and innovation into their curricula. Beyond broad applications toward entrepreneurship, design education inculcates discipline and teaches approaches to help learners better navigate a uniquely complex environment involving the five Ps: patients, physicians, payers, providers, and policymakers.

In the University, innovation is often introduced through structured curricula in design-oriented engineering courses. These typically involve PjBL, particularly in senior capstone design courses in undergraduate programs. Such courses lend authenticity to learning and help students develop problem-solving skills and better appreciate how knowledge may be applied to the real world. Indeed, design is one of the most commonly required courses in BME departments (Linsenmeier and Saterbak 2020). This was partly driven by efforts in the late 1990s, when the Wallace H. Coulter Foundation played a major role in BME education in the United States by spurring the incorporation of content related to entrepreneurship, innovation, and the translation of ideas into biomedical products in biomedical engineering design

DOI: 10.1201/9781003520313-6

courses and programs. It is now recognized that these principles can be even more broadly applied across geographies (Maloney et al. 2025; Xu et al. 2025). In order for education in design to be delivered in a meaningful way, however, suitable frameworks for design instruction are necessary to scaffold learning activities and to help students navigate indeterminacy.

6.1.2 Frameworks for Teaching Design

Common frameworks used to describe approaches to design include the Double Diamond, the five-step design thinking process, and systems design. The five-step model (Empathize, Define, Ideate, Prototype, and Test) originated in the Hasso Plattner Institute of Design (d.school) at Stanford, and is widely used to teach user-centered problem-solving. The Double Diamond framework (developed by the British Design Council) similarly emphasizes divergent and convergent thinking phases that separate problem identification from solution development. In University settings, such models have generally been influential in promoting creativity and structured exploration in both engineering and interdisciplinary education (Lindberg, Meinel, and Wagner 2011; Razzouk and Shute 2012). As a tool, Design Thinking has been shown to foster creative confidence, thoughtful concept development, and empathy-driven approaches to problem-solving (Luka 2014; Noweski et al. 2012). However, other studies have also highlighted various limitations, including inconsistent application, lack of domain specificity, and limited applicability toward downstream phases in development (Glen et al. 2015; Luchs, Swan, and Griffin 2015).

These shortcomings become especially evident in the context of healthcare innovation. While generic design models offer valuable tools to guide design in general, they typically underemphasize essential healthcare-specific constraints. Clinical workflows, regulatory requirements, and reimbursement models are often treated superficially or insufficiently emphasized in the design process. The lack of disciplined interrogation of the clinical need may result in teams jumping forward into premature solutioning, an approach that can undermine both relevance and feasibility of the concepts that they choose to bring forward (Altman, Huang, and Breland 2018). This gap points toward the need for more specialized frameworks that are purpose-built for the healthcare setting. In the next section, we describe how the Biodesign process addresses these limitations through a structured, need-driven approach tailored to meet the unique demands of medical innovation.

6.2 THE BIODESIGN PROCESS

6.2.1 Genesis

Stanford Biodesign was started in 2001 to provide an ecosystem of training and support for aspiring health technology innovators. At the time, design education, particularly human-centered design, was experiencing a resurgence, fueled by the success of design thinking paradigms. However, these approaches could not be directly translated to health technology, in part due to multiple "valleys of death" that exist for such innovations. The Biodesign program was established to bridge this gap through a rigorous, needs-driven approach to innovation, placing understanding clinical needs at the core of the educational experience (Denend et al. 2021; Wall et al. 2017).

The program's flagship offering is the Stanford Biodesign Innovation Fellowship, a year-long full-time training experience for postgraduate professionals from diverse backgrounds in engineering, medicine, and business. Each year, fellows begin their journey with a month-long clinical immersion, generating hundreds of observations that are then researched and filtered into a smaller set of well-characterized, validated unmet needs that represent promising innovation opportunities. Only after this clinical grounding and progressively in-depth research to understand the underlying problem do teams begin generating solution concepts, which are then systematically evaluated for viability (Fuerch et al. 2021; Wall et al. 2017) with the help of guidance from real-world health technology industry experts and healthcare stakeholders.

Biodesign is anchored on the belief that innovation is a discipline that is teachable and repeatable. The emphasis on systematic need identification and characterization, critical analyses (both of needs and potential solutions), and abstraction of learning from the real world reflects this intention. Over time, this methodology has expanded beyond the fellowship to a broader portfolio of offerings (described in Section 6.3) around the world (Augustin et al. 2019; Denend et al. 2021; Kadlowec et al. 2017).

6.2.2 Overview of the Approach

The Biodesign process is structured in three phases (Identify, Invent, and Implement) that outline a systematic, healthcare-specific approach toward user-centric design. While the framework may be applied in full in some postgraduate programs (such as the Stanford Biodesign Innovation Fellowship described earlier), many academic settings emphasize selected components of the Biodesign, depending on intended learning outcomes, institutional resources, and learner level.

In both undergraduate and postgraduate courses, the Identify phase is often the most emphasized. It typically begins with a clinical immersion, where innovation teams are given opportunities to identify clinical problems that can be translated into clinical need statements (Need Identification). Students are trained to generate and iteratively refine need statements, each comprising a problem, target population, and desired outcome, supported by real-world observations and stakeholder interviews. Subsequently, teams conduct research to characterize the need statements in order to uncover insights from understanding the disease state, studying existing solutions (and gaps), analyzing stakeholders, and evaluating the market (Need Selection). This method typically aligns well with BME programs in most universities, where the problem framing exercises form the foundation of both undergraduate design modules and postgraduate innovation tracks. The value of this phase is widely supported in the literature as critical to downstream success in medical innovation (Denend et al. 2021; Yock et al. 2015).

The Invent phase, which focuses on generating and screening solution concepts, may be similarly applied to classroom settings. Students engage in team-based ideation (Concept Generation), using tools such as brainstorming to generate a range of concepts. This is followed by initial concept screening, guided by the need criteria in the preceding stage. Exploration of the generated concepts typically involves early prototyping and technical feasibility assessments, particularly if maker spaces are available. Real-world considerations for health technology innovations, such as IP, regulatory requirements, business models, and reimbursement, are also factored in to this Concept Selection stage (Augustin et al. 2019; Denend et al. 2021).

In contrast, the Implement phase is less frequently addressed in depth within formal BME coursework. This phase covers stages in Strategy Development and culminates in Business Planning. A frequent challenge faced is the breadth and, paradoxically, use-specific nature of the topics, which often exceed the timeframe or scope of academic courses and programs. Even in the Stanford Biodesign Innovation Fellowship, teaching the Implement phase relies heavily on external mentorship (matched to the fellowship team) and often on extended project timelines (Fuerch et al. 2021; Wall et al. 2017). In academic settings, the Implement phase may be introduced through short modules or guest lectures, but students are typically not expected to develop and/or execute on full business and commercialization strategies. Similarly, prototyping is performed to demonstrate initial proof-of-concept, but achieving a viable prototype is typically difficult to achieve within the confines of a time-limited fellowship.

Biodesign is now being taught around the world, where common practices have been observed to converge on a few key components: early and authentic clinical immersion, structured need filtering frameworks, ensuring diversity of ideas, milestone-driven deliverables, and dedicated mentoring. Chua et al. (2024) consolidate evidence from 26 studies across North America, Asia, and Europe, highlighting that the Biodesign framework has been successfully implemented in a wide range of formats, from semester-long courses to a variety of fellowships. The review identifies key factors for successful programs, including immersion-based need identification, cross-disciplinary collaboration, and strong mentorship structures. Notably, the review confirms that programs using the Biodesign process consistently enhance participants' innovation, leadership, and entrepreneurship capabilities, with reported career shifts and commercial product outcomes observed even beyond academic settings.

It should be noted, however, that several challenges exist that hinder these critical learning activities. For example, providing clinical immersion for need identification is increasingly challenging, particularly for undergraduate engineering students and in a post-pandemic world (King and Salvo 2024). Maintaining engagement, particularly across heterogeneous teams, may also pose challenges, particularly in cross-faculty engagements. Finally, integrating regulatory and other commercially-oriented content must be done in a way that is meaningful to learners, without overwhelming them (Augustin et al. 2019; Denend et al. 2021). The latter is further exacerbated by the academia-industry disconnect that is evident in many university settings.

Besides the textbook, recent innovations have been introduced to facilitate effective teaching of the Biodesign process. In their study, Denend et al. (2024) reported the development and evaluation of a structured rubric for assessing student-generated need statements. While the rubric did not demonstrably improve SOs in a short-term setting, implementation of a rubric was shown to more clearly communicate instructor expectations, promote alignment across assessors, and guide the delivery of formative feedback. These insights underscore the need for scaffolding in PjBL environments where outcomes are indeterminate and varied, by shifting some of the focus away from the artifact, getting instructors to instead focus feedback on the process.

Another recent innovation was the introduction of a web resource. *A Student Guide to Biodesign* (https://biodesignguide.stanford.edu/) complements classroom instruction by offering practical advice and examples for students to review. It includes worksheets that guide inquiry-based learning, with annotations that help students recognize the thought process behind their decision-making. Compared to traditional didactic instruction, information is more concisely presented, with a greater focus on experiential learning.

In summary, Biodesign represents an opportunity to incorporate design and innovation in BME education. This structured approach has laid a strong foundation for training health innovators who are technically capable, clinically grounded, and translationally oriented. There is also constant innovation and introduction of new pedagogical tools, reflecting efforts to keep abreast of a rapidly evolving field. The next section explores each phase of the Biodesign process in greater detail, identifying opportunities for integration into BME curricula.

6.2.3 Detailed Description of Each Phase

6.2.3.1 Identify

The Identify phase serves as the starting point of the Biodesign process. Learners are introduced to a "focus and flare" approach of needs finding, followed by screening, leading to the selection of the most compelling needs to bring forward to the next phase. Students are guided through a disciplined and systematic process of conducting deep research of each need based on the principle that successful innovation begins with an in-depth and accurate understanding of the problem.

In traditional Biodesign courses and programs, this phase typically begins with clinical immersions to perform "Needs Finding." Learners shadow care teams, conduct informal interviews, and log their observations of problems they may encounter in the clinic. In academic course settings, however, such clinical immersion is often limited or not feasible. Educators commonly adapt the Identify phase by using clinician-supplied need statements, supplemented with clinical lectures and/or clinician interviews. Other tools being explored for use here include online videos of clinical processes, immersion in simulated environments, and virtual reality (VR) platforms (King and Salvo 2024). While these potentially reduce opportunities for raw need discovery, students may instead focus on problem framing and apply structured tools to characterize a healthcare challenge

Instruction during Identify focuses on helping students deepen their understanding of the unmet needs they have discovered through progressively in-depth research on the disease state, existing solutions, stakeholders' landscape, and market. As this work is conducted, there are three essential tools that students learn. The first is the "need statement" that articulates in a single sentence the problem that most needs to be addressed, the population it most negatively affects, and the outcome that is most desired from solving it (Wall et al. 2017; Yock et al. 2015). The initial need statement is the team's hypothesis based on what has been observed. Through extensive need research, students apply the information uncovered to refine the need statement, experimenting with different problem/population/outcome combinations until they arrive at a "final" need statement that reflects the interest of the most important stakeholders in the need areas.

Once students have multiple well-defined need statements supported by need research, the second key technique is "need filtering." In this exercise, students compare needs against one another to choose the one that represents the most promising innovation opportunity. The first step is to choose a set of objective filters that reflect the team's priorities and then evaluate each need against those filters in a competitive manner to determine which one to focus on. Common filters used in this exercise include factors such as the prevalence of the problem, the magnitude of the impact from solving it, the presence or absence of competition in the need area, and so on.

The third helpful tool is defining "need criteria" for the top project. Using all the information gleaned through need research, students create a list of the most important stakeholder requirements that ***any*** solution to the need must address in order to have a chance of displacing the current standard of care and of being adopted. Such criteria are not product specifications, but solution-independent requirements based on everything that has been learned about the need. They typically are organized into "must-have" and "nice-to-have" categories and address important considerations about the efficacy, cost, safety, and usability of whatever solution the team developed in the next phase of the Biodesign process: Invent.

The value of the Identify phase training, even in short format or constrained settings, has been shown. In a study of an accelerated needs finding course, students who participated in structured observation and guided need characterization reported significant improvements in their ability to analyze stakeholder needs, write effective problem statements, and resist premature development of solutions (Denend et al. 2023). More broadly, such studies suggest that such training is useful in equipping students with problem-solving skills adapted for the medical environment.

6.2.3.2 Invent

The Invent phase of the Biodesign process leads from validated clinical needs into preliminary solution concepts. Using the need criteria as a guide, students are encouraged to explore broadly but remain grounded in the insights and criteria revealed during the Identify phase. It has to be stressed that the Invent phase is never performed in isolation and is instead a "need-driven" process.

Ideation typically begins with brainstorming sessions guided by structured prompts such as "how might we . . ." or "what if . . ." questions based upon the need criteria developed in the Identify phase. A range of tools can be introduced to help generate a diverse portfolio of ideas, and instructors may play roles in getting teams started or even facilitating some sessions.

Following ideation, students are guided to screen concepts, first against the need criteria before moving on to a more thorough evaluation of their top concepts against factors such as the IP landscape, regulatory requirements, business model options, and reimbursement pathway. (Depending on intended learning outcomes, time constraints, and access to resources, instructors may have difficulties covering the full range of topics.) Decision matrices, weighted scoring, or comparative concept tables are commonly used in the concept selection process, further training learners in tools commonly used in product design. Engagements with BME graduates suggest that such training in the topics and design process leaves a strong impression and that such exposure distinguishes them from other engineering disciplines (Department of Biomedical Engineering, NUS).

A frequent challenge experienced by instructors during this phase is managing student expectations around prototyping. Many teams equate prototyping with detailed design or fabrication when, in fact, early prototypes are tools for learning. In this context, the prototypes are more often used to explore assumptions, clarify form or function, and/or as tools to communicate with stakeholders. It is helpful during this phase to help students reframe prototyping as a means of reducing uncertainty or "de-risking" their concepts. Accordingly, this requires students to clearly state the purpose and intent behind each prototype iteration.

The strongest student projects in this phase are often those that preserve the logic chain from need to concept. When students drift from their specified need or attempt to retrofit a preconceived idea, the quality of their innovation and learning is inevitably compromised. Review checkpoints may be embedded that (i) require justification of their design choices and (ii) connect the concept to the need statement. Such a review may help students better recognize the importance of problem-solution fit, prompt reflection, and to reinforce this linkage.

6.2.3.3 Implement

The Implement phase of the Biodesign process focuses on what would be required to translate a promising solution concept that was defined in the preceding Invent phase into a product or service that can reach patients. While full implementation is typically beyond the scope of most academic courses, this phase could provide a rare opportunity to introduce students to industry-relevant topics. The exposure can help them better appreciate common risks and the complex ecosystem into which their solutions must ultimately fit.

In fellowship programs, the Implement phase may span several months (and even beyond the fellowship), with participants working closely with legal, regulatory, and commercial consultants. They develop strategies to bring their solutions to market and assimilate these into a viable business plan that will often be taken forward to spin-off. Going through the activities in this phase of the process provides hands-on exposure to real-world innovation constraints and decision-making.

In contrast to fellowship programs, students in typical university courses often lack time and resources in credit-bearing academic courses to engage deeply in Implement activities. As a result, this phase may often be best taught conceptually through case studies, guest lectures, or simulation exercises. Students may be tasked to formulate and present strategies to address challenges in IP, regulatory, reimbursement, funding, and other commercially-oriented activities. These activities may increase awareness of practical considerations, albeit in a superficial (rather than applied) fashion.

A typical challenge faced in this phase is striking the right balance between realism and depth. Introducing students to too many implementation considerations at once can be overwhelming and/or detract from the technical learning focus of the course. On the other hand, omitting implementation entirely risks giving students a narrow view of what health technology development entails. Ultimately, the goal of teaching the Implement phase is not to turn students into subject matter experts, but to expose them to the multidimensional considerations that define successful innovation in healthcare. Even brief engagement with implementation content helps students develop strategic awareness, fosters respect for the complexity of medical translation, and prepares them to work more effectively with cross-functional teams in their future careers.

6.3 DIFFERENT MODELS FOR TEACHING BIODESIGN IN THE UNIVERSITY SETTINGS

6.3.1 Biodesign at Stanford

Stanford Biodesign has served as a foundational model for need-driven health technology education for roughly a quarter century. At Stanford University, Biodesign is offered as credit-bearing innovation courses at both the graduate and undergraduate levels, using one-quarter (ten weeks) and two-quarter (20 weeks) curricula. Other training offerings from Stanford Biodesign include:

Global Faculty-In-Training Program: an immersive five-month program designed to equip international educators with the tools and strategies to launch and or sustain institution- or university-based programs that teach need-driven health technology innovation using the Biodesign methodology.

Biodesign Faculty Fellowship: an eight-month, part-time program for Stanford-affiliated faculty members to gain hands-on training in the Biodesign process while developing health technology projects in parallel.

Executive Education Workshop: a short-format (three-day) workshop targeted at senior leaders in medtech, healthcare, and academia, focusing on how to implement and support blank-sheet, need-driven innovation inside large organizations.

One important lesson from developing different models for teaching need-driven innovation is to initiate curriculum planning by considering: (1) the skills, level, and motivation of the learner and (2) what the learner should be able to accomplish after completing the relevant program. In general, short programs (e.g., multi-day workshops and short-form courses) are effective at raising awareness and exciting learners to seek additional training. Longer programs (e.g., full-time, multi-month fellowships) have greater potential to lead to content mastery and sustained educational and career benefits. Other success factors include using a teaching approach that blends didactic instruction and hands-on PjBL, providing numerous real-world examples and case studies of how early-stage innovators have overcome common challenges and constraints at the intersection of medicine, engineering, and business, and engaging subject matter experts from the health technology industry in coaching and guiding student projects to keep their work practical and grounded in reality. In combination, these factors are instrumental in building knowledge and skills that extend beyond engineering and equip students to contribute meaningfully to diverse health-related career paths.

6.3.2 Biodesign in Singapore

In Singapore, Biodesign is being taught with a mix of university-led coursework, national fellowship programs, and hospital-based innovation efforts. As observed in the preceding sections, direct clinical immersion is limited outside fellowship or clinical settings. However, the core principles of the Biodesign methodology have been retained and adapted to fit local needs.

For example, at the undergraduate level, one such course in the NUS introduces key Biodesign concepts through structured classroom instruction. Students are provided with pre-scoped clinical needs from local clinicians and are guided to perform need characterization, stakeholder analysis, solution ideation, and early feasibility assessment (prototyping, IP, and regulatory affairs). Although the Identify phase is condensed and based on secondary research and expert interviews rather than first-hand immersion, it remains central to the project structure. Clinician partners remain actively involved as domain mentors, maintaining clinical relevance throughout.

Beyond the undergraduate setting, Singapore Biodesign, hosted at the Agency for Science, Technology, and Research, has built a national platform for health technology innovation training. Singapore Biodesign (an accredited Stanford Biodesign global affiliate) offers a range of programs, including Innovation Fellowships for aspiring innovators, Faculty Fellowships for educators and innovation leaders, design thinking workshops, and short-format bootcamps (Singapore Biodesign).

These initiatives combine PjBL, mentoring, and contextualized implementation frameworks tailored to the Asian medtech environment. They also build capability at different levels of the innovation pipeline, from curriculum integration to product development (Singapore Biodesign). While Singapore's programs differ in structure from Stanford's, they reflect the same pedagogical values and commitment to scalable innovation education.

6.4 OUTCOMES FROM USING THE BIODESIGN APPROACH

6.4.1 Stanford Experience

Studies conducted by Stanford Biodesign have demonstrated measurable educational and career benefits across a variety of course and program formats. Educational outcomes are less well studied than career outcomes. However, across programs, students have reported significant gains in areas such as analyzing clinical needs, developing clinically relevant solutions, and understanding the healthcare landscape (Augustin et al. 2019; Denend et al. 2023). Multiple studies also confirm that the structured approach of Biodesign improves students' confidence and capability in working on open-ended, multidisciplinary healthcare problems. In Stanford University's accelerated undergraduate Biodesign course, for example, students demonstrated statistically significant improvements in core skills related to need characterization (prior to solution development), and interest in health technology innovation (Denend et al. 2023). Importantly, students also reported a better understanding of the importance of rigorous research on clinical needs before jumping into solutioning. The studies suggest the Biodesign framework offers educators a robust scaffold to integrate systematic consideration of healthtech-specific factors with design methodology in a coherent way. Whether used fully or partially, the process-based and modular nature allows alignment with a range of learning objectives by focusing on different sections, ranging from creativity and problem-solving to awareness about market access considerations.

Beyond academic benefits, Biodesign programs have also shown lasting career impact. In a 2021 study of over 180 alumni from a two-quarter graduate-level course, 94% of respondents self-reported that the Biodesign course was useful in their careers, and 84% expressed sustained commitment to working in the health technology field (Denend et al. 2021). Among alumni of the full-time year-long Innovation Fellowship, a 2022 study indicated that 94% of respondents said that they found the fellowship beneficial to their career development and 91% reported that the fellowship was influential on their chosen career trajectory. In support of the hypothesis that Biodesign training excites learners about careers in health and health technology innovation and prepares them for success in pursuing those career pathways, a comparison of alumni to finalists interviewed but not selected for the Fellowship indicated that 98% of alumni remained in health-related positions versus 80% of finalists. Furthermore, 79% of alumni were in leadership roles compared to 57% of finalists (Denend et al. 2022).

In terms of the pathways trainees pursue, those completing Stanford Biodesign training have founded or joined start-ups, advanced health technology development in established companies, or led innovation efforts in clinical and policy settings. From an economic development perspective, as of 2024, 57 companies had been founded based on projects initiated during Biodesign training programs at Stanford University that, in combination, resulted in 2,146 full-time jobs and $1.2B in funding raised. Perhaps most importantly, more than 18 M people had been helped by technologies brought into patient care by these start-ups (Stanford Biodesign 2024).

6.4.2 Singapore Experience

Singapore's experience with Biodesign reflects similar positive outcomes, even with adaptations tailored to local constraints. Between 2011 and 2025, the national-level talent development platform had supported 76 Innovation and Faculty Fellows and trained more than 2,600 learners spanning academia, clinics, and industry. Singapore Biodesign's Innovation Fellowship alumni have founded 15 companies, launched 22 products into the market, raised over S40 million in funding, and created solutions that have impacted 1.78 million lives. In addition to these achievements, Singapore Biodesign-enabled initiatives extended to the broader ecosystem have enabled over 750 projects, unlocked more than S129 million in funding, and generated over 60 start-ups.

While longitudinal career tracking data is still emerging, anecdotal evidence and internal reporting suggest that Biodesign-trained individuals in Singapore are now contributing to strategic innovation roles across hospitals, research institutes, and start-ups. Moreover, by tailoring its offerings to Singapore's medtech landscape, Singapore Biodesign has positioned Biodesign as a foundational pillar in the country's innovation training ecosystem, with all health tech innovators "speaking" a common Biodesign "language."

A notable example of early-stage translational outcome is documented by Dharmawan et al. (2020), who describe an SGH-based Biodesign initiative in head and neck surgery. Their team conducted structured immersion, identified over 100 unmet needs, and ultimately developed KLARO® (https://www.vivo-surgical.com/klaro), a surgical lighting system that reached commercialization. The study highlights not only the success of the process but also regional challenges such as risk aversion and slower adoption timelines.

6.5 CONCLUSION

The Biodesign process provides a robust framework for teaching innovation in health technologies. Its structured, needs-driven approach not only aligns with core biomedical engineering design principles but also provides a framework for learners to appreciate the complexities in navigating real-world considerations in the health and biomedical sector.

Training in Biodesign has led to meaningful educational outcomes, enhanced career trajectories, and real-world impact. Importantly, the success of Biodesign education does not depend on a singular format. Rather, the emphasis is on the need-driven approach toward innovation and a systematic approach to consider health technology-specific factors when analyzing the need and chosen concepts. As interest in health-related innovation education in BME continues to grow, the Biodesign framework stands as a proven, flexible model for cultivating the next generation of impactful health technology innovators.

ACKNOWLEDGMENTS

The authors would like to acknowledge Dr. Lee Phin Peng and Dr. Tan Ee Lim of Singapore Biodesign for contributing toward the "Outcomes" section of this chapter.

REFERENCES

Altman, Micah, Tiffany T. K. Huang, and Jessica Y. Breland. 2018. "Design Thinking in Health Care." *Preventing Chronic Disease* 15: E117. https://doi.org/10.5888/pcd15.180128.

Augustin, Dimitri A., Lyn Denend, James Wall, Thomas Krummel, and Dan E. Azagury. 2019. "The Biodesign Model: Training Physician Innovators and Entrepreneurs." In *Success in Academic Surgery: Innovation and Entrepreneurship*, edited by Mark S. Cohen and Lillian Kao, 71–88. Cham: Springer International Publishing.

Chua, J. Y. X., E. M. Kan, P. P. Lee, and S. Shorey. 2024. "Application of the Stanford Biodesign Framework in Healthcare Innovation Training and Commercialization of Market-Appropriate Products: A Scoping Review." *Journal of Medical Systems* 48 (1): 44. https://doi.org/10.1007/s10916-024-02067-x.

Denend, Lyn, Susie Spielman, Ross Venook, Ravinder D. Pamnani, David Camarillo, James Wall, and Joseph Towles. 2023. "Using an Accelerated Undergraduate Needs Finding Course to Build Skills, Inspire Confidence, and Promote Interest in Health Technology Innovation." *Biomedical Engineering Education* 3 (2): 319–29. https://doi.org/10.1007/s43683-023-00109-3.

Denend, Lyn, Ross Venook, Ravinder D. Pamnani, Kunj Sheth, and Joseph Towles. 2024. "Lessons from Developing a Rubric for Evaluating Need Statements on Health Technology Innovation Projects." *Biomedical Engineering Education* 4 (2): 437–42. https://doi.org/10.1007/s43683-024-00153-7.

Denend, Lyn, Shiqin Xu, Paul Yock, and Ross Venook. 2021. "Biomedical Technology Innovation Education and Its Effect on Graduate Student Careers Over 17 Years." *Biomedical Engineering Education* 1 (2): 291–300. https://doi.org/10.1007/s43683-021-00050-3.

Denend, Lyn, Paul G. Yock, Josh Makower, Dan E. Azagury, and James K. Wall. 2022. "Are We Making a Difference? A Case Study of Assessment in Innovation Training." *The Bridge* 51 (4): 43–51.

Department of Biomedical Engineering, National University of Singapore. n.d. *Self-Reported Data from Alumni Surveys.*

Dharmawan, R., H. Ho, H. H. M. Ng, N. G. Iyer, H. K. Tan, and N. C. Tan. 2020. "Implementing the Biodesign Process for Medical Device Innovation in Head and Neck Surgery." *Surgical Innovation* 27 (6): 653–8. https://doi.org/10.1177/1553350620943796.

Fuerch, Jennifer H., Ping Wang, Robert Van Wert, and Lyn Denend. 2021. "Turning Practicing Surgeons into Health Technology Innovators: Outcomes from the Stanford Biodesign Faculty Fellowship." *Surgical Innovation* 28 (1): 134–43. https://doi.org/10.1177/1553350620984338.

Glen, Roy, Christy Suciu, C. Christopher Baughn, and Robert Anson. 2015. "Teaching Design Thinking in Business Schools." *The International Journal of Management Education* 13 (2): 182–92. https://doi.org/10.1016/j.ijme.2015.05.001.

Kadlowec, Jennifer, Tom Merrill, Sameer Sood, Jane Ryan, Anilchandra Attaluri, and Robert Hirsh. 2017. *Clinical Immersion and Team-Based Design: Into a Third Year.* Presented at 2017 ASEE Annual Conference & Exposition, Columbus, OH, June 24–28, 2017. https://peer.asee.org/28040

King, Christine E., and Dalton Salvo. 2024. "Phenomenological Evaluation of Undergraduate Clinical Needs Finding Skills through a Virtual Reality Clinical Immersion Platform." *Biomedical Engineering Education* 4 (2): 381–97. https://doi.org/10.1007/s43683-024-00139-5.

Lindberg, Tilmann, Christoph Meinel, and Ralf Wagner. 2011. "Design Thinking: A Fruitful Concept for IT Development?" In *Design Thinking: Understand—Improve—Apply*, edited by Christoph Meinel, Larry Leifer, and Hasso Plattner, 3–18. Berlin: Springer.

Linsenmeier, Robert A., and Ann Saterbak. 2020. "Fifty Years of Biomedical Engineering Undergraduate Education." *Annals of Biomedical Engineering* 48 (6): 1590–615. https://doi.org/10.1007/s10439-020-02494-0.

Luchs, Michael G., Scott Swan, and Abbie Griffin. 2015. *Design Thinking: New Product Development Essentials from the PDMA*. Hoboken, NJ: John Wiley & Sons.

Luka, Ineta. 2014. "Design Thinking in Pedagogy." *The Journal of Education, Culture, and Society* 5 (2): 63–74.

Maloney, Lauren M., Christopher Page, Michael Bielski, Annie Rohan, and Wei Yin. 2025. "A Longitudinal and Interdisciplinary Biodesign Internship Program for Biomedical Engineering Undergraduate Students Focused on Medical Device Innovation." *Biomedical Engineering Education.* https://doi.org/10.1007/s43683-025-00174-w.

Noweski, Christine, Andrea Scheer, Nadja Büttner, Julia von Thienen, Johannes Erdmann, and Christoph Meinel. 2012. "Towards a Paradigm Shift in Education Practice: Developing Twenty-First Century Skills with Design Thinking." In *Design Thinking Research: Measuring Performance in Context*, 71–94, Springer, Berlin, Heidelberg. https://doi.org/10.1007/978-3-642-31991-4_5

Razzouk, Rim, and Valerie Shute. 2012. "What Is Design Thinking and Why Is It Important?" *Review of Educational Research* 82 (3): 330–48.

Singapore Biodesign. n.d.a *Singapore Biodesign.* https://www.a-star.edu.sg/sb/training.

Singapore Biodesign. n.d.b *The Health and Medtech Innovation Skills and Competencies Framework.* https://www.a-star.edu.sg/sb/resources

Stanford Biodesign. 2024. *Self-Reported Data.* https://biodesign.stanford.edu/our-impact/trainee-outcomes.html.

Wall, James, Eva Hellman, Lyn Denend, Douglas Rait, Ross Venook, Linda Lucian, Dan Azagury, Paul G. Yock, and Todd J. Brinton. 2017. "The Impact of Postgraduate Health Technology Innovation Training: Outcomes of the Stanford Biodesign Fellowship." *Annals of Biomedical Engineering* 45: 1163–71.

Xu, Chenchen, Zhihao Zhang, Lizhu Wang, Xin Ji, Yue, Xurui Liang, Yufei Han, Jiqin Hou, and Tao Zhang. 2025. "Exploring the New Model of Medical Innovation and Entrepreneurship Talent Training Based on Biodesign in Eastern China." *BMC Medical Education* 25 (1): 388. https://doi.org/10.1186/s12909-025-06870-z.

Yock, Paul G., Stefanos Zenios, Josh Makower, Todd J. Brinton, Uday N. Kumar, F. T. Jay Watkins, Lyn Denend, Thomas M. Krummel, and Christine Q. Kurihara. 2015. *Biodesign: The Process of Innovating Medical Technologies.* 2nd ed. Cambridge: Cambridge University Press.

7 Approaches to Teaching and Assessing Capstone Design Courses

Jennifer R. Amos, Joe A. Bradley, and Holly McIlwee Golecki

7.1 DESIGN CURRICULUM

7.1.1 Topics Fundamental to Design in Engineering

Design experiences are a crucial part of engineering education at both the post-secondary and professional levels and serve as an experiential and concrete way to develop design thinking skills. According to Dym et al., design thinking in the context of engineering education primarily refers to the ability to iterate through the divergent-convergent questioning loop to make design decisions (Dym et al. 2005). Engineering design has been described as "the systematic, intelligent generation and evaluation of specifications for artifacts whose form and function achieve stated objectives and satisfy specified constraints" (Dym 1994).

Design strategies such as understanding the challenge, building knowledge, generating ideas, representing ideas, making decisions, conducting experiments, troubleshooting, iterating, and reflecting on the process distinguish novices from their advanced counterparts in design broadly (Crismond and Adams 2012). Figure 7.1 shows the competencies from the Informed Design Matrix from Crismond and Adams (2012), a synthesis of over 100 empirical studies of designers, as a conceptual framework for understanding the values emphasized in assessments from a variety of design instructors.

7.1.2 Topics Fundamental to Bioengineering Design

More recently, there has been a shift in design education to one of user-centric design. The Biodesign framework (developed from the Stanford Biodesign Fellowship) is focused on design in the context of health technologies (Augustin et al. 2019). The fellowship program initially sought to train interdisciplinary teams of faculty, clinicians, and industry professionals in an iterative innovation process grounded in design thinking methodologies. Now, the curriculum has been adapted for students, providing a framework for progression through design courses. The Biodesign framework puts patients' needs in the clinical setting at the forefront of the design process (Augustin et al. 2021), particularly relevant for biomedical engineering students.

DOI: 10.1201/9781003520313-7

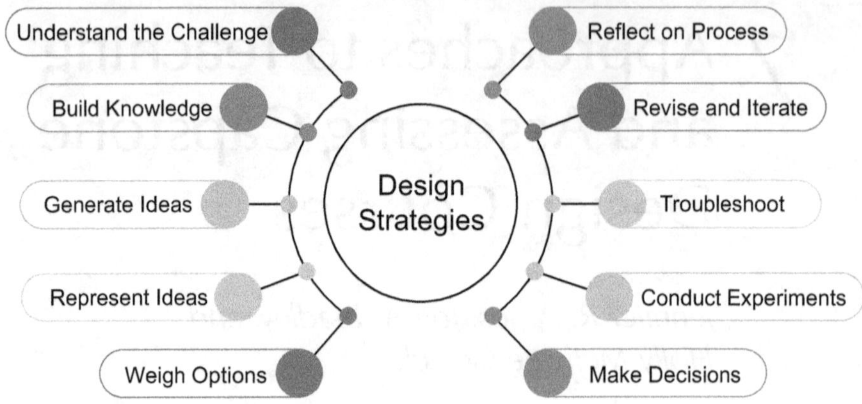

FIGURE 7.1 Graphical representation of Crismond and Adams framework showing the nine design behaviors.

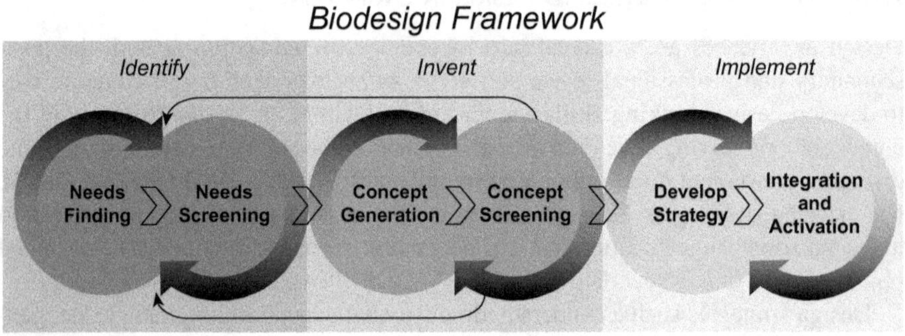

FIGURE 7.2 Biodesign process overview.

After needs finding, teams proceed through three phases of design: identify, invent, and implement, as depicted in Figure 7.2.

The Biodesign process also aligns with the waterfall process shown in Figure 7.3. This quality process is used for product design controls in alignment with the United States Code of Federal Regulations section by the Food and Drug Administration (May-Newman and Cornwall 2012).

New design methodologies, including the more broadly applied human-centered design, also emphasize end-user needs and are especially relevant for biomedical engineers. The Human Centered Design (HCD) Thinking framework, shown in Figure 7.4, emphasizes understanding the user's needs and point of view throughout the commercialization process. Fundamentally, this framework represents a problem-solving approach to creating innovative solutions by empathizing with end users, defining the core problem, ideating concepts, prototyping, testing, and integrating feedback into the final design. The HCD thinking framework focuses on five primary activities: Understand, Synthesize, Ideate, Prototype, and Implement.

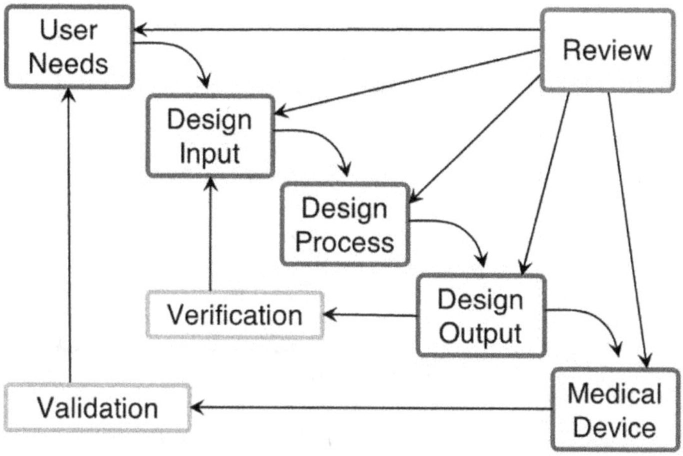

FIGURE 7.3 Waterfall diagram showing design control steps in the quality process

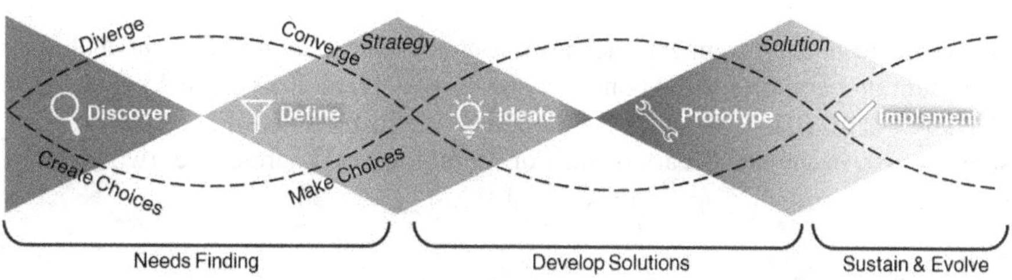

FIGURE 7.4 HCD framework

7.1.3 Where Is Design Taught in the Curriculum?

Design education in biomedical engineering and across engineering disciplines varies widely (Nassersharif and Rousseau 2010). Project features that vary across programs include credit hours and time spent on the project, project sourcing and funding, and design instruction (Nassersharif and Rousseau 2010). In a survey of top universities globally (Ward 2013), there are common features across successful capstone courses. These include (1) scaffolded PBL experiences early in undergraduate curricula as preparation for PjBL in capstone, (2) emphasis on team projects to mimic workplace structure, (3) iterative design cycles (design, build, and test), and (4) industry involvement. With these features in mind, capstone design is operationalized in different ways.

There has been a steady increase in reports of design education in biomedical engineering, as seen in Figure 7.5 (Publication Count n.d.). The steady increase in publications related to design after the year 2000 is likely due to the ABET changes to criteria, known as EC 2000, which focused on outcomes-based learning and a new definition of design (Gassert et al. 2006). Best practices in engineering education

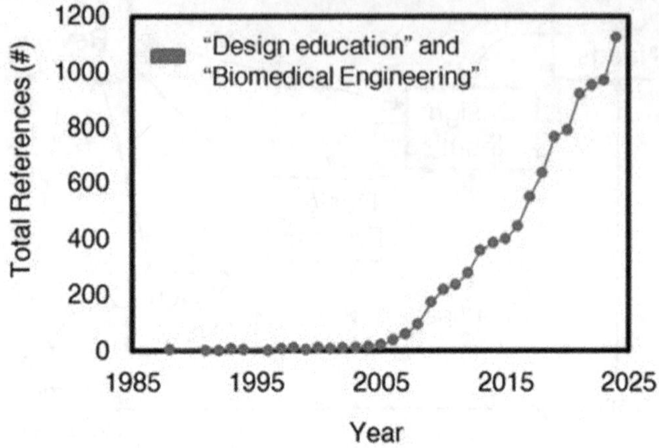

FIGURE 7.5 Publications including "design education" and "biomedical engineering" since 1985.

now cite scaffolded design experiences throughout the undergraduate curriculum as important preparation for capstone design courses (Ward 2013; Golecki et al. 2024; Cvetkovic et al. 2024). However, most engineering institutions still do offer one capstone course in the later years of the curriculum, offered across one, two, or three semesters.

7.1.4 Course Structure: Lecture, Studio, Lab, and so on

Documentation from a meeting of BME educators summarized findings from a survey of BME departments (Cvetkovic et al. 2024). They found that "manufacturing (17%)" and "verification and validation (14%)" were the areas that departments feel need the most attention in BME design education (Cvetkovic et al. 2024). This finding highlights the importance of scaffolded design and prototyping experience early in the curriculum for BME students (White et al. 2020; Bethke, Ansari, Amos et al. 2024). One study showed that continuous exposure to hands-on design curricula results in significant gains in Design Self-Efficacy (Carberry et al. 2010) for BME students, further emphasizing the importance of this continued exposure in courses but also in extracurricular experiences (Higbee and Miller 2020). Additionally, engineering identity is reinforced through senior design courses, but multiple, authentic design projects through an undergraduate curriculum have shown further support for the development of strong engineering identities (Ju and Zhu 2023).

7.1.5 Common Deliverables in Design Courses

Common deliverables in capstone design courses include written reports, presentations, multimedia recordings, and prototypes. A study on industry perspectives on professional and design skills of BME students in capstone revealed that presentation skills were the highest-ranked skills that students demonstrated in their design projects (Khojah et al. 2024). The interdisciplinary nature of the field necessitates that students understand and describe engineering technologies across content areas in a clear and effective manner. Design output is often captured across multiple modes of presentation. While there is an abundance of content from which to assess students, the team-based and open-ended nature of the BME capstone presents challenges for instructor assessment of design output.

7.2 ASSESSMENT OF DESIGN

7.2.1 Team Versus Individual Assessment

Since capstone projects are typically framed as a team project, the assessment of student performance can be approached through both team-based and individual-based methods.

Team assessments focus on evaluating the collective output and dynamics of the group, emphasizing collaboration, communication, and the integration of diverse skills (Bethke, Ansari, Bradley et al. 2024). This approach encourages students to develop essential teamwork competencies, which are critical in real-world biomedical engineering projects. Additionally, a well-scoped project will challenge team members to persist through challenges and coordinate their efforts. Therefore, design faculty should strive to provide an authentic training experience that emulates industry teams, where each member contributes diverse and complementary expertise to a complex, real-life problem (Golecki et al. 2023).

Conversely, individual assessments aim to evaluate each student's personal contribution and understanding of the project (Borrego et al. 2013). In a recent review of recent capstone-focused papers from a 5.5-year period from 2007 to 2013, "social loafing" was cited as the single most cited negative outcome from team projects (Karau and Williams 1995). In the paper, social loafing is defined as "the tendency of individuals to exert less effort when working collectively than when working individually" (Karau and Williams 1995). There are several strategies suggested in the literature to reduce social loafing, but many of them rely on requiring an individual evaluation. Studies have shown that by implementing strategies that capture individual contributions, social loafing is reduced or even eliminated. Methods such as Individual Peer Assessment of Contribution have been developed to address issues like social loafing and ensure fairer marks by providing individual feedback and grades based on peer evaluations (Grammenos et al. 2019). This dual approach ensures that while teamwork is fostered, individual accountability and learning are also maintained.

7.2.2 Journey Versus the Destination

In the context of capstone design courses, assessing the journey versus the destination involves evaluating both the process and the final product. Journey assessment focuses on the steps taken by students throughout the project, including their problem-solving strategies, iterative design processes, and adaptability to challenges.

This approach highlights the importance of learning and growth during the project. Courses that foster this approach opt to teach a structured design process and grade students on how well they follow the process (Denayer et al. 2003). Courses may also use specifications or standards-based grading where students are provided with multiple opportunities for feedback and revision in order to meet a learning outcome (Atwood et al. 2014; Fernandez et al. 2020).

On the other hand, destination assessment evaluates the final outcome of the project, such as the functionality, innovation, and impact of the designed solution (Voß et al. 2016). While the final product is crucial, emphasizing the journey allows educators to recognize and reward the efforts and learning experiences that students undergo, which are equally valuable in their professional development (Proc. 4th World Conf. Des. n.d.).

7.2.3 Cognitive Assessments Versus Affective Assessments

Given that capstone design courses are often one of the last courses that students take in a curriculum, assessments of SO attainment are often performed in these courses. While much of the curriculum can support the assessment of technical skills like a student's "ability to identify, formulate, and solve complex engineering problems by applying principles of engineering, science, and mathematics," few courses offer an opportunity to assess a student's "ability to apply engineering design to produce solutions that meet specified needs with consideration of public health, safety, and welfare, as well as global, cultural, social, environmental, and economic factors" or "ability to function effectively on a team whose members together provide leadership, create a collaborative environment, establish goals, plan tasks, and meet objectives" (Criteria for Accrediting Engineering Programs, 2025–2026 n.d.).

Cognitive assessments focus on evaluating students' intellectual abilities and knowledge acquisition. Bloom's Taxonomy is often employed to design assessments that range from basic recall of information to higher-order thinking skills such as analysis and creation (Krathwohl 2002). Affective assessments, on the other hand, measure students' attitudes, values, and emotional responses toward their learning experiences. This domain includes aspects such as motivation, teamwork, and ethical considerations, which are essential for holistic development in biomedical engineering. Bloom's Taxonomy provides a similar framework for the affective domain. Additionally, tools like Krathwohl's Affective Domain taxonomy can be used to structure these assessments. Integrating both affective and cognitive assessments provides a comprehensive evaluation of students' capabilities, ensuring that they are well-prepared for the multifaceted challenges of biomedical engineering.

Capstone courses are an ideal place to measure the affective domain due to the open-ended, client-driven projects. Unlike many other courses in the biomedical engineering curriculum, capstone courses are loosely scaffolded, and students work on longer projects than in previous courses. Due to this, students need to rely more on team communication and motivation to meet the client's expectations. Additionally, since the products may be commercialized after the completion of the course, the product development needs to meet industry standards for ethical considerations as well as social and environmental impacts (Biomedical Ethics for Engineers 2007).

Affective assessment can take place across a variety of contexts, including team contracts, team self- and peer-evaluation, and writing assignments, individual or team. In team contracts, the team is setting the stage for how the team will operate and interact (Howe 2010). A team contract offers an opportunity for students to reflect on past team experiences and discuss team attributes and individual strengths and weaknesses (Howe 2010). Additionally, having the team revisit the team contract frequently can help to reset expectations within the team.

Team self- and peer-evaluations allow students to identify strengths and weaknesses across a set of behavioral attributes of teamwork as discussed in Section 7.2.1. Requiring short written progress updates can force students into metacognitive steps to set goals and assess performance on meeting their goals. Additionally, many studies of capstone teams suggest including a section on team member contributions and progress in written progress updates (Davis et al. 2023). These sections allow students to evaluate their own and the overall team's contributions and discuss how they can regulate future actions to work together as a cohesive team.

7.3 OUTCOMES OF DESIGN

7.3.1 BME Design Competitions

Due to the nature of the capstone experience being tied to a course, many projects that could have commercial potential sit on shelves or are tossed away after the course ends. Students in capstone courses are often graduating and leaving to careers or pursuing further education, so there is little incentive to continue working on the project. Student design competitions attempt to bridge this gap by providing substantial support to student teams to continue their development and provide mentoring and training opportunities to help them determine if their products are commercially viable.

VentureWell was launched in 1995 to test an audacious proposition: if creative students are given the opportunity to pursue invention and taught how to turn their ideas into scalable businesses, we can solve the world's most pressing problems (*Transforming the World through Innovation* n.d.). For nearly 30 years, VentureWell has worked to support, train, and foster networks to ensure that the next generation of science and technology innovators realize—and maximize—their potential in bringing their ideas to impact.

The National Institute of Biomedical Imaging and Bioengineering (NIBIB) and VentureWell have come together to support and expand the Design by Biomedical Undergraduate Teams (DEBUT) Challenge, a competition that recognizes undergraduate excellence in biomedical design and innovation (National Institute of Biomedical Imaging and Bioengineering (NIBIB) and VentureWell Have Come Together to Support and Expand the Design by Biomedical Undergraduate Teams (DEBUT) Challenge n.d.). DEBUT is a competition open to undergraduate student teams working on innovative solutions to unmet health and clinical problems. Each team can win up to $20,000 in prize funds to continue development and pursue commercialization of their product under the guidance of experts.

In addition to the DEBUT award, VentureWell has a program that focuses on the development of products with a global impact. VentureWell is supporting delivery of the US Department of State's Global Innovation through Science and Technology initiative, which empowers young innovators through networking, skills building, mentoring, and access to financing to develop start-up solutions that address economic and development challenges (Global Innovation Through Science and Technology Initiative n.d.).

These design competitions and awards provide opportunities for students to continue developing their capstone projects after the course has ended. The awards are due in June each year, allowing opportunities for semester-long and year-long projects to submit their work for the awards.

Additionally, research has shown that participation in technological innovation and entrepreneurship competitions correlates positively with students' development of engineering identity, competence, and performance in design activities (Ju and Zhu 2023).

7.3.2 Commercialization of BME Products

Commercialization creates the vital linkage between a need and the solution. The transition from a need statement to ideas to concepts to products is oftentimes a winding path to success or maybe an opportunity to learn from failures. The commercialization of biomedical products—medical devices, biologics, and pharmaceuticals—typically includes design and development, regulatory compliance, marketing, sales, manufacturing, launch, and post-market surveillance (Scanlon and Lieberman 2007). The design and development steps help ensure that the product meets its design specification and meets end-user needs. Regulatory compliance may require navigating the complexities of the regulatory agencies to receive product approvals. The launch phase introduces the new product to the market. Marketing and sales are critical in increasing the awareness of the products and generating revenue and profit. Manufacturing and production represent the process of turning the "raw material" inputs into final products. Post-market surveillance monitors the performance of a product after it has been released to ensure that the product continues to meet required standards.

Decision-making during the commercialization process is critical. There are several tools that have been developed and implemented to support the commercialization activities: stage-gate, business model canvas (BMC), quality functional deployment (QFD), business readiness level (BRL), and technology readiness level (TRL). Table 7.1 outlines the steps or phases of each tool for ease of comparison.

The stage-gate process consists of five sequential phases/gates that span identification of the opportunity to product launch and post-launch (Pietzsch et al. 2009). In order to advance to the next stage, there are milestones that must be obtained during the commercialization steps, as shown in Figure 7.6.

The BMC is a visual tool that illustrates the business model of an organization (Wiley.Com n.d.). As depicted in Figure 7.7, the model is defined by nine building blocks. Each of these nine blocks can be segmented into four sub-categories—Value Focus, Customer Focus, Operations Focus, and Financial Focus (Fritscher and Pigneur 2014). In addition to the BMC methodology, another supportive approach is

TABLE 7.1
Stages or levels for commercialization of BME products

Stage-Gate	BMC	QFD	BRL	TRL
1. Initiation (opportunity and risk analysis)	1. Customer Segments (customer needs)	1. Customer requirements (voice of the customer)	1. Basic idea of a venture or innovation	1. Basic principles of the concept are observed and reported
2. Formulation (concept and feasibility)	2. Customer Relationships (acquire and retain customers)	2. Technical requirements (how)	2. Problem-solution fit, identifying a problem and proposing a solution	2. Technology concept and/or application formulated
3. Design and development (verification and validation)	3. Channels (communication strategies)	3. Relationship matrix (strength of the relationship between the customer and technical requirements)	3. Building a team and developing a basic plan	3. Analytical and experimental critical function and/or proof-of-concept
4. Final validation (product launch preparation)	4. Value Propositions (connecting product to customer)	4. Correlation matrix (interaction amongst technical requirements)	4. Defining the target customer segment	4. Component and/or validation in a laboratory environment
5. Product launch and post-launch assessment	5. Key Partners (strategic market partners)	5. Importance ratings (rating of the importance of the customer requirements)	5. Testing hypotheses about the business model	5. Component and/or validation in a simulated environment
	6. Key Activities (organizational tasks)	6. Target values (determine the technical specifications based on importance and relationships identified)	6. Launching an MVP and gathering feedback	6. System/subsystem model or prototype demonstration in a simulated environment
	7. Key Resources (critical resources—human, financial, intellectual)		7. Refining the product or service based on feedback	7. Prototype ready for demonstration in an appropriate operational environment
	8. Cost Structure (operating costs)		8. Scaling the business beyond the MVP	8. Actual technology completed and qualified through tests and demonstrations
	9. Revenue Stream (price points and revenue generation)		9. Achieving a fully embedded and sustainable business model	9. Actual technology proven through successful deployment in an operational setting

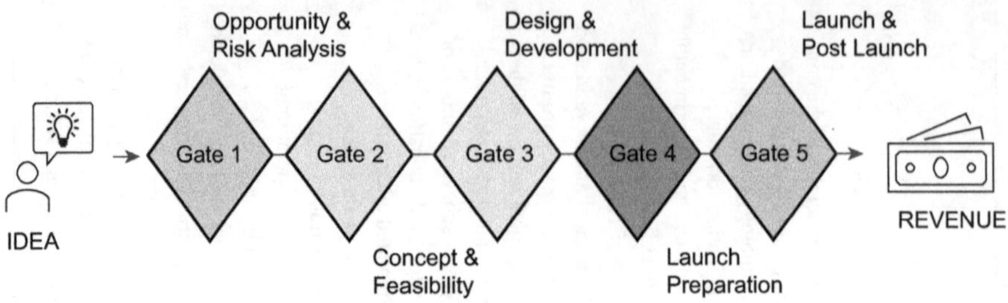

FIGURE 7.6 Stage-gate diagram

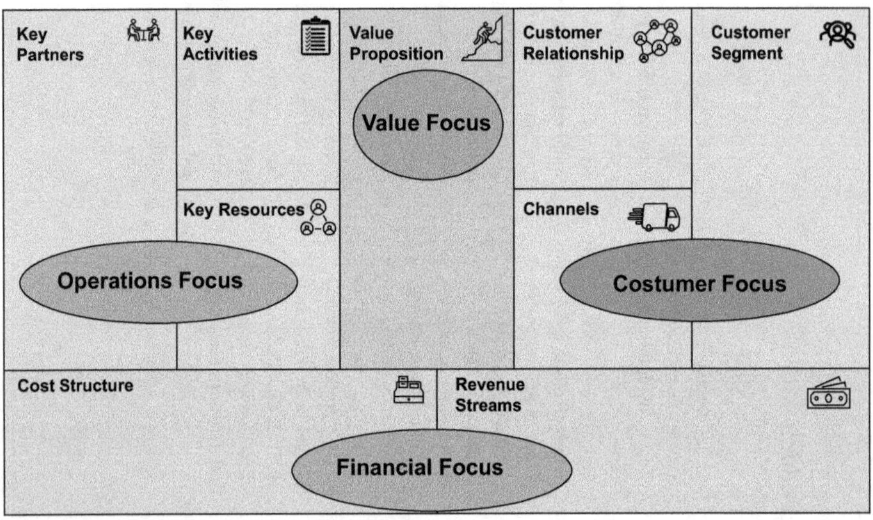

FIGURE 7.7 Business model canvas

the quality function deployment (QFD) methodology. This method, along with its House of Quality tool, depicted in Figure 7.8, is discussed in the following section.

The QFD methodology was invented in the Japanese automobile industry. This methodology is effective at ensuring that customer needs are focused on by all the cross-functional teams involved in the commercialization process. A key tool within this methodology is the House of Quality (Rosenau 1993). The House of Quality identifies six components to support commercialization decision-making (Practical Manual of Quality Function Deployment | SpringerLink n.d.).

Two other tools that are helpful in the commercialization decision process are the TRL scale and the BRL scale. The TRL scale was developed at the NASA in the 1970s to be a consistent measure to quantify technology maturity. The readiness level has a range from 1 to 9 (Hirshorn 2016). The TRL starts at level 1, which represents a technology in a basic theoretical form. After a series of design and

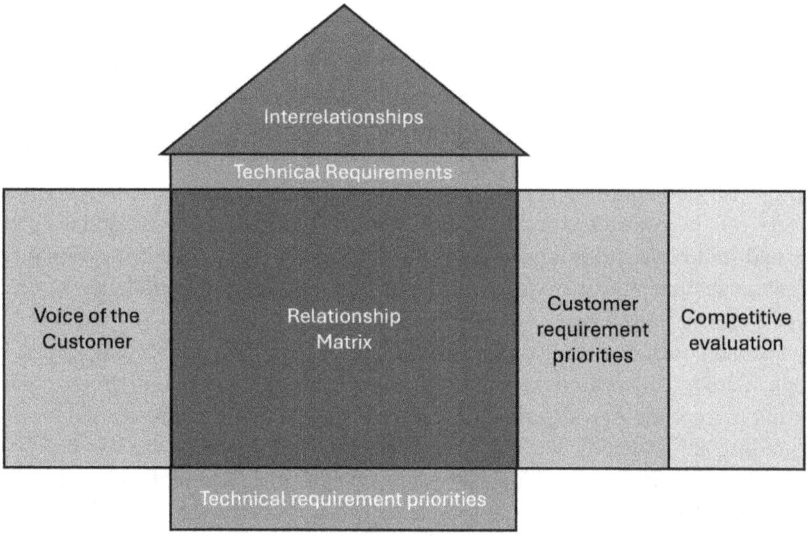

FIGURE 7.8 House of quality diagram showing the relationship between the "what" and the "how" of the design project.

development activities, a progression to level 9 represents a technology that has been proven in the operating environment. The TRL nine-level scale provides an assessment of the maturation of the technology toward successful operations and commercialization (Olechowski et al. 2020)—the BRL scale. Similar to the TRL, BRL focuses primarily on the evolution of the business side of the solution during the commercialization process. The readiness level also has a range from 1 to 9. A BRL at level 1 is an initial concept. This may be an idea in its very early stages that is not fully formed. By BRL, level 9 represents a product that may be fully embedded into the market (Francese and King 2024).

The commercialization of a biomedical product is a complex landscape. Identifying the most important healthcare need or challenge to address is only the first step. It is critical to identify experts to help develop a (1) regulatory strategy, (2) clinical strategy, (3) manufacturing strategy, and (4) project plan. These experts can help you save time and identify the appropriate next steps and resources. Additionally, it is important to establish early communication with the required regulatory agencies. Early communication can (I-Corps Medical Jumpstart n.d.):

1. Facilitate the product development pathways;
2. Provide critical feedback on development plans;
3. Provide insight and assistance with determining product designations (i.e., device, drug, or combination product);
4. Create a regulatory proposal based on regulatory strategy, manufacturing strategy, and clinical strategy;
5. Support review of a reimbursement path.

7.4 CONCLUSION

Capstone courses provide students with a culminating experience to integrate knowledge gained throughout the curriculum. Capstone experiences bridge the gap between theoretical learning and real-world scenarios, allowing students to tackle complex problems, develop solutions, and gain valuable hands-on experience. Due to the project-based nature of capstone courses, they provide an opportunity to include industry-related concepts not often covered in core courses, such as regulatory pathways and standards. Additionally, by simulating the demands of a professional environment, capstone courses equip students with the skills and confidence needed to navigate careers in industry.

Capstone courses present unique challenges to instructors. Instructors must lead groups of students working on different projects through a common process and on a common timeline. Additionally, flexible assessment strategies are needed to ensure fair grading across teams working on different projects.

There is no perfect model for instructing design. Instructors of capstone courses should carefully consider the strategies described in this chapter for teaching, assessing, and promoting projects beyond the classroom when designing the capstone experience.

REFERENCES

ABET. n.d. "Criteria for Accrediting Engineering Programs, 2025–2026." Accessed August 21, 2025. https://www.abet.org/accreditation/accreditation-criteria/criteria-for-accrediting-engineering-programs-2025-2026/.

Atwood, Sara A., Matthew T. Siniawski, and Adam R. Carberry. 2014. *Using Standards-Based Grading to Effectively Assess Project-Based Design Courses: 121st ASEE Annual Conference and Exposition: 360 Degrees of Engineering Education*. January 1. http://www.scopus.com/inward/record.url?scp=84905168425&partnerID=8YFLogxK.

Augustin, Dimitri A, Glenn M Chertow, and Dan E Azagury. 2021. "Innovation in Hemodialysis: Using the Biodesign Process to Identify Unmet Needs." *The Journal of Vascular Access* 22 (4): 509–14. https://doi.org/10.1177/1129729820913692.

Augustin, Dimitri A., Lyn Denend, James Wall, Thomas Krummel, and Dan E. Azagury. 2019. "The Biodesign Model: Training Physician Innovators and Entrepreneurs." In *Success in Academic Surgery: Innovation and Entrepreneurship*. Cham: Springer. https://doi.org/10.1007/978-3-030-18613-5_7.

Bethke, Eliot, Ali Ansari, Jennifer Amos, Joe Bradley, Ruth Ochia, and Holly Golecki. 2024. "Bridging Extracurricular Skill Needs in Bioengineering Capstone Design with Just-in-Time Workshops." In *2024 ASEE Annual Conference & Exposition Proceedings* (Portland, Oregon), 48410. https://doi.org/10.18260/1-2-48410.

Bethke, Eliot, Ali Ansari, Joe Bradley, Jennifer Amos, and Holly Golecki. 2024. "An Adaptive Scaffolding Approach Based on Team Dynamics in an Integrated Masters and Undergraduate Bioengineering Capstone Design Course." In *2024 ASEE Annual Conference & Exposition Proceedings* (Portland, Oregon), 46542. https://doi.org/10.18260/1-2-46542.

Biomedical Ethics for Engineers. 2007. https://shop.elsevier.com/books/biomedical-ethics-for-engineers/vallero/978-0-7506-8227-5.

Borrego, Maura, Jennifer Karlin, Lisa D. McNair, and Kacey Beddoes. 2013. "Team Effectiveness Theory from Industrial and Organizational Psychology Applied to Engineering Student Project Teams: A Research Review." *Journal of Engineering Education* 102 (4): 472–512. https://doi.org/10.1002/jee.20023.

Carberry, Adam R., Hee-Sun Lee, and Matthew W. Ohland. 2010. "Measuring Engineering Design Self-Efficacy." *Journal of Engineering Education* 99 (1): 71–9. https://doi.org/10.1002/j.2168-9830.2010.tb01043.x.

Crismond, David P., and Robin S. Adams. 2012. "The Informed Design Teaching and Learning Matrix." *Journal of Engineering Education* 101 (4): 738–97. https://doi.org/10.1002/j.2168-9830.2012.tb01127.x.

Cvetkovic, Caroline, Sarah Lindley, Holly Golecki, and Robert Krencik. 2024. "Biofabrication of Neural Organoids: An Experiential Learning Approach for Instructional Laboratories." *Biomedical Engineering Education* 4 (2): 409–19. https://doi.org/10.1007/s43683-024-00145-7.

Davis, Denny, Michael Trevisan, Paul Leiffer, et al. 2023. "Reflection and Metacognition in Engineering Practice." In *Using Reflection and Metacognition to Improve Student Learning*. 1st ed., edited by Danielle LaVaque-Manty, Deborah Meizlish, Naomi Silver, Matthew Kaplan and James Rhem. Routledge. https://doi.org/10.4324/9781003448570-4.

Denayer, I., K. Thaels, J. Vander Sloten, and R. Gobin. 2003. "Teaching a Structured Approach to the Design Process for Undergraduate Engineering Students by Problem-Based Education." *European Journal of Engineering Education* 28 (2): 203–14. https://doi.org/10.1080/0304379031000079031.

Dym, Clive L. 1994. *Engineering Design: A Synthesis of Views*. Cambridge University Press.

Dym, Clive L., Alice M. Agogino, Ozgur Eris, Daniel D. Frey, and Larry J. Leifer. 2005. "Engineering Design Thinking, Teaching, and Learning." *Journal of Engineering Education* 94 (1): 103–20. https://doi.org/10.1002/j.2168-9830.2005.tb00832.x.

Fernandez, Todd, Kaela Martin, Richard Mangum, and Cristi Bell-Huff. 2020. "Whose Grade Is It Anyway?: Transitioning Engineering Courses to an Evidence-Based Specifications Grading System." In *2020 ASEE Virtual Annual Conference Content Access Proceedings*, June, 35512. https://doi.org/10.18260/1-2-35512.

Francese, Simona, and Roberto S. P. King, eds. 2024. *Driving Forensic Innovation in the 21st Century: Crossing the Valley of Death*. Springer International Publishing. https://doi.org/10.1007/978-3-031-56556-4.

Fritscher, Boris, and Yves Pigneur. 2014. "Visualizing Business Model Evolution with the Business Model Canvas: Concept and Tool." In *2014 IEEE 16th Conference on Business Informatics*, July, 151–8. https://doi.org/10.1109/CBI.2014.9.

Gassert, John D., John Denis Enderle, Amy Lerner, Samantha Jacques, and Peter Katona. 2006. "Design Versus Research; Abet Requirements for Design and Why Research Cannot Substitute for Design." *2006 Annual Conference & Exposition Proceedings*, June, 11.412.1–10. https://doi.org/10.18260/1-2-663.

Global Innovation Through Science and Technology Initiative. n.d. Accessed May 13, 2024. https://venturewell.org/gist/.

Golecki, Holly M., Jennifer Amos, and Joe Bradley. 2023. "Designing Capstone Experiences for Interdisciplinarity in Biomedical Engineering Education." In *2023 ASEE Annual Conference & Exposition Proceedings*, June, 42977. https://doi.org/10.18260/1-2-42977.

Golecki, Holly M., Jason Robinson, Caroline Cvetkovic, and Conor Walsh. 2024. "Empowering Students in Medical Device Design: An Interdisciplinary Soft Robotics Course." *Biomedical Engineering Education*, ahead of print, April. https://doi.org/10.1007/s43683-024-00143-9.

Grammenos, R., M. Garcia Souto, I. Chester, and L. Albelda Gimeno. 2019. "Peer Assessment of Individual Contribution in Group Work: A Student Perspective." In *Proceedings Paper.* https://Www.Sefi.Be/Wp-Content/Uploads/2019/10/SEFI2019_Proceedings. Pdf, European Society for Engineering Education (SEFI), September 20. https://doi.org/10/3/Grammenos_Peer%20assessment%20of%20individual%20contribution%20in%20group%20work.%20A%20student%20perspective_AAM.pdf.

Higbee, Steven, and Sharon Miller. 2020. "Biomedical Engineering Students Gain Design Knowledge and Report Increased Confidence When Continually Challenged with Integrated Design Projects." In *2020 ASEE Virtual Annual Conference Content Access Proceedings*, June, 34217. https://doi.org/10.18260/1-2-34217.

Hirshorn, Steven R. 2016. *Expanded Guidance for NASA Systems Engineering. Volume 1: Systems Engineering Practices*, March 1. https://ntrs.nasa.gov/citations/20170007238.

Howe, Susannah. 2010. "Where Are We Now? Statistics on Capstone Courses Nationwide." *Advances in Engineering Education* 2 (1). https://eric.ed.gov/?id=EJ1076085.

"I-Corps Medical Jumpstart." n.d. *NSF I-Corps Hub: Great Lakes Region.* Accessed August 21, 2025. https://www.greatlakesicorps.org/event/i-corps-medical-jumpstart/.

Ju, Tongjie, and Jiabin Zhu. 2023. "Exploring Senior Engineering Students' Engineering Identity: The Impact of Practice-Oriented Learning Experiences." *International Journal of STEM Education* 10 (1): 48. https://doi.org/10.1186/s40594-023-00439-2.

Karau, Steven J., and Kipling D. Williams. 1995. "Social Loafing: Research Findings, Implications, and Future Directions." *Current Directions in Psychological Science* 4 (5): 134–40. https://doi.org/10.1111/1467-8721.ep10772570.

Khojah, Reem, Alyssa Taylor, and Isgard Hueck. 2024. "Industry Perspectives on Professional and Design Skills of Bioengineering Senior Students." In *2024 ASEE Annual Conference & Exposition Proceedings*, June, 47618. https://doi.org/10.18260/1-2-47618.

Krathwohl, David R. 2002. "A Revision of Bloom's Taxonomy: An Overview." *Theory Into Practice* 41 (4): 212–18. https://doi.org/10.1207/s15430421tip4104_2.

May-Newman, Karen, and G Bryan Cornwall. 2012. "Teaching Medical Device Design Using Design Control." *Expert Review of Medical Devices* 9 (1): 7–14. https://doi.org/10.1586/erd.11.63.

Nassersharif, Bahram, and Carl-Ernst Rousseau. 2010. "Best Practices in Assessing Capstone Design Projects." In *Capstone Conference.* capstonedesigncommunity.org.

National Institute of Biomedical Imaging and Bioengineering (NIBIB) and VentureWell Have Come Together to Support and Expand the Design by Biomedical Undergraduate Teams (DEBUT) Challenge, n.d. Accessed May 13, 2024. https://venturewell.org/debut/.

Olechowski, Alison L., Steven D. Eppinger, Nitin Joglekar, and Katharina Tomaschek. 2020. "Technology Readiness Levels: Shortcomings and Improvement Opportunities." *Systems Engineering* 23 (4): 395–408. https://doi.org/10.1002/sys.21533.

Pietzsch, Jan B., Lauren A. Shluzas, M. Elisabeth Paté-Cornell, Paul G. Yock, and John H. Linehan. 2009. "Stage-Gate Process for the Development of Medical Devices." *Journal of Medical Devices* 3 (2): 021004. https://doi.org/10.1115/1.3148836.

"Practical Manual of Quality Function Deployment | SpringerLink." n.d. Accessed August 21, 2025. https://link-springer-com.proxy2.library.illinois.edu/book/10.1007/978-3-319-08521-0.

Proceedings of the 4th World Conference on Design. n.d. "Innovative Grading for Design Exercises—A Case Study from Aerospace Engineering." Accessed May 13, 2024. https://wwhttps://ris.utwente.nl/ws/files/5398987/IASDR2011_book_of_abstracts_and_programme.pdfw.researchgate.net/publication/303824784_Innovative_Grading_for_Design_Exercises_-_A_case_Study_from_Aerospace_Engineering.

Publication Count. n.d. Web of Science Platform | Clarivate. Accessed March 1, 2025. https://clarivate.com › research-discovery-and-referencing.

Rosenau, Milton D. Jr. 1993. *Managing the Development of New Products: Achieving Speed and Quality Simultaneously Through Multifunctional Teamwork by Milton D. Rosenau and John J. Moran*. John Wiley & Sons Inc.

Scanlon, Kevin J., and Mark A. Lieberman. 2007. "Commercializing Medical Technology." *Cytotechnology* 53 (1–3): 107–12. https://doi.org/10.1007/s10616-007-9056-5.

Transforming the World Through Innovation. n.d. Accessed May 13, 2024. https://venturewell.org/venturewell-celebrating-25-years-ideaimpact/.

Voß, Markus, Hulusi Bozkurt, and Thorsten Sauer. 2016. "Grading Engineering Design Projects—Let Products Give Feedback!" In *DS 83: Proceedings of the 18th International Conference on Engineering and Product Design Education (E&PDE16), Design Education: Collaboration and Cross-Disciplinarity, Aalborg, Denmark, 8th–9th September 2016*, 442–7. https://www.designsociety.org/download-publication/39105/GRADING+ENGINEERING+DESIGN+PROJECTS+–+LET+PRODUCTS+GIVE+FEEDBACK!

Ward, Thomas A. 2013. "Common Elements of Capstone Projects in the World's Top-Ranked Engineering Universities." *European Journal of Engineering Education* 38 (2): 211–18. https://doi.org/10.1080/03043797.2013.766676.

White, John A., Donald P. Gaver, Robert J. Butera, et al. 2020. "Core Competencies for Undergraduates in Bioengineering and Biomedical Engineering: Findings, Consequences, and Recommendations." *Annals of Biomedical Engineering* 48 (3): 905–12. https://doi.org/10.1007/s10439-020-02468-2.

Wiley.Com. n.d. *Business Model Generation: A Handbook for Visionaries, Game Changers, and Challengers | Wiley*. Accessed August 21, 2025. https://www.wiley.com/en-ie/Business+Model+Generation%3A+A+Handbook+for+Visionaries%2C+Game+Changers%2C+and+Challengers-p-9780470876411.

8 Problem-Based Learning in Biomedical Engineering

Emily Cook, Fiona Truscott, and Jennifer Griffiths

8.1 INTRODUCTION: PBL

PBL is a type of experiential-learning pedagogy in which students learn through facilitated problem-solving. Its origins were in medical sciences education, with focused, clinical problems (e.g., formulate a diagnosis from some clinical data) used as the basis for student learning. It is a pedagogical approach that emphasizes the student's role in the learning process. By engaging with real-world problems, students develop critical thinking and problem-solving skills. This method encourages active learning and collaboration among students, making the learning experience more dynamic and engaging.

PBL in its purest form poses real-world problems, from which students work collaboratively to define learning objectives, identify knowledge gaps, and propose a solution to the problem (Hmelo-Silver 2004), though many structures have been reported for PBL integration across different institutions and courses (Chen, Kolmos, and Du 2020). However, when implemented, PBL is fundamentally a student-centered, facilitated approach, with the aim to support students to acquire knowledge independently, and often through a social-learning setting (Bandura 1977), rather than through direct instruction. PBL is not just a teaching method; it is a philosophy that fosters a deeper understanding of the subject matter. By working on real-world problems, students learn to apply theoretical knowledge in practical situations. This approach also helps students develop essential skills such as teamwork, communication, and self-directed learning.

PBL has similarities to PjBL, and the terms are indeed often used synonymously. They share the use of real-world applications to frame problems, emphasize group work and the social construction of knowledge, and have a diverse range of assessment strategies depending on the required output of the problem-solution or project deliverable. However, PjBL has a focus on developing professional skills, often applying knowledge, skills, and theoretical concepts taught previously, as well as the production of deliverables, while PBL is itself the means of knowledge acquisition for the students. In engineering, PjBL often also overlaps with design-based challenges, whereas PBL has a broader range of potential problem-solving approaches and outputs, such as a hypothesis or a recommendation rather than a design or

 DOI: 10.1201/9781003520313-8

physical artifact (Linsenmeier and Saterbak 2020). It is a pedagogical approach that emphasizes the student's role in the learning process.

PBL aims not just to help students acquire knowledge, but to make deep connections as the knowledge has been acquired in response to a challenge and socially constructed with group members; Long, Dragich, and Saterbak (2022) showed that students reported PBL as the sole pedagogy they experienced that supported their confidence in achieving the skills linked to the higher levels of Bloom's taxonomy. PBL also aims to ensure that knowledge can be retrieved and applied in a range of professional settings. In addition, students develop problem-solving and lifelong learning skills by practicing the process of asking questions and seeking answers independently. By working in ways that are more aligned with practice in the real world, PBL also provides experiences of engineering in action and provides the space for students to develop the skills needed for the world beyond university (Schön 1992).

Biomedical engineering, with its strong links to both medical sciences and engineering, two areas that have seen significant implementation of, and innovation within, PBL, is inherently suited to being taught via PBL approaches. Given its nature as a fast-evolving field addressing complex health-related challenges, traditional teaching methods focused on knowledge transfer can easily become out of date, as well as failing to capture the complex interaction of factors that need to be considered when working within Biomedical Engineering. PBL focuses on skills development, providing the students with the tools to tackle problems, work with others, and update their own knowledge, as well as providing a space to bring in the complexity of real-world problems. PBL is an essential way to address the future needs of biomedical engineers and provide a mechanism to bring authenticity into biomedical engineering programs (Graham 2018). This interdisciplinary field combines principles of engineering and biological sciences to develop technologies and systems that improve healthcare. The integration of PBL in biomedical engineering education helps students understand the complexities of medical problems and develop innovative solutions.

As an inherently interdisciplinary subject, biomedical engineering requires its practitioners to work across disciplines, integrating knowledge and navigating non-technical frameworks. Simply designing a medical device is not enough; practitioners must understand how clinicians will use it, how to get legal approval, and what patients will think of it. Working in an interdisciplinary manner such as this is not an easy proposition; there is a lack of a common formula for integrating different topics or even a lack of shared language or goals across disciplines (de Ruiter, Wittingslow, and Chiu 2024). Working across disciplinary boundaries requires the ability to translate and communicate between different topics as well as an understanding of your work's purpose within the whole complex project and respect for others' contributions and expertise (Dalton, Wolff, and Bekker 2022). PBL, alongside PjBL, is an effective way to bring interdisciplinarity into the classroom, providing a space for students to develop the skills needed to cross disciplinary boundaries and integrate knowledge from different areas (Van den Beemt et al. 2020). This interdisciplinary field combines principles of engineering and biological sciences to develop technologies and systems that improve healthcare. The integration of PBL in biomedical engineering education helps students understand the complexities of medical problems and develop innovative solutions.

Nevertheless, PBL can bring challenges with it regardless of the discipline in which it is implemented (Chen, Kolmos, and Du 2020). These include the need for training instructors, creating effective assessments that reliably and validly evaluate the wide range of skills students learn through PBL, preparing a diverse student cohort for a style of learning that may be new to them, and resourcing in terms of time and facilities available.

8.2 EXAMPLES OF PBL IN BME

The inherently interdisciplinary nature of biomedical engineering allows for many different implementations of PBL theories, methods, and processes. This interdisciplinary field combines principles of engineering and biological sciences to develop technologies and systems that improve healthcare. The integration of PBL in biomedical engineering education helps students understand the complexities of medical problems and develop innovative solutions. In this chapter, we will explore examples of applications of:

1. Reframing questions
2. Scenario-based learning
3. Design-based problems
4. Case studies
5. Simulation-based learning

8.3 REFRAMING QUESTIONS

Traditional lecture-based teaching often starts by introducing theoretical concepts, then moves on to provide simple examples, and later relates the theory to applied situations. PBL reverses this and starts by posing a problem, which then forms the basis for students, usually working in groups, to explore the problem, develop the knowledge and skills to suggest solutions, and present and discuss these solutions. According to Hmelo-Silver (2004), the problem posed by the instructor should be realistic and ill-structured, forming a basis for students to explore the topic and identify their knowledge gaps. This complexity in problem formation is crucial as it is estimated that engineering students solve more than two thousand "problems" in the course of a four-year degree (Warnock and Mohammadi-Aragh 2015), though the vast majority of these are merely applications of known processes and formulae and do not develop critical thinking skills or the ability to approach problems which contain ambiguity. Thus, students, encountering PBL for the first time, struggle with the idea that there is not just one correct answer, or indeed that there are multiple ways to interpret the problem. It is only by repeating the process of tackling ill-structured problems that students develop the skills and confidence to approach new, open-ended challenges. It is a pedagogical approach that emphasizes the student's role in the learning process. By engaging with real-world problems, students develop critical thinking and problem-solving skills. This method encourages active learning and collaboration among students, making the learning experience more dynamic and engaging.

The starting point of PBL is therefore the problem itself, which can be large and complex or a simple reframing of a learning outcome. To provide an example from BME, consider how a learning outcome in fluid mechanics, such as "apply fundamental conservation laws of fluid mechanics to biomedical problems," can be converted into a question such as "how does the viscosity of blood affect flow rates in the large arteries?" Students in their facilitated groups can break down the question into constituent components and identify what knowledge they need to be able to answer the question, approaching the need to understand fundamental conservation laws of fluid dynamics for themselves. The relevant theory can be discovered through self-directed learning, with targeted input from the facilitator, or through separate direct learning, but the process of asking the question highlights the relevance of the theory and its application to a real-life example, making the learning process meaningful for the students.

An example from the literature of reframing content as a question was described by Newstetter et al. (2010). The authors undertook a comparative study of two approaches to delivering a Systems Physiology unit. The control was a traditional delivery method that focused on providing students with step-by-step instructions on how to perform analytical tests. In comparison, the PBL delivery method reframed the lab with an initial prompt, "what species of animal is this serum sample from?" and provided no step-by-step instructions to the processes, or even guidance as to which processes would be suitable. Facilitators guided students, but often allowed them to follow a path they themselves could identify as wrong, to provide students with the opportunity to learn from their unsuccessful attempts. Students worked in teams of five, as opposed to pairs in the control lab, emphasizing the social collaborative learning aspects of PBL, and had access to more equipment and supplies than needed to force them to systematically consider their experimental design. The assessment items (quizzes, lab books, reports, presentations, and end-of-term test) were the same items for both groups and showed similar outcomes in terms of knowledge acquisition, with the PBL students having statistically significantly higher scores for oral presentation and the end-of-term comprehension test compared to the traditionally taught control group.

8.4 SCENARIO-BASED LEARNING

Teaching and learning environments within universities are usually very different from the clinical and real-world settings in which biomedical engineering students will ultimately work in or design for. This disconnect can hinder students' ability to transfer theoretical knowledge into practical, impactful solutions. Thus, in addition to posing a problem to students that requires them to understand the logistical, socio-cultural, or socio-economic constraints of a system or environment, there is also a need to provide experiential learning experiences that allow students to explore the problem space and generate contextually informed solutions.

A critical skill required in all fields of engineering, but particularly for biomedical engineers, is that of empathy. Before commencing a design, there is a need to understand the problems faced by the end user, both physical and often also psychological, and the context of its use. Developing a piece of equipment that may meet technical specifications, but is too ugly/heavy/expensive for its target audience, is unlikely to succeed in practice. Scenario-based PBL addresses this challenge by fostering empathy through experiential engagement. This can be achieved through theoretical personas, direct interactions with end users, or immersive simulations and role-playing scenarios. It can also be an opportunity to engage a class in sharing their own lived experience where appropriate, enriching the learning environment with diverse, relevant, and real perspectives. This peer-to-peer exchange can be particularly valuable in multicultural classrooms where students bring varied insights into healthcare systems, patient expectations, and cultural norms. PBL is not just a teaching method; it is a philosophy that fosters a deeper understanding of the subject matter. By working on real-world problems, students learn to apply theoretical knowledge in practical situations. This approach also helps students develop essential skills such as teamwork, communication, and self-directed learning.

An example of a scenario-based biomedical devices unit was presented by Singh, Ferry, and Mills (2018). The unit involved both nursing and biomedical engineering students working in pairs, and the learning environment was a simulation laboratory designed to mimic a clinical setting, but with the ability for instructors or peers to observe and record interactions via a camera in the room to provide a debrief and feedback on the simulation. Student groups took part in simulated challenges, where they had to solve a problem. Examples of problems included an actor waiting to be diagnosed with a beeping intravenous device, a mannequin that was showing signs of distress while being hooked up to gas, and a mannequin admitted to the emergency room with blurred vision, for which the student team was to make a diagnosis of his condition, administer the required medication, and offer the correct treatment option. The learning from this problem-based scenario was both related to communication and critical thinking skills and developing familiarity with a clinical setting pre-placement.

Research supports the efficacy of this scenario-based approach (Long, Dragich, and Saterbak 2022), and the competencies developed are those outlined in the Washington Accord and "Engineer of 2020" vision, which emphasize the importance of addressing complex, ill-defined problems in uncertain environments.

8.5 DESIGN-BASED PROBLEMS

These problems require students to apply their knowledge and creativity to develop solutions to complex challenges. By working on design-based problems, students learn to think critically and develop innovative solutions. This approach also helps students understand the importance of considering various factors, such as user needs, technical constraints, and regulatory requirements, when developing solutions. Design is a key feature of BME and is defined by Lerner et al. (2006) as follows:

> Design in biomedical engineering means the conception, creation and/or fabrication of devices, instruments, fixtures, procedures, methods, algorithms or simulations intended

> to benefit health and wellness, including means to interrogate, analyze or otherwise define operating or physical parameters.

Design-based learning focuses on problem-solving through iterative processes, including brainstorming, prototyping, and testing solutions. It emphasizes both empathy as discussed previously, understanding the problem space, and creativity in generating solutions. Examples might include designing a prosthetic limb or wearable monitoring device, or creating a simple user-friendly app or assistive tool.

Griffiths, Yerworth, and Hatten (2017) presented an example of a design problem where students initially approached a problem in a task- and product-oriented manner but then had to pivot to embrace a more iterative process as the need for debugging and testing became apparent.

In this example, students were tasked with the broad and open-ended challenge of creating an item of "smart clothing" for an athlete within a financial budget and a timeframe of one academic week (35 hours of lab time). Their brief was that the clothing should measure an appropriate physiological parameter for a sport of their choice and should give a warning if that parameter falls out of a pre-set range that they should decide upon, and justify, themselves.

Design challenges can be used as problems in PBL, and although this initial brief can be seen as a "design an X to do . . .," the open nature of the task, with students having agency in choice of athlete, sport, item of clothing, and measurable parameter, meant that the challenge became centered around "How can we . . .?" It is notable that all student teams in this study of second-year undergraduates began by attempting to construct an entire clothing, monitoring, and warning system before the realities of creating a tangible product led to them needing to take a more step-by-step iterative approach to their design and build. Students were asked to write a reflection on their teams' work, focusing on how they deviated from their original design plans and why. Over 60% of students mentioned debugging, troubleshooting, and the need for iterative processes in design in their reflections.

The act of experiential learning in design-based PBL—actually taking part in the design process—built students' understanding of practical aspects of the process in a way that their theoretical education had not.

Alongside de-bugging, design-based PBL can strengthen students' understanding of multi-disciplinary systems engineering. Pennes et al. (2023) described a short (90-minute) assignment in mechatronics where students are required to assemble a syringe pump, calculate the appropriate patient dose, program the pump, and evaluate their pump's dispensing performance. This requires integration of different aspects of biomedical engineering, practical mechatronic skills, and teamwork in order to complete all aspects of the design brief within the timeframe of the lab session. A syringe pump was chosen due to its prevalence in clinical settings, showing relevance to students' interests and future career aspirations. PBL provides space to foster deeper understanding as well as bring in authenticity and relevant real-world experiences. By working on real-world problems, students learn to apply theoretical knowledge in practical situations. This approach also helps students develop essential skills such as teamwork, communication, and self-directed learning.

8.6 CASE STUDIES

Case studies provide students with an opportunity to analyze real-world problems and develop solutions based on their understanding of the subject matter. This approach helps students develop critical thinking and problem-solving skills. By working on case studies, students learn to apply theoretical knowledge in practical situations and develop a deeper understanding of the subject matter.

Early PBL practices have been credited to have evolved from CBL, particularly within Law at Harvard University in the 19th century (Schmidt 2012), where legal reasoning was taught through engagement with real judicial decisions. This pedagogy then influenced other disciplines and found a particular space in business and medical education.

In BME education, case-study-based PBL offers an authentic learning experience. By engaging with real-life scenarios—especially those drawn from biomedical start-ups and small enterprises—students are exposed to the breadth of challenges that professionals in the field face. These case studies setting up PBL often involve technical, ethical, regulatory, and commercial dimensions, providing a narrative giving a holistic and real view of biomedical engineering innovation and the broader ecosystem in which biomedical engineers operate.

One key strength of case-study-based PBL is its ability to showcase the complexity and ambiguity of real-world problems. There is often no single clear-cut answer. Nor indeed even necessarily a "good" answer. Students are required to navigate complex and incomplete information, conflicting stakeholder interests, and uncertain outcomes. This mirrors the reality for many commercial interests where engineers must make decisions under pressure and with limited data. Students learn to frame a problem, evaluate alternatives, and justify their decisions, balancing technical expertise, business acumen, and regulatory awareness.

A case-based approach means that after the event, students are also often able to then compare their decisions with the final real outcomes of the case study. The learning experience can often be enhanced further by incorporating guest speakers from industry into the classroom to talk through their real experiences in the case studies.

Case studies are a classic technique for teaching ethics and, when combined with PBL, prove to be an effective demonstration for students of real-world ethical decision-making, as Lewis, Van Hout, and Huang-Saad (2010) show. Within teams, students acted as a fictional company that developed implantable medical devices. These devices are the subject of a potential product quality problem, and so the teams have to develop a plan for how the company proceeds. Once teams had presented their company's approach, the problem was put into context through the presentation of real similar recall cases and a capstone discussion.

8.7 SIMULATION-BASED LEARNING

This approach uses computer-based simulations to provide students with a realistic learning experience. By working on simulations, students can develop their problem-solving skills in a controlled environment. This approach also helps students understand the complexities of real-world problems and develop innovative solutions.

Here, we separately categorized scenario-based challenges, in which the problems were experiential and involved physical learning environments or people, from the simulation-based learning discussed here. Simulation-based learning, as defined here, uses physical models, computer programs, or virtual realities to replicate real-world problems to enable students to experiment and learn in a controlled and safe environment that is often replicable, allowing for repeat attempts at solving a problem. This is of particular relevance to biomedical engineering, where students may not have ready access to patients or specialist equipment. For instance, Harvey and Dean (2025) discuss an electrophysiology simulation tool that "allows students to perform virtual patch clamp experiments without the needs for complex laboratory equipment, training, or prior knowledge in mathematical modelling." This interdisciplinary field combines principles of engineering and biological sciences to develop technologies and systems that improve healthcare. The integration of PBL in biomedical engineering education helps students understand the complexities of medical problems and develop innovative solutions.

Simulation-based learning can also bolster creativity, whereby the abstract environment of some simulations allows for playful learning and exploration of ideas. Harvey and Dean (2025) give a short example of a student posing a hypothesis about Blake Mamba snake venom—which would be very challenging to test in the lab, but is entirely possible in a simulation environment.

Clinical immersion is an effective tool to prepare biomedical engineers for the challenges of professional work. While effective, it can be difficult to implement at scale for large cohorts. VR simulations are one way of providing an experience of a clinical setting without having large classes on field trips to hospitals or the logistics of arranging multiple clinical placements. An example of applying VR to biomedical engineering is simulation-based training for teaching communication in a clinical environment (Singh et al. 2020), where students working on medical device-related problems compared VR immersion to watching 2D videos of an interdisciplinary team interacting. The students indicated in post-event surveys that they felt more immersed in real-world clinical scenarios when using VR compared to video, and there were also indications that VR is a promising alternative to "in-person" real-world observation. The students also indicated that they felt better prepared for operating room visits after using VR.

VR and augmented reality (AR) can also be used for exploring places not accessible in a classroom, for example, inside the human body to explore physiology, visualizing chemical reactions, or investigating material properties.

8.8 CONCLUSION

PBL has proven to be a highly effective and adaptable pedagogical approach, particularly well-suited to the demands of biomedical engineering. As this chapter has demonstrated, PBL not only supports the acquisition of technical knowledge but also fosters the development of critical professional skills such as communication, collaboration, empathy, and systems thinking. These are essential attributes for biomedical engineers, who must navigate complex, interdisciplinary environments and address real-world challenges that rarely have straightforward solutions. It is a pedagogical approach that emphasizes the student's role in the learning process. By engaging with real-world problems, students develop critical thinking and problem-solving skills. This method encourages active learning and collaboration among students, making the learning experience more dynamic and engaging. This is reflected in the six recommendations made by the Learning Environments track of the Fourth BME Education Summit in 2019, all of which can be facilitated via active learning pedagogies such as PBL (Billiar et al. 2022).

BME is a fast-paced and evolving discipline that sits at the intersection of engineering, medicine, and the life sciences. It requires practitioners to integrate knowledge across domains, communicate effectively with diverse stakeholders, and design solutions that are technically sound, clinically relevant, and socially responsible. Traditional knowledge-transfer models, while still valuable in some contexts, often fall short in preparing students for this complexity. PBL, by contrast, offers a skills-focused, experiential learning environment that mirrors the realities of professional practice. PBL is not just a teaching method; it allows teaching to mirror real-world applications and environments, giving students a realistic experience of their future careers. By working on real-world problems, students learn to apply theoretical knowledge in practical situations. This approach also allows space for students to develop essential skills such as teamwork, communication, and self-directed learning.

One of the key advantages of PBL is its flexibility. As illustrated throughout this chapter, PBL can be implemented in a variety of forms—from reframing questions and scenario-based learning to design challenges, case studies, and simulation-based experiences. This adaptability allows educators to tailor PBL to the specific needs of their students, institutions, and subject matter. Whether the goal is to deepen understanding of fluid mechanics, foster empathy through clinical simulations, or explore ethical and commercial considerations via case studies, PBL provides a robust framework for engaging students in meaningful, context-rich learning.

Moreover, PBL creates a safe and supportive environment for students to learn through iteration, experimentation, and reflection. It encourages them to take intellectual risks, confront ambiguity, and develop resilience in the face of failure—experiences that are invaluable in preparing for the uncertainties of real-world engineering practice. By working collaboratively to solve open-ended problems, students also develop the interpersonal and teamwork skills that are critical for success in multidisciplinary teams.

Importantly, PBL supports a systems engineering approach to learning. It enables students to bring together diverse strands of knowledge and apply them in an integrated, holistic manner. This is particularly relevant in BME, where solutions must account for technical, clinical, ethical, and economic factors. Through PBL, students learn not only how to solve problems but also how to define them, frame them within broader contexts, and evaluate the implications of their decisions.

The chapter has also highlighted the growing body of evidence supporting the effectiveness of PBL in engineering education. Studies have shown that PBL enhances student engagement, improves learning outcomes, and increases confidence in applying knowledge to complex, real-world situations. These benefits are especially pronounced in interdisciplinary fields like BME, where the ability to translate across areas of expertise and work collaboratively is essential for professional progression and can only be learnt through experience of interdisciplinary practice.

In conclusion, PBL goes beyond a teaching method—it is a philosophy of learning that aligns closely with the goals and realities of biomedical engineering. It equips students with the knowledge, skills, and mindset needed to thrive in a rapidly changing world, and it provides educators with a versatile and impactful tool for fostering deep, authentic learning. As BME continues to evolve, so too must our approaches to education—and PBL offers a compelling model for preparing the next generation of biomedical engineers to meet the challenges and opportunities that lie ahead.

REFERENCES

Bandura, Albert. 1977. "Self-Efficacy: Toward a Unifying Theory of Behavioral Change." *Psychological Review* 84 (2): 191–215. https://doi.org/10.1037/0033-295X.84.2.191.

Billiar, Kristen, Donald P. Gaver, Kenneth Barbee, Anita Singh, John D. DesJardins, Beth Pruitt, Joe Tranquillo, Glen Gaudette, Beth Winkelstein, Linda Makowski, Jennifer R. Amos, Ann Saterbak, Joseph LeDoux, Brian Helmke, Michael Grimm, Paul Benkeser, Lisa D. Segan, Beth Pfister, David Meaney, Treena Arinzeh, and Susan Margulies. 2022. "Learning Environments and Evidence-Based Practices in Bioengineering and Biomedical Engineering." *Biomedical Engineering Education* 2: 1–16. https://doi.org/10.1007/s43683-021-00062-z.

Chen, Jun, Anette Kolmos, and Xiangyun Du. 2020. "Forms of Implementation and Challenges of PBL in Engineering Education: A Review of Literature." *European Journal of Engineering Education* 46 (1): 90–115. https://doi.org/10.1080/03043797.2020.1718615.

Dalton, Alice, Karin Wolff, and Ben Bekker. 2022. "Interdisciplinary Research as a Complicated System." *International Journal of Qualitative Methods* 21: 1–13.

De Graaf, Erik, and Anette Kolmos. 2003. "Characteristics of Problem-Based Learning." *International Journal of Engineering Education* 19 (5): 657–62.

de Ruiter, Naomi, Ross Wittingslow, and Raymond Chiu. 2024. "Making Strange." In *Strange Bedfellows: An Experiment in Student-Directed Interdisciplinary Research*, edited by Naomi de Ruiter, Ross Wittingslow and Raymond Chiu. Groningen: University of Groningen Press.

Graham, Ruth. 2018. *The Global State of the Art in Engineering Education*. Cambridge, MA: Massachusetts Institute of Technology.

Griffiths, J. A., R. J. Yerworth, and E. Hatten. 2017. "Connecting Staff Expectations and Student Understanding of Professional Engineering Skills in a Multidisciplinary Design Challenge." In *Proceedings of the 45th SEFI Conference*, 585–92. SEFI: Azores, Portugal. https://discovery.ucl.ac.uk/id/eprint/10064700/

Harvey, T. G., and Daniel Dean. 2025. "CellSpark: A Simulation Tool to Spark Discovery Learning of Electrophysiology." *Biomedical Engineering Education* 5: 95–9.

Hmelo-Silver, Cindy E. 2004. "Problem-Based Learning: What and How Do Students Learn?" *Educational Psychology Review* 16: 235–66.

Lerner, Aaron L., Bruce H. Kenknight, Alan Rosenthal, and Paul G. Yock. 2006. "Design in BME: Challenges, Issues, and Opportunities." *Annals of Biomedical Engineering* 34: 200–8.

Lewis, Scott, Wouter Van Hout, and Aileen Huang-Saad. 2010. "Teaching Biomedical Engineering Ethics: A Case-Based Approach." In *2010 IEEE Frontiers in Education Conference (FIE)*, Arlington, VA. 2010, S3E-1–S3E-5. https://doi.org/10.1109/FIE.2010.5673545

Linsenmeier, Robert A., and Ann Saterbak. 2020. "Fifty Years of Biomedical Engineering Undergraduate Education." *Annals of Biomedical Engineering* 48 (6): 1590–615.

Long, Joseph, Emily Dragich, and Ann Saterbak. 2022. "Problem-Based Learning Impacts Students' Reported Learning and Confidence in an Undergraduate Biomedical Engineering Course." *Biomedical Engineering Education* 2: 209–32.

Newstetter, Wendy C., Elham Behravesh, Nancy J. Nersessian, and Barbara B. Fasse. 2010. "Design Principles for Problem-Driven Learning Laboratories in Biomedical Engineering Education." *Annals of Biomedical Engineering* 38: 3257–67.

Pennes, Andrew, Kristina Mendez, Nikhil Hanumara, Ellen T. Roche, Giovanni Traverso, Daniel Custer, and Grace Hom. 2023. "A Hands-On Medical Mechatronics Exercise to Pump Up Student Learnings." *Biomedical Engineering Education* 3: 235–42.

Schmidt, Henk G. 2012. "A Brief History of Problem-Based Learning." In *One-Day, One-Problem*, edited by Gabriel O'Grady, Ee Ling Yew, Kaycheng Soh Goh and Henk Schmidt. Singapore: Springer.

Schön, Donald A. 1992. *The Reflective Practitioner: How Professionals Think in Action*. London: Routledge.

Singh, Anita, Daniel Ferry, and Simon Mills. 2018. "Improving Biomedical Engineering Education through Continuity in Adaptive, Experiential, and Interdisciplinary Learning Environments." *Journal of Biomechanical Engineering* 140 (8): 081009. https://doi.org/10.1115/1.4040359.

Singh, Anita, Daniel Ferry, Arun Ramakrishnan, and Shankar Balasubramanian. 2020. "Using Virtual Reality in Biomedical Engineering Education." *Journal of Biomechanical Engineering* 142 (11): 111013. https://doi.org/10.1115/1.4048005.

Van den Beemt, Antoine, Miles MacLeod, Jeroen Van der Veen, Anouk Van de Ven, Suzanne van Baalen, Rob Klaassen, and Maarten Boon. 2020. "Interdisciplinary Engineering Education: A Review of Vision, Teaching, and Support." *Journal of Engineering Education* 109 (3): 508–55.

Warnock, James N., and M. J. Mohammadi-Aragh. 2015. "Case Study: Use of Problem-Based Learning to Develop Students' Technical and Professional Skills." *European Journal of Engineering Education* 41 (2): 142–53. https://doi.org/10.1080/03043797.2015.1040739.

9 Clinical Immersion in Biomedical Engineering Education

William H. Guilford, Miiri Kotche, and Rachael H. Schmedlen

9.1 INTRODUCTION AND HISTORY

Clinical immersion experiences for biomedical engineering (BME) students have been a significant topic of discussion and research over the past two decades, building upon foundational concepts that emerged prior to the turn of the century. The practice dates back at least to the 1950s and 1970s in rehabilitation engineering. According to Childress (Childress 2002), "Engineers and orthotists were integrated into clinical teams. . . . These programs again produced technical innovations for persons with reduced limb and upper body function due to neuromuscular disease and resulting dysfunction." Likewise, engineering students sometimes participated in co-op programs and internships at Veterans Administration hospitals in the United States, gaining firsthand experience with clinical environments and patient care (Hays 2019). These experiences emphasized an understanding of the environment in which medical equipment was used and contributed to the evolution of clinical immersion programs in engineering education. Today, the design of medical devices is strengthened when biomedical engineers observe how users in the clinical environment interact with devices and patients, as well as the decision processes involved in diagnosis and treatment.

The modern-day emphasis on clinical immersion experiences for students may have been inspired by the Stanford Biodesign Program, also known simply as "Biodesign" (Brinton et al. 2013). The Biodesign program is described in three steps—*Identify*, *Invent*, and *Implement*. A relatively novel aspect of this process is in the *Identify* step, wherein Fellows engage with healthcare providers and other stakeholders and typically are immersed in clinical settings, aiming to uncover unmet medical needs. Prior to the dissemination of the Biodesign approach around 2001, engineering design was dominated by "technology push," anecdotal reports of needs, and incremental improvements on existing designs. In these paradigms, a user-centered approach is not emphasized, and therefore, clinical observation is not a critical component of the process. While others noted the tension between technology push and "market pull" (unmet needs) at the time (Dixon 2001), Paul Yock and his colleagues at Stanford Biodesign certainly impacted modern biomedical engineering

DOI: 10.1201/9781003520313-9

design education by focusing on identifying unmet clinical needs through promoting clinical immersion and observation. When biomedical engineering students work in collaboration with end users and other stakeholders (e.g., clinicians, clinical engineers, and patients), they are empowered to identify unmet needs and opportunities for innovation. In this way, clinical immersion programs help develop students' ability to communicate across discipline boundaries and understand why designs must meet multiple realistic constraints.

9.2 WHAT IS CLINICAL IMMERSION IN ENGINEERING?

Design thinking is a human-centered, iterative approach to problem-solving that emphasizes understanding the needs of users, creatively generating ideas, prototyping, and testing solutions. This approach has significantly transformed engineering design education by shifting the focus from purely technical problem-solving to human-centered innovation. Clinical immersion experiences have been a part of this process, emphasizing the importance of gaining a deep understanding of unmet clinical needs, behaviors, and context in which medical devices will be used. That said, neither the goals nor the approach to clinical immersion is limited to design contexts.

Clinical immersion is a term used across several professional education fields, but its definition and purpose vary widely. The Biodesign approach uniquely emphasizes immersion as a means to identify unmet clinical needs, which is a focus not shared by all BME programs or by other fields such as nursing, medicine, or psychology. These latter three emphasize skill development and direct patient interaction over longer durations, and they are instrumental in bridging the theory-to-practice gap and supporting students in their transition from academic settings to clinical environments (Fowler, Knowlton, and Putnam 2018; Moore et al. 2023). Even within BME, programs differ in patient contact, educational level, duration, and goals. For example, NIH defines clinical immersion as "a 6- to 10-week program, where students engage full-time in the hospital or other clinical environment becoming familiar with the language, issues, and problems that can benefit from an engineering approach" ("PAR-10–140: Team-Based Design in Biomedical Engineering Education (R25)," n.d., 10–140). This, too, is limiting.

Clinical immersion experiences for engineering students are multi-dimensional in how they seek to meet the goals of understanding the clinical environment, identify unmet clinical needs, enhance human-centered design skills, facilitate innovative thinking, and strengthen interdisciplinary collaboration and communication. There is no unique characteristic of these programs, courses, and experiences.

9.2.1 Definition

We propose the following as a definition in the context of BME education:

> Clinical immersion in biomedical engineering education involves sustained, structured engagement in real clinical settings to observe and interact with healthcare professionals, patients, systems, and technologies, with the goals of identifying and validating unmet needs, understanding end users and the social, cultural, and economic factors

that contribute to medical decision-making, enhancing interdisciplinary communication, and developing engineering solutions tailored to real-world clinical environments.

These experiences contribute to the development of students' professional identity and problem-solving capabilities, though these may or may not be immediate goals of the experience. Our definition is consistent not only with the baselines established by Biodesign and by nursing programs but also with the authors' findings about BME clinical immersion programs broadly (William H. Guilford, Kotche, and Schmedlen 2023; Kotche et al. 2020).

Our definition reflects an ideal state, not necessarily the state of every BME clinical immersion experience as it exists today. An ideal clinical immersion experience happens at the intersection of engineering education and the clinical environment (Figure 9.1). However, the real world of clinical immersion in biomedical engineering is more nuanced and includes a partial union of these two environments—academic and clinical. On the academic side of the intersection, we find "clinic-adjacent" experiences in which students are exposed to real clinicians or real problems, but not to the clinical environment itself. For example, a clinician may visit a BME class and talk about their clinical practice and the problems they encounter. Student chapters of the US-based organization, Engineering World Health (EWH) (Malkin and Calman 2014), are another example (now merged with Engineers Without Borders USA). Students work in a real-world, under-resourced setting to repair medical equipment, but their exposure to clinicians, patients, and treatment settings is often limited. The unmet need is the broken piece of equipment before them, not a broader challenge to be analyzed and addressed.

On the clinical side of the intersection are "engineering-adjacent" experiences. Engineering-adjacent experiences involve scenarios where non-engineering participants (clinicians or patients) are exposed to engineering concepts, tools, or methodologies. This exposure can occur through collaborative projects, educational programs including clinical immersion or capstone experiences, or participation in design processes. These, too, have their roots in rehabilitation engineering and Biodesign, where clinicians are in teams with engineers. Despite their long history and their positive impact on innovation, the benefits of engineering exposure to the clinicians themselves are understudied (Zhou, Li, and Li 2021).

9.2.2 Characteristics

Clinical immersion programs are multidimensional, as we wrote earlier, and can include both clinic-adjacent and engineering-adjacent experiences. If we were to build a more nuanced classification system for clinical immersion experiences for biomedical engineering (BME) students, the principal dimensions might include setting, duration, focus, and level of engagement.

9.2.3 Setting

9.2.3.1 Clinic and Hospital-Based Immersion Experiences

Students are placed directly in clinical settings, such as operating rooms, intensive care units, or outpatient clinics. Examples include shadowing physicians, nurses,

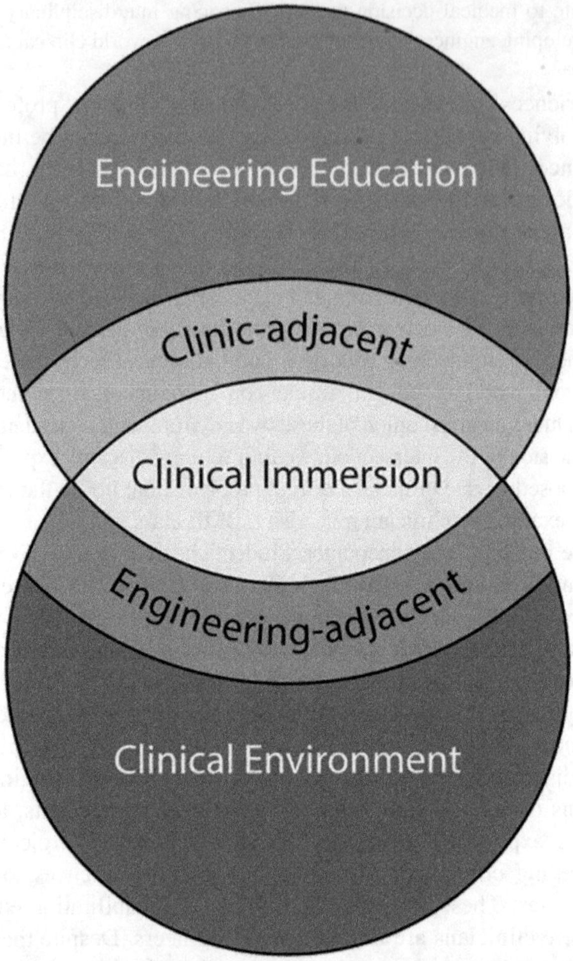

FIGURE 9.1 Depiction of clinical immersion in BME education. The central overlap represents the ideal clinical immersion experience, characterized by sustained, structured engagement in real clinical settings to foster understanding and develop tailored engineering solutions. This ideal is contextualized by "clinic-adjacent" experiences (academic focus with clinical exposure) and "engineering-adjacent" experiences (clinical focus with engineering exposure), illustrating the nuanced reality of BME clinical immersion

medical students, or technicians, observing surgeries, or collaborating with medical staff in a clinical environment to identify unmet clinical needs or to understand clinical operations. These experiences might include understanding patient care in low-resource environments (community health immersions), observing how engineering solutions are implemented outside of traditional hospital settings, and understanding process workflow.

9.2.3.2 Clinical Labs and Support Units

These include maintenance, infection control, clinical engineering, hospital labs, quality control, or any other units that work in support of the clinical mission. Interactions with patients, doctors, nurses, and other clinical staff may be limited.

9.2.3.3 Classroom-Based Clinical Perspectives

This clinic-adjacent approach brings clinicians, typically with self-identified clinical problems, into a traditional classroom setting. The students do not have direct or prolonged exposure to a clinic or clinical support unit.

9.2.3.4 Remote, Recorded, or Simulated Clinical Environments

Simulated clinical scenarios mimic real-world healthcare challenges, using procedural/task trainers, advanced mannequins, VR, and other technologies. Recordings, remote presentations, and simulations were prominent during the pandemic and may still be in use today, though they do not qualify as clinical immersion by our definition.

9.2.4 Duration of Immersion Experience

9.2.4.1 Extensive Experiences

With > 80 hours of direct immersion in the clinical environment, these are typical of dedicated clinical immersion programs. For example, these experiences may take place during academic breaks or as part of required clinical internships.

9.2.4.2 Medium-Length Experiences

With 20–80 hours of clinical immersion exposure, these are typical of credit-bearing clinical immersion courses.

9.2.4.3 Short-Term Experiences

Highly focused, short-duration experiences of 20 hours or less introduce students to clinical workflows and problem-solving, often as a prelude to design experiences. These are relatively common in capstone design projects. These can also include structured site visits to clinics.

9.2.5 Focus

9.2.5.1 Unmet Needs and Problem Definition

Programs centered on either identifying unmet clinical needs through observation and interaction with healthcare professionals or better defining a problem that has already been identified. The goal is to gather data for subsequent engineering design projects.

9.2.5.2 Device Testing and Feedback

Experiences that allow students to see how prototypes or medical devices are tested and used in clinical settings.

9.2.5.3 User-Centered Design

The emphasis is on understanding patient and caregiver experiences, including interactions with technology and care systems, to inform design.

9.2.5.4 Systems Perspective

The emphasis is on a high-level understanding of the complexities of the healthcare system to place design requirements in the context of the unmet need, market opportunity, insurance reimbursement, device regulation, and other considerations.

9.2.5.5 Interdisciplinary Collaboration

Some programs emphasize a mixed-discipline approach in order to foster stronger communication and collaboration between engineering, design, business, medical, and/or nursing students.

9.2.6 Level of Engagement

9.2.6.1 Collaboration

Students work as part of a team with clinicians and other stakeholders to solve real-world problems. This is often a hallmark of senior capstone projects or research-focused programs.

9.2.6.2 Participation

Students contribute actively, such as assisting in data collection, research, interviewing clinicians, or participating in multidisciplinary team meetings.

9.2.6.3 Passive Observation

Students shadow medical professionals and observe clinical workflows without direct involvement. These experiences provide foundational knowledge of clinical processes. This framework, spanning setting, duration, focus, and level of engagement, is helpful because it provides a structured way to understand, compare, and design clinical immersion experiences in biomedical engineering education. By organizing programs along these dimensions, educators can tailor experiences to meet specific learning goals, ensure alignment with curricular outcomes, and assess program depth and impact.

9.3 BME CLINICAL IMMERSION AROUND THE WORLD

Adoption of clinical immersion programs in BME education varies globally due to factors such as regional educational structures, healthcare partnerships, resource availability, and cultural differences. Unfortunately, the prevalence of these programs is unknown. Outside the United States, they are often unreported in the literature, even on institutions' websites. We therefore offer here a few observations and notable examples of programs as they can be found today.

9.3.1 Clinical Immersion in the United States and North America

Clinical immersion is a well-established component of BME education in the United States, though it is far from being a core component of the curriculum. Many universities offer structured programs that integrate students into clinical settings to observe medical procedures, identify unmet clinical needs, and develop engineering solutions.

To date, North American clinical immersion programs are the only such programs widely reported in the literature. Here, we summarize the results of our own survey of those programs (William H. Guilford, Kotche, and Schmedlen 2023). Fifty-two clinical immersion courses and programs were identified in the United States, 14 of which were previously or currently funded by the NIH. Those programs engaged an average of 27 students per year, with participation ranging from 2 to 160 students. The duration of the immersion experiences varies significantly, from as short as 3 hours to as long as 400 hours. The primary objectives of these programs included identifying clinical problems, developing engineering solutions, and learning clinical procedures. Although some evidence suggests that these experiences impact student learning, motivation, professional identity, and career paths, more investigation is needed (Schmedlen et al. 2019).

The rapid growth of clinical immersion programs for BME in the United States was probably driven by the R25 grant funding program of the NIBIB titled "Team-Based Design in Biomedical Engineering Education." The aim of this program is to support the development and implementation of TBL experiences that engage students in solving real-world biomedical engineering challenges. The program focuses on enhancing educational practices that promote collaboration, innovation, and problem-solving skills in biomedical engineering. This program was founded in 2009 to address two goals—first, to promote design education in BME because many graduates of BME were going into industry, and second, to incentivize the foundation of additional BME bachelor's degree programs at a time that was already seeing rapid growth. Clinical immersion is highlighted in the program announcement as a possible mechanism toward this goal, but it is not the focus of the program. Nevertheless, clinical immersion spoke to a trend at a time of multidisciplinary training and experiential learning, and the program appears to have prompted many immersion programs (Guilford, Kotche, and Schmedlen 2023).

In Mexico, the Universidad Autónoma de Querétaro offers a semester-long clinical immersion program for biomedical engineering students that emphasizes real-world exposure to healthcare environments (Montesinos, Salinas-Navarro, and Santos-Diaz 2023). An interesting aspect of this program is that it trains students not so much for the development of healthcare technologies through clinical observations, but for administration and systems improvement through immersion in non-clinical areas of the hospital. Through observations in areas such as maintenance, sterilization and disinfection, and clinical laboratories, students identify unmet needs and propose context-appropriate technological solutions. The program uses a PBL framework and is implemented in collaboration with local medical institutions, enabling students to develop socially responsive design skills and a deeper understanding of the challenges within the Mexican healthcare system.

We are not aware of clinical immersion programs for biomedical engineering students in Canada, though there is at least one program with immersion components for academic faculty—the Western Medical Innovation Fellowship at Western University (Western Medical Innovation Fellowship, n.d.).

9.3.2 Clinical Immersion Outside North America

It is difficult to report on BME clinical immersion programs outside the United States, although this is not to say that these programs do not exist. They do, at least anecdotally, and we assume them to be prevalent! As previously mentioned, however, they are not well represented in literature and are not always featured on university websites. Here we summarize what we know.

9.3.3 Clinic Immersion in Europe

Comprehensive data on the prevalence of clinical immersion programs across Europe is limited. There is a clinic-adjacent program in Portugal at the Faculty of Engineering of the University of Porto (Maia and Claro 2014). They adapted the Biodesign program for their master's level program but have so far been unable to include a clinical immersion step. They instead sourced biomedical technologies under development at the university, and it is thus clinic-adjacent. Biodesign Finland includes clinical immersion, but it is geared toward faculty and does not include students ("Biodesign Finland—Programme" n.d.).

9.3.4 Clinic Immersion in Asia

In Asia, the integration of clinical immersion into BME curricula is emerging. While some institutions may have begun to incorporate clinical experiences, the practice is not yet widespread, and detailed information on specific programs is scarce. Others have noted, "Although engineering students' presence in clinical settings is increasingly common in U.S.-based healthcare facilities, it is still a relatively unusual practice in sub-Saharan Africa and China" (Sienko et al. 2018).

There are historical and cultural reasons for this. For example, at the NUS, clinical immersion opportunities for biomedical engineering undergraduates have become increasingly limited since the onset of the COVID-19 pandemic. Pandemic-related restrictions heightened hospital security protocols, limiting access to clinical environments. As a result, direct patient interaction has been largely replaced by controlled, simulation-based exposure within existing academic courses, particularly design-oriented ones modeled loosely on the Biodesign framework. Instead of immersion, clinicians present authentic clinical needs, and students engage in role-play and device analysis to support needs identification. These semester-long experiences are targeted at the undergraduate level. While limited in scale, some students have access to global health immersion experiences, including fieldwork in East Timor. Thus, cultural and systemic factors in Singapore significantly influence the structure and feasibility of clinical immersion—factors including concerns for infection control—that have led NUS to focus primarily on clinic-adjacent experiences

(Chong n.d.). However, a growing institutional interest in service learning and assistive technologies has the potential to evolve both these clinical-adjacent and global immersion experiences in the future.

9.3.5 Clinical Immersion in Africa

In many parts of Sub-Saharan Africa, the inclusion of clinical immersion within institutions of higher education is beginning to gain traction. Many of these institutions still embrace the traditional lecture-based model of learning and have been slower to adopt active-learning pedagogies, including in the engineering design process. Furthermore, many biomedical engineering programs prepare their students for clinical engineering positions that are more prevalent in African countries than the biomedical engineering jobs found in the medtech industry in other parts of the world. To encourage active learning and design thinking, organizations like the Rice360 Institute for Global Health Technologies offer training workshops for African faculty and an "Invention Education Toolkit for African Universities" with a wide range of resources to develop curricula, support translation of invention, foster faculty development, and cultivate partnerships. Some institutions have already started implementing design and using clinical immersion as a means of needs identification for design projects. A couple of examples are provided here.

At Mbarara University of Science and Technology in Uganda, biomedical engineering undergraduates participate in structured clinical immersion experiences integrated directly into their academic curriculum. According to Eng. Dr. Johnes Obungoloch, students complete two hospital-based "workshop practice" courses during their second and third years, each totaling 60 hours. These experiences are designed to build practical skills, foster collaboration between biomedical engineers and clinical staff, and support the identification of unmet clinical needs that may inform future design work. Unlike many programs that operate as extracurricular or informal experiences, Mbarara's clinical immersion is a formalized part of the undergraduate program. (Obungoloch 2025).

At Makerere University in Uganda, biomedical engineering undergraduates engage in both curricular and extracurricular clinical immersion experiences designed to expose them to real-world healthcare challenges and support problem-driven innovation. As part of the academic program, students complete eight- to ten-week-long hospital-based internships during their second year, and optionally during their third year, with approximately 30 students participating annually. These internships focus on identifying clinical problems and building context-sensitive engineering solutions. In addition to these in-curriculum experiences, Makerere partners with Duke University through the Duke-Makerere Summer Design Fellowship, an eight-week collaborative program that pairs eight students from each institution to work directly with hospital-based health workers. Together, teams identify unmet needs and co-develop potential solutions. These programs reflect a strong commitment to experiential learning in clinical environments and emphasize the value of international collaboration.

Clinical immersion programs within Africa exist for non-African students (e.g., US students) that partner with clinics and/or academic institutions to solve healthcare problems in resource-constrained settings. These experiences range from repairing medical equipment (clinic-adjacent), conducting needs finding and assessment, to prototype implementation (clinical immersion). Examples of such programs include the Global Health Design Initiative from the University of Michigan, Rice360 Global Health Technologies Summer Internship Program, Duke-Makerere University BME Partnership, Case Western Reserve University collaboration with Makerere University, and the Northwestern University Center for Innovation in Global Health Technologies collaboration with the University of Cape Town, South Africa, University of Ibadan, and the University of Lagos, both in Nigeria (Ploss et al. 2017; Sienko et al. 2014).

9.3.6 Clinic Immersion in the Caribbean, Central, and South America

Information about clinical immersion experiences in the Caribbean and Latin America is sparse. As the sole example we can find, at Universidad Finis Terrae, a private university in Chile, clinical exposure is required for undergraduate study in BME. Specifically, in their penultimate semester, *Práctica Inicial en campus clínico* is required, and another semester (*Práctica Profesional en campus clínico*) is required to earn the BME professional title.

US universities have developed partnerships with clinics in this region, which have provided clinical immersion experiences for US undergraduate students. Beyond Traditional Borders, a program out of Rice University, develops healthcare technologies for under-resourced parts of the world, such as Haiti and Ecuador (Richards-Kortum, Gray, and Oden 2012). While students rely on clinical partners in those countries to identify the problems (clinic-adjacent), some outstanding designs and their student inventors find their way to that country, sometimes to implement their solution (clinical immersion and intensive). Michigan Health Engineered for All Lives, a student co-curricular organization at the University of Michigan, also emphasizing healthcare technology development using an interdisciplinary, human-centered approach, has worked with healthcare professionals in the Dominican Republic, Nicaragua, and Peru to identify problems and/or confirm unmet needs, as well as test and receive feedback on prototypes.

9.3.7 Clinic Immersion in Oceania

At the UNSW in Australia, a suite of clinical immersion and health technology innovation programs has recently been developed to provide structured, translational experiences for biomedical engineering students. The curricular sequence includes three courses: the first focuses on identifying and validating unmet clinical needs through limited clinical shadowing (approximately ten hours across five weeks); the second, currently being piloted, supports solution development; and a third, pending approval, will emphasize translation and commercialization in collaboration with the business faculty. These courses are modeled on the Biodesign process and are designed to be interdisciplinary and scalable within the constraints of UNSW's ten-week academic terms.

In addition to these credit-bearing courses, UNSW supports more immersive, service-oriented extracurricular experiences through the Assistive Technology Hub.

These include international, PjBL programs in the Solomon Islands and Tonga, where students co-develop assistive technologies in collaboration with local stakeholders. Many of these projects are housed within UNSW's Vertically Integrated Projects program, allowing sustained, multi-year student involvement. While the integration of students into clinical settings is constrained by administrative and regulatory barriers, UNSW has leveraged its proximity to a major hospital and cross-faculty partnerships to facilitate access. UNSW's programs stand out in the Australian context for their degree of formalization and alignment with global clinical immersion models, despite broader regional challenges in program visibility and dissemination. (Kark 2024).

There is likewise a Biodesign Innovation program at the University of Melbourne in which teams of Master of Business Administration (MBA) and M.Eng. students collaborate with hospital clinicians to design medical devices to meet important clinical needs.

9.3.8 Volunteer Clinical Experiences Not Specific to BME

Not all immersion experiences occur within an academic setting. Some require that students pay for experiential services or meet certain fundraising targets. There are other programs that are not specific to BME. Furthermore, while they may offer volunteer clinical immersion to a broad array of engineers and others, they do not necessarily require participants to draw broader meaning, identify needs, or otherwise meet our working definition of clinical immersion.

EWH is a clinic-adjacent organization that offers opportunities for students to work in hospitals in low-resource countries, often repairing equipment or improving workflows. Their Summer Institutes are open to university students from all over the world. Medical Brigades is part of Global Brigades—a fundraise-to-participate model with university chapters across the United States, the United Kingdom, Europe, and Central America. Students who participate in Brigades experience a weeklong clinical immersion with professional caregivers in under-resourced clinics in Honduras, Ghana, Panama, Greece, Guatemala, and Belize (Global Medical Brigades 2024). Projects Abroad is a non-profit for-fee service that places students with professionals to work on projects, some of them clinical, in under-resourced environments (Projects Abroad US, Volunteer Abroad Programs & Internships n.d.). Finally, Global Medical Training blends these two models, using university chapters as organizational structures, yet relying on a for-fee model (Global Medical Training 2015). We are aware of at least one student engineering team that volunteered with this organization, conducted a study, and produced a manuscript (Guilford, Downs, and Royce 2008).

9.3.8.1 A Caveat

All this is not to say that clinical *exposure* is rare. Take, for example, the case of the Instituto de Ingeniería Biológica y Médica, Pontificia Universidad Católica de Chile:

> In our BME capstone course, students work with a clinical mentor, and they find or refine a need in the mentor's area. While we do not have a course wide generic clinical

> rotations for needs finding, almost all teams perform clinical visits with their mentors where they work on refining their need and learning more about their clinical problem to complement their investigations from literature. But the arrangement of these rotations is managed by the student teams, and at the discretion of the clinical director of the department in question, many times outside our institution. Since most times the clinical mentors organize these visits with high interest and high specificity, we have preferred to keep doing this instead of trying to organize generic clinical visits in our institution as part of the program.
>
> (Parot 2024).

These sorts of exposures are presumably not uncommon. They are the norm at the institutions of the authors. These push the boundaries of what constitutes "clinical immersion" through the dimensions of duration, focus, and level of engagement. Tracking them would be impractical since they take place at the level of individual mentors and students rather than being implemented through courses or programs.

9.4 BEST PRACTICES

What have we collectively learned about clinical immersion programs that others can use—current practitioners and those wishing to create immersion programs of their own?

Others have offered best practices stemming from their own experiences (Kotche et al. 2020; Moravec et al. 2023; Sienko et al. 2018; Sood et al. 2015). Based on the published literature, our examination of clinical immersion programs in the United States (Guilford, Kotche, and Schmedlen 2023) and our own experiences, we offer the following recommendations:

9.4.1 Build and Sustain Institutional Partnerships

The success of clinical immersion programs depends on the strength and sustainability of institutional relationships. For new programs, identifying clinical or academic partners can be challenging! Long-term partnerships with clinicians, department heads, administrative staff, and leadership—at both home and host institutions—create the foundation for effective and sustainable program delivery. When students are hosted at locations beyond the home institution, the host site selection should align with institutional strategy and consider logistical feasibility, shared educational missions, and the local context. When thoughtfully cultivated, these partnerships foster trust, continuity, and a culture that welcomes engineering students in clinical settings. Regular feedback from clinical partners, on what works, and what aspects of the program can be strengthened can ensure mutually beneficial outcomes.

9.4.2 Manage Expectations

Partnerships must be built on mutual understanding, especially around expectations. In most cases, clinical stakeholders should not anticipate polished, patient-ready solutions from student participants. Instead, they should recognize the value in exposing engineering students to authentic clinical challenges and providing feedback on prototypes of potential solutions. It is not uncommon for outputs from clinical immersion programs to be further developed in capstone design courses. Programs that are modeled on Biodesign may come closer to producing polished deliverables, but this typically occurs on extended timescales.

Clinical immersion programs also provide an opportunity for biomedical engineering students to strengthen their interpersonal communication skills when working with clinicians and other stakeholders. Providing context to the needs-finding process and defining vocabulary helps clinicians understand the approach and allows students to communicate across disciplines. In addition, programs should ensure that students recognize the privilege and responsibility of observing patient care. Situations arise where sensitivity and discretion are necessary. Engineering students must be reminded that although they are participating in a program that seeks to identify unmet clinical needs, patient care always takes priority.

For those programs with global health partnerships, students will gain cultural and social awareness and should receive appropriate training prior to the experience. In addition, partnerships should be cultivated in a way that is mutually beneficial for both partners and is grounded in a sincere commitment to build a sustainable framework for the clinicians, faculty, and students in the host country.

9.4.3 Establish Clear Administrative Processes

Managing the logistical and compliance-related aspects of clinical immersion requires proactive planning and efficient administrative systems. Student documentation, such as vaccination records and background checks, must be collected well in advance, often weeks before the immersion begins. Trainings such as mask fitting, gowning, patient privacy, and bloodborne pathogens also need to be organized well in advance and fully documented. A program administrator who has existing relationships across hospital departments can streamline operations, particularly in sensitive environments like operating rooms. In practice, having two administrators—one who understands the academic side of the program, and one who understands the clinical side—is advantageous.

9.4.4 Integrate Feedback and Reflection

A hallmark of effective clinical immersion is the inclusion of regular, structured opportunities for feedback and reflection. Students benefit immensely from weekly or even daily check-ins to help them process what they observe, navigate challenges as they arise, and iteratively refine their thinking. Faculty should ensure that learning is guided and intentional. These feedback mechanisms "close the loop" on experiential learning, allowing students to engage in cycles of observation, inquiry, and refinement.

Clinical practitioners may be tempted to provide students with specific learning targets or problems to examine. We find that this is not necessary if feedback, reflection, and iteration of clinical observation are integrated into the program.

9.4.5 Plan for the Long-Term Sustainability of the Program

For clinical immersion programs to persist and grow, they either need continued financial support or must be embedded into the academic curriculum. Programs that are optional enhancements dependent on external funding are destined to be short-lived. The NIH R25 programs in the United States may have expanded access to clinical immersion programming, but this is a fragile model; most of these programs do not persist beyond their initial five years of funding. Integrating immersion into coursework ensures that programs are structurally supported by the institution. Curricular integration also allows for ongoing evaluation of educational impact, promoting continuous improvement, long-term success, and a better scholarly understanding of these programs. We previously highlighted examples of clinical immersion experiences around the world that exist as credit-bearing courses. Potential limitations of this approach are that it may limit the duration of clinical immersion or limit the number of students who can participate. Extended immersions are necessary when needs identification is the goal of the program, whereas shorter observations can work for validating unmet needs or solutions.

9.4.6 Maximize Clinical Exposure and Maintain Post-Immersion Engagement

Effective clinical immersion allows students enough time to absorb and explore clinical problems through repeated cycles of observation, reflection, and inquiry. As mentioned earlier, immersions that are too brief limit students' ability to develop meaningful insights, iterate on ideas, filter information, and learn how to observe effectively. We recommend targeting 80 hours of immersion in each clinical unit to effectively identify and evaluate unmet clinical needs that can be adopted as viable design projects.

Ideally, students should have multiple opportunities to revisit clinical sites or to maintain communication with clinical partners as they transition back to the academic environment and begin design work. Indeed, we strongly recommend that, alongside their clinical observations, students also catalog the people with whom they interacted. Continued engagement ensures that solutions remain grounded in clinical reality and that students can validate their assumptions and refine their designs with stakeholder input throughout the design process.

9.4.7 Additional Best Practices for Special Circumstances

Scale can be a challenge, depending on the size of the educational program and the clinical environments available to it. It may not be practical for all students to participate if, for example, annual enrollments are in the hundreds. A practice employed by two institutions to get around this scaling problem is to embed participants in the immersion program with non-participants when it comes to capstone design teams. The participants share their first-hand knowledge, enthusiasm, and clinical contacts with their teammates (Sienko et al. 2018; Guilford et al. 2019).

When possible, it is best to provide an array of immersion environments, typically several clinical units, and to offer students some freedom of selection among them. Immersing students collectively in a broad range of clinical units results in a similarly broad range of identified unmet clinical needs and cross-fertilization of experiences and ideas to draw from. In addition, providing students with agency is generally thought to improve individual SOs (Stenalt and Lassesen 2022). Finally, specialized single-field immersion programs anecdotally have a harder time recruiting students, presumably because they appeal only to a subset of the available pool. Of course, not all host institutions have the benefit of offering a broad range of options.

When immersion programs are narrowly focused, it offers the opportunity to deepen students' understanding of underlying science. For example, a clinical immersion program in nephrology offers remarkable learning opportunities in ion transport, electrophysiology, and biotransport. When the connections are clear, clinical immersion programs should incorporate educational scaffolding that is structured and relevant. Case-based instruction in related topics offered before, during, or after the immersion provides contextualized learning.

9.5 CHALLENGES AND OPPORTUNITIES

9.5.1 Challenges

Clinical immersion in biomedical engineering education faces significant challenges, even though it is not new and promises enormous benefits to students and clinicians alike. These challenges were mentioned throughout this chapter.

First, achieving scalable and consistent access to clinical environments is difficult; programs often struggle to accommodate large student numbers while maintaining patient safety and workflow. Compounding this, establishing and sustaining robust partnerships between academic faculty and healthcare providers is challenging and is often hampered by misaligned expectations, administrative complexities, and the demanding schedules of clinical staff.

Further complicating the landscape is a lack of standardized outcomes and rigorous assessment methods; thus, even after decades of clinical immersion experiences, it remains difficult to make any quantitative statements about the educational impact of immersion programs and advocate for their long-term sustainability.

Finally, and most notably, there persists a global disparity in program documentation and dissemination. This limits the exchange of best practices, hinders the widespread adoption of effective clinical immersion models, and leaves us without an answer to the most fundamental question of them all—how common is clinical immersion in biomedical engineering education?

9.5.2 Opportunities

Opportunities mirror challenges. We conclude this chapter with ways that we might collectively overcome these obstacles and propose other directions that we may find clinical immersion may develop in the coming years.

9.5.2.1 Integrate Contemporary and Emerging Technologies for Scalable Access

It may never be the case that every biomedical engineering student can be offered the opportunity to be immersed in a clinical environment. In addition to remote observation of procedures (e.g., surgeries), the innovative use of VR and AR potentially offers appealing alternatives to the inherent challenges of access and scalability in clinical immersion. By creating immersive digital environments, programs can provide high-fidelity observational experiences for a much larger student body, overcoming limitations of physical space, hospital regulations, and geographic barriers. This allows for repeated exposure to diverse clinical scenarios, preparing students more effectively for their future roles while democratizing access to crucial clinical insights. In combination with generative AI, it may be possible for every student to have a unique experience that nonetheless accurately reflects the real-world challenges of clinical environments.

9.5.2.2 Broaden the Scope of Programs to System-Level Needs

Most clinical immersion experiences for biomedical engineering students result in devices, and those devices tend to be directly related to patient care. Moving beyond the sole focus on direct patient care and devices, there is a significant opportunity to immerse students in the wider healthcare ecosystem. This includes immersion experiences in hospital support units (e.g., medical imaging labs, clinical cleaning and sterilization, clinical labs, and supply chain management) and situations where systems and processes are at issue rather than a particular device. This expanded scope would allow students to identify unmet needs in reducing inefficiencies, improving workflows, and developing solutions that contribute to overall operational excellence and patient safety. Indeed, systems engineers have contributed greatly to the solution of specific healthcare challenges, and we are aware of one program where systems engineers experienced clinical immersion (Watts et al. 2015). There is a great opportunity in interdisciplinary training of biomedical engineers in systems engineering, particularly in the context of clinical immersion and needs identification (Ferreira et al. 2023).

9.5.2.3 Cultivate Longitudinal and Horizontal Integration

There may be value in establishing sustained, multi-semester or multi-year clinical engagements that bridge the gap between initial clinical observation, iterative design, and refined product. Such longitudinal integration (also known as vertical integration) may ensure that identified unmet needs are not merely observed but are deeply explored, validated, and prototyped with continuous feedback from clinicians and end users, leading to more relevant and impactful engineering solutions, improved skills, and a stronger professional identity for students. At least one study has shown value in this approach in mechanical engineering (Swenty, Dymond, and Ojard 2019). Horizontal integration (Balkos et al. 2017), in which a clinical immersion experience would be integral to multiple courses taken in the same semester or year, may also have outsized value.

9.5.2.4 Integrate Immersion With the Academic Curriculum and Use Standardized Assessment

To ensure the long-term sustainability of clinical immersion, these experiences must be embedded directly into the required BME curriculum rather than relying on optional, externally funded programs. In the United States, the federally funded grant programs that fueled a rapid expansion of clinical immersion experiences may be ending, and there are few alternative funding mechanisms. If external funding ends and unless long-term donors can be found, the only mechanism for continuation is curricular integration. Integration brings with it the opportunity to formalize robust assessments of these programs. We lack a general understanding of the impacts of these diverse immersion programs for lack of assessments, standardized or otherwise. Curricular integration with standardized assessment instruments will enable educators to measure the impact on student learning outcomes, such as problem-solving skills, interdisciplinary communication, professional identity, and understanding of healthcare disparities. This will provide the evidence needed to continuously improve and justify these valuable programs.

9.5.2.5 Share Knowledge Globally

Perhaps most importantly, the current literature is heavily biased to programs based in the United States. There is an immense opportunity for global knowledge sharing and adaptation of clinical immersion models. By documenting and disseminating successful programs from regions such as Africa, Latin America, and Oceania, institutions worldwide can learn from diverse approaches to overcome local resource constraints, cultural nuances, and healthcare system structures. We urge broader publication of these programs and reporting of them at educational conferences. Even broader documentation of their existence on public-facing websites would improve the global dialogue. This dialogue can lead to innovative, context-appropriate clinical immersion strategies that are responsive to specific regional needs, strengthening the global BME community and its ability to address healthcare challenges on a wider scale.

9.6 CONCLUSION

From extensive hospital- and clinic-based internships to clinic-adjacent classroom experiences, clinical immersion programs seek to provide authentic experiences that vary in setting, duration, focus, and engagement. Despite the diversity of experiences, each program demonstrates the shared commitment to experiential learning, interprofessional collaboration, and innovation across regions and institutions.

Clinical immersion in biomedical engineering education is a valuable means to bridge the gap between engineering and healthcare delivery. Students develop a deeper understanding of healthcare challenges, collaborate with other disciplines, and are empowered to identify and address unmet clinical needs through human-centered design. Best practices emphasize the importance of strong institutional partnerships, clear administrative processes, structured reflection, and curricular integration. Challenges remain—particularly in scaling access, sustaining programs, and assessing impact—yet these programs provide significant benefits and present opportunities to leverage emerging technologies, broaden the scope of immersion to include systems-level needs, and foster global knowledge exchange.

To ensure the long-term sustainability and effectiveness of clinical immersion in BME education, it is essential to incorporate these experiences within the curriculum, develop standardized assessment tools, and document programs more broadly. Doing so will not only enhance student learning and professional development but also contribute to a more responsive and innovative global healthcare system.

As the field continues to evolve, educators, institutions, and students must work collaboratively to expand access to these programs and deepen their impact to ensure that biomedical engineers are equipped to meet the complex challenges of modern healthcare.

REFERENCES

Balkos, Kyle Daniel, Benjamin Dow, Shoeleh Shams, Rania Al-Hammoud, Monica B. Emelko, Scott Walbridge, and Chris Bachmann. 2017. "Pedagogical Skill Development Through the Horizontal Integration of a Second-Year Engineering Curriculum." In *ASEE Annual Conference & Exposition*. https://peer.asee.org/pedagogical-skill-development-through-the-horizontal-integration-of-a-second-year-engineering-curriculum.

Biodesign Finland. n.d. *Biodesign Finland—Programme*. Accessed December 4, 2024. https://www.biodesignfinland.fi/programme.

Brinton, Todd J., Christine Q. Kurihara, David B. Camarillo, Jan B. Pietzsch, Julian Gorodsky, Stefanos A. Zenios, Rajiv Doshi, et al. 2013. "Outcomes from a Postgraduate Biomedical Technology Innovation Training Program: The First 12 Years of Stanford Biodesign." *Annals of Biomedical Engineering* 41 (9): 1803–10. https://doi.org/10.1007/s10439-013-0761-2.

Childress, Dudley S. 2002. "Development of Rehabilitation Engineering Over the Years: As I See It." *Journal of Rehabilitation Research and Development* 39 (6 Suppl): 1–10.

Chong, Seow Khoon Mark. n.d. Personal communication.

Dixon, Jon. 2001. "The Market Pull Versus Technology Push Continuum of Engineering Education." In *ASEE Annual Conference & Exposition Proceedings*, 6.1027.1–15. https://peer.asee.org/the-market-pull-versus-technology-push-continuum-of-engineering-education.

Ferreira, Susan, Eleanor Phelps, Shannon Abolmaali, Gary Reed, and Philip Greilich. 2023. "Opportunities to Apply Systems Engineering to Healthcare Interprofessional Education." *Frontiers in Medicine* 10 (September). https://doi.org/10.3389/fmed.2023.1241041.

Fowler, Susan M., Mary C. Knowlton, and Amy W. Putnam. 2018. "Reforming the Undergraduate Nursing Clinical Curriculum Through Clinical Immersion: A Literature Review." *Nurse Education in Practice* 31 (July): 68–76. https://doi.org/10.1016/j.nepr.2018.04.013.

Global Medical Brigades. 2024. *Global Medical Brigades*. Accessed May 31, 2024. https://medical.globalbrigades.org/get-involved/.

Global Medical Training. 2015. *Global Medical Training*. Accessed January 22, 2015. https://gmtonline.net/.

Guilford, William H., Kara Elizabeth Downs, and Trevor Joseph Royce. 2008. "Knowledge of Prenatal Health Care Among Costa Rican and Panamanian Women." *Revista Panamericana de Salud Pública* 23 (6): 369–76. https://doi.org/10.1590/S1020-49892008000600001.

Guilford, William H., Meg Keeley, Brian P. Helmke, and Timothy E. Allen. 2019. "Work in Progress: A Clinical Immersion Program for Broad Curricular Impact." In *ASEE Annual Conference & Exposition Proceedings*. https://peer.asee.org/work-in-progress-a-clinical-immersion-program-for-broad-curricular-impact.

Guilford, William H., Miiri Kotche, and Rachael H. Schmedlen. 2023. "A Survey of Clinical Immersion Experiences in Biomedical Engineering." *Biomedical Engineering Education* 3 (2): 113–22. https://doi.org/10.1007/s43683-023-00107-5.

Hays, Marguerite T. 2019. *A Historical Look at the Establishment of the Department of Veterans Affairs Research & Development Program*. Washington, DC: VA Office of Research & Development.

Kark, Lauren. 2024. Personal communication.

Kotche, Miiri, Anthony E. Felder, Kimberlee Wilkens, and Susan Stirling. 2020. "Perspectives on Bioengineering Clinical Immersion: History, Innovation, and Impact." *Annals of Biomedical Engineering* 48 (9): 2301–9. https://doi.org/10.1007/s10439-020-02508-x.

Maia, Catarina, and João Claro. 2014. "Biodesigning with European Undergraduates: Adaptation, Trade-Offs, and Outcomes." In *Proceedings of the National Collegiate Inventors and Innovators Alliance Annual Conference*, 1–10. https://www.proquest.com/openview/7f1457839ee1f4b074fd6ef6ba68b8ff/1?cbl=38283&pq-origsite=gscholar.

Malkin, Robert, and Leslie J. Calman. 2014. "Service-Learning in Biomedical Engineering: Engineering World Health (EWH)." *International Journal for Service Learning in Engineering, Humanitarian Engineering and Social Entrepreneurship*, December: 39–47. https://doi.org/10.24908/ijsle.v0i0.5542.

Montesinos, Luis, David Ernesto Salinas-Navarro, and Alejandro Santos-Diaz. 2023. "Transdisciplinary Experiential Learning in Biomedical Engineering Education for Healthcare Systems Improvement." *BMC Medical Education* 23 (April): 207. https://doi.org/10.1186/s12909-023-04171-x.

Moore, Wendy, Andrea Palerino, Katie Pawloski, Martha Desmond, Barbara Erickson, and Marsela Salkic-Mehkic. 2023. "The Effects of Clinical Immersion on Readiness for Nursing Practice." *Journal of Nursing Education* 62 (1): 47–50. https://doi.org/10.3928/01484834-20221109-08.

Moravec, Katherine R., Emily L. Lothamer, Amy Hoene, P. Mike Wagoner, Daniel J. Beckman, and Craig J. Goergen. 2023. "Clinical Immersion of Undergraduate Biomedical Engineering Students: Best Practices for Short-Term Programs." *Biomedical Engineering Education*, February: 1–7. https://doi.org/10.1007/s43683-022-00097-w.

National Institutes of Health. n.d. *PAR-10-140: Team-Based Design in Biomedical Engineering Education (R25)*. Accessed July 20, 2022. https://grants.nih.gov/grants/guide/pa-files/par-10-140.html.

Obungoloch, Johnes. 2025. Personal communication.

Parot, Vincente. 2024. Personal communication.

Ploss, Brittany, Tania S. Douglas, Matthew Glucksberg, Elsie Effah Kaufmann, Robert A. Malkin, Janet McGrath, Theresa Mkandawire, et al. 2017. "Part II: U.S.—Sub-Saharan Africa Educational Partnerships for Medical Device Design." *Annals of Biomedical Engineering* 45 (11): 2489–93. https://doi.org/10.1007/s10439-017-1898-1.

Projects Abroad. n.d. *Projects Abroad US: Volunteer Abroad Programs & Internships*. Accessed December 30, 2024. https://www.projects-abroad.org/.

Richards-Kortum, Rebecca, Lauren Vestewig Gray, and Maria Oden. 2012. "Engaging Undergraduates in Global Health Technology Innovation." *Science* 336 (6080): 430–1. https://doi.org/10.1126/science.1213947.

Schmedlen, Rachael, Jin Woo Lee, Prateek Shekhar, and Jan Stegemann. 2019. "The Clinical Peer Mentors Program: Student Motivations, Skills and Knowledge Acquisition, and

Influence on Career Path." In *ASEE Annual Conference & Exposition Proceedings.* https://peer.asee.org/the-clinical-peer-mentors-program-student-motivations-skills-and-knowledge-acquisition-and-influence-on-career-path.

Sienko, Kathleen H., Elsie Effah Kaufmann, Moses E. Musaazi, Amir Sabet Sarvestani, and Samuel Obed. 2014. "Obstetrics-Based Clinical Immersion of a Multinational Team of Biomedical Engineering Students in Ghana." *International Journal of Gynecology and Obstetrics* 127 (2): 218–20. https://doi.org/10.1016/j.ijgo.2014.06.012.

Sienko, Kathleen H., Margaret R. Young, Elsie Effah Kaufmann, Samuel Obed, K. A. Danso, H. S. Opare-Addo, A. T. Odoi, C. A. Turpin, and T. Konney. 2018. *Global Health Design: Clinical Immersion, Opportunity Identification and Definition, and Design Experiences.* http://ugspace.ug.edu.gh/handle/123456789/31471.

Sood, Sameer, Michael Short, Robert Hirsh, Jennifer Kadlowec, and Thomas Merrill. 2015. *Biodesign Through Clinical Immersion.* https://venturewell.org/open/wp-content/uploads/2013/10/SOOD.pdf.

Stenalt, Maria Hvid, and Berit Lassesen. 2022. "Does Student Agency Benefit Student Learning? A Systematic Review of Higher Education Research." *Assessment & Evaluation in Higher Education* 47 (5): 653–69. https://doi.org/10.1080/02602938.2021.1967874.

Swenty, Matthew, Benjamin Z. Dymond, and Sara Ojard. 2019. "Longitudinal Integration of the Same Design Project in Multiple Structural Engineering Courses." In *126th ASEE Annual Conference & Exposition: Charged Up for the Next 125 Years.* ASEE. http://www.scopus.com/inward/record.url?scp=85078786556&partnerID=8YFLogxK.

Watts, Bradley V., Brian Shiner, Jeffrey A. Cully, Stuart C. Gilman, James C. Benneyan, and William Eisenhauer. 2015. "Health Systems Engineering Fellowship: Curriculum and Program Development." *American Journal of Medical Quality* 30 (2): 161–6. https://doi.org/10.1177/1062860614523033.

Western University. n.d. *Western Medical Innovation Fellowship.* Accessed June 5, 2025. https://brainscan.uwo.ca/programs/medical_innovation_fellowship/index.html.

Zhou, Ying, Zheng Li, and Yingxin Li. 2021. "Interdisciplinary Collaboration Between Nursing and Engineering in Health Care: A Scoping Review." *International Journal of Nursing Studies* 117 (May): 103900. https://doi.org/10.1016/j.ijnurstu.2021.103900.

10 Practical Design of Laboratory Modules in Biomedical Engineering Undergraduate Curriculum

David A. Rubenstein

10.1 INTRODUCTION

Laboratory modules, incorporated through core and elective courses, play a critical role in the biomedical engineering undergraduate curriculum. When designed effectively, laboratory modules serve as a bridge between theoretical knowledge and practical applications. These modules provide students with hands-on experience that reinforces and extends lecture concepts, cultivates independent problem-solving skills, and enhances students' ability to think critically about real-world practical engineering challenges. Traditional, full-semester, laboratory courses often focus on general laboratory techniques, statistics, data analysis, and experimental design principles, which are applicable across various engineering and science disciplines. Traditional lab courses provide value to students via foundational and professional skills development. In contrast, laboratory modules integrated into specific courses, which build on and extend the skills developed in traditional lab courses, must be designed to align with the course material and to ensure that students develop both conceptual understanding and relevant technical competencies. In many cases, these modules allow students to freely explore concepts they are learning in class, instead of constraining them to a predetermined experimental process/outcome.

There are many considerations that should be weighed when deciding where in the curriculum and how to integrate laboratory modules within biomedical engineering courses. From student-centric and curriculum modernization perspectives, the addition of lab modules is typically driven by the need to create more engaging and application-oriented learning environments, which help to retain and train students in practical skills related to specific fields of biomedical engineering. By embedding practical experiments directly into coursework, students gain exposure to key principles in a way that mirrors real-world problem-solving. Furthermore, these modules are strategically developed to complement theoretical instruction, allowing students

DOI: 10.1201/9781003520313-10

to see immediate, tangible applications of the concepts they study. From a pedagogical standpoint, the addition of laboratory modules reinforces classroom learning but also prepares students for advanced coursework, research opportunities, and professional careers in the biomedical field. Therefore, there is a wide range of benefits to the careful and clear addition of lab modules into the biomedical engineering undergraduate curriculum.

One of the primary learning objectives that should be considered when developing lab modules is how the incorporation of this work will enhance students' ability to transfer their knowledge to practical scenarios. These objectives should focus on the application, analysis, and evaluation of knowledge. Rather than simply acquiring procedural laboratory skills, as is more typical with traditional laboratory courses, students should be asked to engage in the experiments and projects in a way that promotes interdisciplinary collaboration, analytical thinking, and innovation. By placing lab modules parallel with traditional course material, educators can offer students an enriched learning experience that goes beyond and reinforces passive instruction. This contextualized learning ensures that students build a strong foundation in biomedical engineering while developing the transferable skills necessary for success in graduate education, research, industry, and beyond. For those engineering programs that seek ABET accreditation, these approaches can help address the emphasis on and requirements for lifelong learning.

As educational institutions continue to evolve and emphasize experiential learning, the incorporation of laboratory modules in biomedical engineering education will become increasingly essential. These modules serve to deepen students' understanding of fundamental concepts and play a pivotal role in shaping their ability to tackle complex real-world biomedical challenges. Through a structured and well-integrated design, laboratory modules provide an effective means to prepare students for the dynamic and multidisciplinary nature of biomedical engineering (Prestigiacomo, Chan, and Kark 2024). Here, we will outline practical steps, considerations, and resources needed to implement lab modules into the biomedical engineering undergraduate curriculum.

10.2 THE ROLE OF LABORATORY MODULES IN BIOMEDICAL ENGINEERING UNDERGRADUATE EDUCATION

The biomedical engineering curriculum is well-defined and covers a wide array of theoretical skills that are required for students to effectively enter engineering or parallel professions (Prestigiacomo, Chan, and Kark 2024). In developing these curricula, laboratory courses have traditionally been included in one of two ways: (1) an introductory course designed to cover a wide range of common biomedical engineering laboratory techniques and (2) lab courses that are integrated with introductory foundational courses (e.g., physics, biology, and/or chemistry) (Leo et al. 2025). While these approaches are extremely valuable and generally lead to the required capstone engineering design course, it is atypical for students to see the connectivity of these laboratory courses with the larger curriculum. Furthermore, many times the growth of knowledge from these courses feels disjointed from the curriculum, except in the rare cases when there is a more comprehensive advanced laboratory course, which follows and requires the introductory lab course(s). In these instances, the advanced laboratory course is typically an elective course and not a core degree requirement.

In contrast, a well-designed and integrated set of laboratory modules serves as an essential link between theoretical instruction and hands-on application for biomedical engineering education in a more focused and direct manner. These types of modules allow students to directly apply their in-class knowledge to real-world projects, enhancing the overall understanding and retention of the course material (Osta 2024) through the introduction of reinforcing practical experiments. Studies have shown that with this approach, students gain a deeper understanding of complex concepts in parallel to developing the necessary skills to apply these skills (de Reviere et al. 2024). Finally, these modules enable students to visualize and manipulate biomedical engineering principles, fostering a more intuitive and experiential learning process.

Beyond reinforcing theoretical knowledge developed in class, well-designed and incorporated laboratory modules play a crucial role in fostering teamwork, problem-solving, and critical thinking skills (Saeidi and Earthman 2024; de Reviere et al. 2024). The biomedical engineering profession requires students to analyze intricate systems, how these systems interact with, replace, or augment biological systems, interpret experimental data, communicate findings, and optimize innovative solutions. By engaging in structured laboratory experiences that parallel developing coursework, students learn to troubleshoot issues, adapt to unexpected challenges, refine their experimental approaches, and apply theoretical skills in unique and creative ways. These skills are critical for their success in senior design courses, honors programs, undergraduate research projects, transition to graduate or professional skills, and professional job placements in biomedical and related industries.

One challenge that many educators face when adding laboratory modules into their curriculum is what content to remove to fit the new lab modules into the course. We believe that this decision should be framed by not only what the lab module adds to the curriculum, but also a deep reflection into identifying the redundancies that sometimes exist within the curriculum. In many instances, material is reviewed in several classes, perhaps due to its prerequisite nature (e.g., review of calculus principles), its importance to the identity of the department (e.g., a molecular biology oriented biomedical engineering department, may cover this material in multiple courses), or due to local modifications to courses (e.g., when new faculty modify an existing course to more align with their expertise). By identifying these redundancies and balancing where in the curriculum the material should be developed, it is possible that the addition of lab modules would not compete with conventionally covered content. Furthermore, we also suggest that faculty think of new creative ways to examine student comprehension, to open class periods for lab modules. For instance, providing three to four major exams throughout the semester allows students a more balanced opportunity to earn credits in individual courses. However, this approach also requires a significant amount of class time to administer and hold review sessions for the exams. Also, take-home, open-ended, and/or self-paced project-based exams may provide instructors with similar means to assess student learning, in lieu of the traditional in-class exam format (Das 2020; Mayled et al. 2019).

To maximize the impact of incorporated laboratory modules, these modules should be strategically aligned with both course-specific and broader program-level objectives. This suggests that individual instructors and courses may need to reimagine these learning objectives with a more modern, student-centric, and active learning framing. This process is important as the field of biomedical engineering and the need for our students to be trained with current practical skills continue to evolve. One of the key goals when integrating lab activities with specific course content is to develop specialized technical competencies relevant to their field of study. These competencies should be founded in and can be used to reinforce the course content. Studies have shown that with this approach, students can more effectively attain and retain course learning outcomes, even with online or virtual labs (Moyaki, Dunmoye, and May 2025).

When revisiting learning outcomes at the program level, laboratory modules can contribute to the overarching goals of biomedical engineering education by systematically building competencies across multiple courses. This can ensure that students develop a cohesive skill set across the breadth and/or depth of biomedical disciplines that evolve throughout their academic journey. Thoughtful sequencing of lab activities across introductory and advanced courses can help scaffold student learning and reinforce key engineering principles over time. These activities can converge at the capstone course level, where design teams are built from students with broad and diverse expertise (perhaps even across majors). The capstone project can be enhanced and tuned to market or clinical needs in a more effective and productive way. To help programs begin to ideate how lab modules can be integrated throughout the curriculum, we have developed a few case studies that could be relatively easily integrated into many biomedical engineering undergraduate degree programs (see Section 10.6). When developing lab modules tailored to your program's course sequence, it is important to remember that the overarching goal of integrating laboratory modules is to provide students with structured opportunities to apply theoretical knowledge in meaningful ways, while fostering deeper learning and preparing them for professional pursuits in a range of biomedical engineering careers.

10.3 GUIDING PRINCIPLES FOR LABORATORY MODULE DESIGN

We propose four key guiding principles to consider, in order to ensure the successful implementation of laboratory modules into the biomedical engineering undergraduate curriculum. These principles are Alignment with Course and Program Learning Outcomes, Practical Feasibility, Student Preparation, and TA and Professional Staff Preparation. Incomplete preparation in one of these principles may lead to a failure of the lab module, which can have a significant impact on student learning. It is also important for programs to initiate a continuous assessment, review, and modification process to ensure that learning outcomes are set appropriately and are being attained by each cohort. As new technologies develop and are integrated into common practice, student preparation and expectations may be different; thus, the lab modules must evolve with the student preparation.

To ensure that laboratory modules are effective, they must be aligned with both course-specific and broader program-level learning outcomes. When degree programs have course sequences, these modules can also be integrated within sequence learning goals. Well-defined learning objectives can highlight both the theoretical knowledge gained and the practical skills that will be developed in the course. Specific experiment modules or techniques can then be mapped directly to these objectives. Assessment of attainment of learning objectives within the lab modules would need to be undertaken in a clear and comprehensive manner. This alignment may require revising learning outcomes and the assessment of the outcomes to better integrate laboratory components.

At the program level, laboratory modules should be designed to build toward key competencies across multiple courses within the curriculum. Some modules may be integrated into prerequisite chains to ensure progressive skill development, while others may be structured to run concurrently in different courses to reinforce interdisciplinary connections. A critical focus should be placed on fostering transferable skills such as analytical thinking, collaboration, and innovation rather than merely procedural knowledge. Finally, student progression of learning can be assessed with this approach, and final core degree competencies can then be assessed in the final capstone element.

To ensure the success of laboratory modules, they must be practically feasible. While individual universities and departments will have their own unique constraints, there are a few considerations that are commonly considered. These include resource availability (which includes equipment, professional staff, TAs, and space), maintenance costs, and instructional time. In terms of resources, a large up-front institutional investment may be required at the department, college, or university level. In the absence of physical space that meets all local safety codes or equipment, the implementation of hands-on lab modules will be difficult. Staff to set up, order consumables, and troubleshoot may also be essential. Appropriate TA staff, to help during lab sessions and assignment grading, may also be required, especially to maintain an appropriate student-to-instructor ratio in this setting. While staff and TAs may not be essential to the implementation of lab modules, as programs begin to scale lab modules throughout the curriculum, these resources may become more essential. Scalability should also be considered to accommodate different class sizes, with approaches tailored for small, medium, and large groups. Standardized lab protocols and accessible instructional resources can further support module feasibility across the curriculum. In the absence of a large investment, it is possible for programs to begin to implement virtual modules. While this approach can begin to address data interpretation and reporting skills, the true hands-on active learning strategies would require a more thorough investment.

Equipment, maintenance costs, and the availability of funds to replace worn equipment need to be considered. If monetary resources can only be provided at start-up, the feasibility of developing long-term hands-on modules reduces, since it is inevitable that equipment will break down, wear out, or need replacing. Furthermore, as mentioned earlier, instructional time must be considered. Students cannot be expected to participate in experiments that take longer than their scheduled instructional time, as they will have other responsibilities. It may also be challenging to divide experiments into multiple smaller pieces, since this may take too much time away from the formal lecture-based instructional time. Therefore, to properly introduce laboratory modules into the curriculum, many aspects need to be considered and balanced for an impactful approach.

Students must be adequately prepared and trained when incorporating lab modules into the curriculum. In an ideal situation, students' foundational laboratory skills would be assessed in an introductory lab course. This course can cover all safety regulations and typical biomedical engineering skills. For instance, introductory skills may include pipetting, microscopy, and basic circuit design. In the lab module, prerequisite knowledge should be clearly communicated to students, and review sessions can be developed and scheduled as needed. If your program does not have an introductory lab course or when prior coursework does not adequately prepare students, alternative instructional methods such as prerequisite workshops or online modules should be considered. It is critical that students are adequately prepared so that they can realize the learning objectives and make the most of the offered laboratory module.

Finally, for the efficient implementation of lab modules, trained and knowledgeable TAs and professional staff are critical. Their assumed knowledge base and prerequisite expertise must be well-defined prior to hiring or assigning TAs to the lab module. Course instructors must clearly communicate the expectations for assisting students during the lab period. This staff must be trained in appropriate lab safety procedures and how to supervise students in a lab setting. Their previous knowledge of and training in experimental techniques should be discussed. If deficiencies are identified, it is possible that training plans are put into place prior to enrolled students conducting the modules. However, this approach becomes risky as lab modules should be run efficiently at the scheduled time during the semester, so that enrolled students gain the most from the opportunity. Prior to the beginning of the semester, staff training should include safety protocols and pedagogical strategies to ensure a smooth and effective learning experience for students. We recommend the development of lab protocols and standard operating procedures to ensure consistency between course offerings.

10.4 FRAMEWORK FOR LABORATORY MODULE DEVELOPMENT

Developing effective laboratory modules requires a structured framework. A well-planned laboratory module should balance technical rigor, accessibility, and student engagement. To begin, instructors must consider the duration of the module and its scheduling in the semester. The modules that we describe in this chapter can be structured as standalone experiments within a single lecture cycle, multi-week projects, or semester-long assignments. There are advantages to each of these approaches. Single lecture modules provide students with a range of short, structured assignments, whereas multi-week projects provide students with a more realistic view of the length for an experiment. Semester-long projects would focus more on team dynamics and addressing more relevant questions in the field. Some of the disadvantages to these approaches are that single lecture modules can lose the innovation aspects and tend to be more predetermined procedural-based tasks. Multi-week projects can become challenging depending on the time of the semester, other responsibilities, and the logistics of retaining experimental setups for an extended period. A semester-long project can be too complex for the depth of knowledge expected from the students.

Labs should be strategically scheduled to reinforce key concepts introduced in lectures. Aligning experiments with lecture content ensures that students apply theoretical knowledge in a timely manner, reinforcing learning through active engagement. Students should be provided with time to digest the theoretical concepts prior to initiating the module. The frequency should also be considered. Some courses may benefit from weekly lab modules, while others may incorporate periodic lab activities alongside lectures. Modules should be flexible enough to accommodate different teaching styles and institutional constraints while maintaining pedagogical effectiveness. Students do not want to feel like these modules are rushed or function as an afterthought to the course material. It is critically important to design modules that are relevant to both the course and the broader biomedical engineering curriculum. Lab modules should reflect real-world challenges that can include the design of relevant biomedical devices, analysis of physiological data, or work with biological materials. Reviewing the course outcomes and program learning objectives can help identify clear links on how the modules contribute to overarching program goals.

Instructors should also consider the optimal team configuration, in terms of both size and responsibilities. Assigning team roles based on previous experiences or rotating roles may be an effective strategy. Along these lines, some experiments lend themselves to team-based assessments, while others may be better suited for individual evaluation. Assignments should strike a balance between collaborative problem-solving and personal accountability. Regardless of the approach, clear rubrics should be communicated to the students. The complexity of the module should be balanced with accessibility to all students, where it is important to make the module as realistic as possible. However, you do not want the challenge to overwhelm students who are less familiar with the basic techniques. All modules should be inclusive and considerate of diverse learning needs. Ensuring that all students have access to necessary resources, accommodating alternative learning needs, and avoiding unnecessary financial burdens (e.g., requiring costly personal lab kits) are essential in promoting equity in education. By adhering to these structured design principles, laboratory modules can effectively complement lecture-based learning, enhance student engagement, and ensure that biomedical engineering education remains hands-on, practical, and aligned with industry needs.

10.5 PRACTICAL CONSIDERATIONS

Successfully implementing laboratory modules requires careful consideration of practical factors that affect their feasibility, effectiveness, and sustainability. Biomedical engineering is inherently interdisciplinary, drawing from fields such as mechanical engineering, electrical engineering, materials science, biological sciences, and the medical sciences. Effective laboratory modules should reflect this interdisciplinary nature by engaging faculty from multiple disciplines and incorporating industry perspectives. Collaborating with faculty from different departments can ensure that laboratory modules remain comprehensive and relevant to the broad scope of biomedical engineering. For example, a bioinstrumentation module may benefit from insights from both electrical engineering faculty (circuit design) and physiology faculty (biomedical signal interpretation). Furthermore, partnering with industry professionals can provide students with exposure to real-world applications and the opportunity for students to work on projects related to emerging trends.

There are numerous potential logistical challenges that need to be addressed to successfully implement laboratory modules. Biomedical engineering laboratories often require specialized equipment such as cell culture incubators, motion capture systems, and bioelectronic sensors. Maintaining and replenishing consumables can be costly and require careful planning. Institutions must consider strategies for optimizing resource use, such as shared lab spaces, bulk purchasing agreements, and periodic audits of inventory. Furthermore, as education environments continue to evolve, adapting laboratory modules for hybrid or online learning environments can present additional challenges or opportunities. Virtual labs that use simulation software to model experimental procedures can potentially address some of the intrinsic financial challenges to implementing lab modules. Take-home customizable remote lab kits can be purchased at nominal costs, allowing students to conduct experiments on the go. Instructors can develop video demonstrations of complex techniques followed by data analysis exercises.

In some cases, proprietary out-of-the-box systems may be an optimal approach. These systems have many benefits, which include their stable data acquisition, cost-effectiveness (especially when purchasing a substantial number of kits), accessibility, and online resources. However, these systems also minimize some aspects of laboratory work, such as troubleshooting experimental setups. A major aspect of firsthand professional experiences is learning that, in many instances, the design does not work as originally expected. This is critically important for students to learn.

Finally, instructors will need to ensure adherence to institutional and legal safety standards when developing lab modules. Depending on the nature of the lab module, these standards can take different forms. However, we thought that it would be valuable to highlight some common considerations that biomedical engineering instructors may face when implementing lab modules. Students and TAs must receive the appropriate mandatory safety training before participating in laboratory activities. This can include proper handling of biological materials, electrical safety protocols, general lab safety, emergency procedures, and reporting processes. The importance of compliance with biosafety regulations and adherence to the Occupational Safety and Health Administration and Environmental Protection Agency guidelines for chemical and waste disposal should also be discussed as appropriate. This is especially true when one of the goals of the work would be to train students for entrance into the workforce. Instructors must also ensure the availability of personal protective equipment (PPE) and must enforce the proper use of lab coats, gloves, eye protection, and other PPE to maintain a safe learning environment while instructing students about the expected norms of working in a laboratory environment. By addressing these considerations, institutions can create laboratory modules that are both educationally effective and operationally sustainable, ensuring that students receive high-quality, hands-on training.

10.6 CASE STUDIES: PRACTICAL APPLICATIONS OF INCORPORATING LAB MODULES INTO THE BIOMEDICAL ENGINEERING UNDERGRADUATE CURRICULUM

The following case studies illustrate examples of how one can implement laboratory modules in a few common areas taught in the biomedical engineering curriculum. Each case study outlines the module's objective, learning outcomes, and prerequisite knowledge, with the goal of demonstrating how hands-on experiments reinforce theoretical concepts and develop critical technical skills. By integrating these modules into biomedical engineering courses, educators can create a more immersive and application-driven learning environment that prepares students for future careers in industry, research, and healthcare innovation.

10.6.1 Case Study 1: Biomaterials Module

The objective of this module is to focus on the characterization of materials used in biomedical implants. Students will evaluate the mechanical properties of various biomaterials to understand their suitability for medical applications. If possible, students may synthesize materials to explore their impact on mechanical behavior. Instructors will need access to tensile testing capabilities for various biomaterials, including polymers and metals, and for the comparison of commercially available biomaterials (e.g., titanium alloys and biodegradable polymers) with experimental materials produced by students (if facilities allow). At the completion of this module, students will be able to obtain a better understanding of the stress-strain behavior in biomaterials, relate mechanical properties to biomedical applications, and gain hands-on experience with material testing equipment. To obtain the most out of this module, students should be familiar with the fundamentals of engineering mechanics, particularly stress and strain concepts, and material science, including polymer and metal properties in biomedical contexts.

10.6.2 Case Study 2: Bioinstrumentation Module

The objective of this module is to have students design, build, and assess a basic electrocardiogram (ECG) circuit to understand bioelectrical signal acquisition, processing, and interpretation. Instructors will need to provide students with access to Arduino microcontrollers (or similar) and operational amplifiers to build a basic ECG circuit. Electrodes will be placed on volunteers to record bioelectrical signals. Signal processing techniques, such as filtering and amplification, will be implemented to refine the ECG waveform. Students will analyze ECG data, identify key waveform components, and troubleshoot issues such as noise interference. At the completion of this module, students will gain experience with biomedical instrumentation design, develop proficiency in signal acquisition, filtering, and analysis, and understand the physiological basis of the ECG and its clinical relevance. To obtain the most out of this module, students should be familiar with bioelectrical signal fundamentals, the basics of circuit design, and knowledge of cardiovascular physiology and ECG interpretation.

10.6.3 Case Study 3: Cellular/Molecular Biology Module

The objective of this module is to allow students to analyze cellular behavior in response to engineered environments. Students can fabricate biomaterial scaffolds, culture cells, and evaluate cellular responses. Instructors will need access to facilities that allow for the fabrication of various biomaterial scaffolds, culturing of mammalian cells on different biomaterial surfaces, and the use of a fluorescent microscope. At the completion of this module, students will be able to apply cell biology concepts to tissue engineering/regenerative medicine, gain hands-on experience with cell culture and biomaterial characterization, and develop skills in quantitative biological analysis and experimental design. To obtain the most out of this module, students should be familiar with the fundamentals of cell biology and the practical considerations of tissue engineering and biomaterial interactions.

10.6.4 Case Study 4: Biomechanics Module

The objective of this module is to allow students to analyze human joint mechanics to understand kinematic principles in real-world applications such as rehabilitation and prosthetics design using motion capture technology. Instructors will need access to motion capture cameras and force plates to analyze gait cycles and force distribution during normal and simulated injury conditions. Instructors can relate this to the improvement of prosthetic and orthotic devices. At the completion of this module, students will be able to develop an understanding of human motion analysis techniques, apply kinematic principles to real-world scenarios, and interpret biomechanical data to inform medical and engineering decisions. To obtain the most out of this module, students should be familiar with the fundamentals of engineering mechanics in biological contexts, have had an introduction to kinesiology and biomechanics principles, and understand motion analysis techniques and force measurement.

10.7 CONCLUSION AND FUTURE DIRECTIONS

Well-designed and integrated lab modules provide students with invaluable hands-on experience, bridging the gap between theoretical knowledge and practical application. These modules enhance conceptual understanding, foster critical thinking, and develop essential technical and problem-solving skills. By aligning lab activities with course and program-level learning outcomes, students gain relevant, real-world experience that prepares them for careers in industry, research, and healthcare innovation. Despite these clear benefits, implementing laboratory modules comes with challenges. Logistical constraints such as equipment availability, faculty and staff training, and curriculum scheduling must be addressed to ensure successful execution. Additionally, adapting lab experiences for varying class sizes and online learning environments requires innovative approaches to maintain educational quality.

As biomedical engineering education continues to evolve, educators must continuously refine and expand laboratory experiences to align with emerging trends, ensuring that students remain competitive in a rapidly advancing field. Emerging technologies, such as VR and AR, may provide additional opportunities for immersive lab simulations. These technologies may allow students to interact with complex biomedical concepts in a controlled, digital environment. Surgical procedures, molecular interactions, and biomechanics experiments can all be simulated, providing a cost-effective alternative to expensive physical setups. AI can be leveraged to assist students in analyzing experimental results, providing real-time feedback, predictive modeling, and automated grading for lab reports.

As online and hybrid learning models become more prevalent, institutions can explore remote-access labs, where students can control physical lab equipment through cloud-based platforms. Pre-recorded or live-streamed demonstrations, combined with data analysis exercises, can offer flexible alternatives for students without direct access to laboratory facilities. Furthermore, lab modules can be co-scheduled with other departments to enhance and promote interdisciplinary applications. For example, mechanical engineering, electrical engineering, or computer science students can work side by side with biomedical engineering students while investigating biomedically relevant topics.

Well-equipped laboratory spaces can additionally serve as a recruitment tool to attract prospective students. Outreach initiatives can increase community engagement and can be used to highlight the role of biomedical engineering in solving healthcare challenges. When developing these modules, we recommend that the modules continue to evolve and improve, using a continuous assessment procedure through student evaluations, faculty observations, and performance metrics. As resources permit, adjustments to lab design, equipment usage, and instructional materials can be made to enhance student engagement and learning outcomes. By embracing these strategies, we hope that educators can maximize the impact of laboratory modules, ensuring that biomedical engineering students receive a dynamic, industry-relevant education that prepares them for the challenges and opportunities of the future.

REFERENCES

Das, Dillip Kumar. 2020. "Civil Engineering Students' Perceptions of Conventional and Alternative Assessment Methods." *African Journal of Research in Mathematics, Science and Technology Education* 24 (1): 116–28.

de Reviere, Arno, Bram Jacobs, Ingeborg Stals, and Jeriffa De Clercq. 2024. "Cross-Curricular Project-Based Laboratory Learning Enables Hands-On Interdisciplinary Education for Chemical Engineering Students." *Education for Chemical Engineers* 47: 1–9.

Leo, Chuen How, Navin Sockalingam, Michelle X. Tan, Yimin Zhu, and Xin Khoo. 2025. "Instructional Design and Implementation of an Inquiry-Based Laboratory Class for Undergraduate Engineering Students." *Biomedical Engineering Education*. https://doi.org/10.1007/s43683-025-00188-4.

Mayled, Lindy Hamilton, Lydia Ross, Casey Jane Ankeny, and Jay Oswald. 2019. "Effects of Alternative Course Design and Instructional Methods in the Engineering Classroom." In *2019 ASEE Annual Conference & Exposition Proceedings*. https://peer.asee.org/effects-of-alternative-course-design-and-instructional-methods-in-the-engineering-classroom.

Moyaki, D., I. Dunmoye, and D. May. 2025. "Students' Perceived Usefulness of Virtual Reality Laboratories." In *Online Laboratories in Engineering and Technology Education*, edited by D. Auer, M. E. May and A. Kist. Cham: Springer. https://doi.org/10.1007/978-3-031-xxxxxx.

Osta, Anu. 2024. "Encouraging Student Participation in Developing Custom-Built Lab Modules in Undergraduate Engineering and Science Course." In *2024 ASEE Annual Conference & Exposition Proceedings*. https://peer.asee.org/encouraging-student-participation-in-developing-custom-built-lab-modules.

Prestigiacomo, Rita, Chun Chuen Chan, and Lauren Kark. 2024. "A Biomedical Engineering Curriculum Development: A Qualitative Study Engaging Four Stakeholders." *European Journal of Education* 59 (2): e12632. https://doi.org/10.1111/ejed.12632.

Saeidi, Amir, and James C. Earthman. 2024. "Innovations in an Undergraduate Laboratory to Increase Engagement." In *2024 IEEE Frontiers in Education Conference (FIE) Proceedings*. https://doi.org/10.1109/FIE58676.2024.xxxxx.

11 Embedding Ethics Within Bioengineering Education

Brit Shields, Aria Zheyuan Huang, and Disha Vaswani

11.1 INTRODUCTION

A robust body of literature offers insight into the wide variety of approaches to engineering ethics education. Curriculum offerings include standalone ethics courses as well as an embedded ethics approach. Valuable resources for those building engineering ethics curricula for biomedical engineering students may find the National Academy of Engineering (NAE) publications, as well as additional secondary literature, informative. In 2016, the NAE published a valuable collection of "exemplars in engineering ethics education" that featured innovative lesson plans and educational programming, often entailing active learning components, ethics content that connect directly to technical content, and replicable or scalable approaches (National Academy of Engineering 2016). The following year, the NAE published the proceedings of a workshop on "Overcoming Challenges to Infusing Ethics into the Development of Engineers" (National Academy of Engineering 2017). A systematic review of US engineering ethics approaches offers further insight into decisions around curriculum strategies (standalone courses versus across the curriculum versus outside of the curriculum programming), format options, rationalization and justification, pedagogical choices in student activities and assignments, engagement with different approaches including philosophy and case studies, and quantitative and qualitative assessment models (Hess and Fore 2018).

Among this landscape of options for teaching engineering ethics within biomedical engineering is embedded ethics, also known as ethics across the curriculum. The secondary literature expands upon the importance of institutional context when embarking on this approach, reflecting on examples of success, failure, and challenges (Mitcham and Englehardt 2019). Mitcham and Englehardt, for example, conclude that the ethics across the curriculum approach largely depends on: "grass roots faculty interest, administrative receptivity, and interdisciplinary leadership" (Mitcham and Englehardt 2019).

The rationale for embedding ethics across the curriculum includes allowing for ethics content placed in relation to advanced, discipline-specific content as well as normalizing sociotechnical approaches to engineering practice. The Harvard

DOI: 10.1201/9781003520313-11

Embedded EthiCS faculty shared that "embedding ethical reasoning throughout the entire CS curriculum has the potential to habituate students to thinking ethically as they develop algorithms and build systems, both in their studies and as they pursue technical work in their careers" (Grosz et al. 2019).

Engineering ethics material is broad, and the topics are expansive, which may include interdisciplinary studies of risk and safety, moral philosophy, and sustainability considerations, and can be tailored to the specific needs of an institution and curriculum. The approach can be flexible, as ethics can be emphasized through themes that persist throughout a curriculum, such as value-sensitive design, or consist of individually curated modules in each course. The content can be developed by a team that offers interdisciplinary perspectives or by the course instructors themselves (Grosz et al. 2019; Hess et al. 2024).

Various biomedical and bioengineering departments have published on their institution's embedded ethics approach. Indiana University-Purdue University Indianapolis faculty reflected on their goal that the ethics material presented in their technical courses will "better equip our students with reflection methods that will help them recognize ethical issues related to the BME profession," as well as on the challenges, including tentative course instructors, concerns of ethics coursework being too distant from the technical material, or diverse expectations for ethics education (Miller et al. 2020, 3). Duke University has introduced a "snail progression" of ethics education within its biomedical engineering curriculum, introducing a distinct multidisciplinary framework for each of the four years of the curriculum: "humility, curiosity, imagination, and complexity" (Bucholz et al. 2024, 1). In an earlier paper, Chan et al. (2023, 1) from Duke wrote that "we believe that an iterative 'ethics everywhere' approach to engineering education supports students in their development and scaffolds important ethical principles in identifying ethical dilemmas and will provide value in their prospective careers." At Duke, ethics modules are embedded into a first-year design course, several sophomore-level and junior-level courses, and all senior design courses, covering content such as foundational bioethics frameworks, moral philosophy, and risk analyses (Chan et al. 2023). Other institutions, such as Arizona State University and Pennsylvania State University, have implemented comparable embedded ethics approaches (Frow et al. 2017; Tang et al. 2020).

11.2 IN PRACTICE AT THE UNIVERSITY OF PENNSYLVANIA

Our team utilizes embedded ethics as a pedagogical approach to incorporate sociotechnical material along with technical content. As students are honing their technical skills, they are also acquiring the knowledge and skill sets necessary to understand and navigate the societal context of engineering practice. At Penn, our aim is twofold: to allow for ethics content to connect directly to discipline-specific advanced technical content and to normalize sociotechnical thinking (STT) as part of the engineering design process.

Following a semester-long faculty-led committee to assess ethics and writing education within the engineering school in which Shields participated, it was determined that our students would benefit from both a standalone ethics course *and* embedded ethics content. Engineering students were already required to take a standalone ethics course, which provides them with foundational content in ethics. The addition of ethics modules within technical courses would address discipline-specific ethical challenges as well as normalize societal considerations in engineering practice. Launched in 2020, Shields has led the engineering ethics initiative to embed ethics content within core required technical courses. A pilot was run to introduce ethics modules with an introductory bioengineering course and a graduate-level computer science course. It was then determined, in consultation with school and department leadership, to build the engineering ethics initiative vertically within the Department of Bioengineering. Reflections on this process were published in the American Society of Engineering Education conference proceedings (Tonn et al. 2025).

After conducting background research on pedagogical models and examples from other institutions, we aimed to expand an embedded engineering ethics pilot within the Department of Bioengineering. Inspired by Harvard's success in embedding ethics into the computer science curriculum, we took a similar approach in our practice in bioengineering (Grosz et al. 2019). We first approached faculty members within the department to gauge their interest in incorporating ethics materials into the existing classes. With the goal of weaving ethics throughout the four-year curriculum, we proposed a four-year ethics roadmap outlining the learning objectives for each year, identifying required core technical courses where we would embed ethics.

Through our conversations with the faculty, we decided that we would carry out a gradual implementation, developing and implementing ethics material into one or two courses per academic year, with the goal of having a robust embedded ethics curriculum fully implemented by year five of the pilot program. The first portion of the engineering ethics initiative, rolled out in the Fall 2020 semester, was in the first-year introductory course. The engineering ethics initiative team developed both asynchronous modules and led synchronous discussions intended to help students establish a foundation in societal considerations of engineering practice. After the pilot year, the department recognized the tremendous value in the continued incorporation of ethics teaching into additional core BE classes. Building on the success of the first-year class, the rest of the engineering ethics initiative components were implemented sequentially. Ethics within a sophomore lab class rolled out in the Spring 2022 semester, followed by two junior labs in Spring 2023 and Fall 2023, and finally senior design in Fall 2024.

We established a partnering strategy to develop ethics modules based on technical teaching across the four-year curriculum. The engineering ethics initiative team reviewed the existing bioengineering course lesson plans and assignments and identified topics that intersected with potential ethical discussions. The team then compiled a menu of learning objectives around relevant topics (i.e., animal research, biocontainment, and health data privacy) and collaborated with the class instructors to select the topics. Additionally, we decided that our pedagogical approach should be tailored to the stage of student development and teaching staff capacity. The first-year course's ethics modules entail asynchronous homework assignments as well as in-class discussions. Due to the lab format of the sophomore and junior courses, we found that it would be most effective to distribute ethics modules as part of the written assignments. Through an iterative process in collaboration with the course instructors, the engineering ethics team designed written assignments that seamlessly integrate into the existing lab assignments.

The senior design material includes an interactive, team-based student activity as well as a compilation of resources accessible as needed for either students or instructors. Importantly, the ethics material produced by the engineering ethics initiative team was meant to supplement and not replace any existing efforts by individual instructors to include the ethical and societal context of engineering practice in the coursework. The material was developed with a four-year ethics roadmap in mind, ensuring that foundational material was introduced early in the curriculum and that more project-based material was introduced in senior design.

One highlight of the engineering ethics initiative is the diverse teaching team. One of the critical aspects of our practice is that we highly value interdisciplinary expertise and perspectives among the team members. The initiative lead has training in the history and sociology of science and brings a humanities perspective into the department. We then appointed graduate student engineering ethics fellows from diverse disciplinary backgrounds, such as bioengineering and law. The student engineering ethics fellows contribute significantly to reviewing the technical lab instructional materials, providing multidisciplinary pedagogical resources, and developing lesson plans drawing from diverse fields such as legal studies, engineering design, and the history of technology. The success of this program has greatly benefited from having team members contributing from the sociological, technical, and legal perspectives.

As the ethics modules were rolled out, we conducted assessments focusing on four main aspects: class participation (first-year only), written work (first-year through senior year), end-of-semester surveys (first-year through junior years), and informal instructor feedback. The ethics team reviewed student performances in in-class discussions and written responses to identify areas for curriculum improvement. We also performed informal evaluations vertically by comparing student work across the four years that we oversee. By taking internal and external feedback every semester, we were able to update the four-year ethics curriculum regularly to better represent the shifting landscape in the field. As a final touch, we also designed an additional senior survey in collaboration with the undergraduate curriculum chair to evaluate the "readiness" of our graduates in their ethical training. This allows us to further quantify the impact of the four-year ethics roadmap in a systematic manner.

11.3 BIOENGINEERING ETHICS ROADMAP AND CURRICULUM EXAMPLES

The ethics roadmaps detailing the technical content and the associated ethics content for each of the core bioengineering courses are described in Tables 11.1–11.5. The engineering ethics initiative includes ethics modules within an introductory course, three bioengineering laboratory courses throughout the sophomore and junior years, and senior design. On the whole, the learning objectives for each course scaffold upon each other to form a cumulative ethics education.

The first-year course focuses on foundational content such as principles of bioethics and professional responsibility (see Table 11.1). Some of the detailed lesson plans have been published in *Biomedical Engineering Education* (Shields 2023). In the sophomore and junior laboratory courses, students explore the applications of these foundational concepts to the development processes of specific technologies (see Tables 11.2–11.4). Finally, the senior design sequence emphasizes general concerns of professional ethics that students are likely to encounter in their post-graduate careers (see Table 11.5).

TABLE 11.1
Bioengineering ethics roadmap for BE 1000: introduction to bioengineering

Technical Content	Ethics Content
Synthetic biology	The role of ethics education and democratic deliberation in bioengineering practice
Neuroengineering	Principles of biomedical ethics and moral philosophy as applied to biomedical engineering
Biomedical devices	Equitable and inclusive medical technologies
Medical imaging and radiation biology	Cancer screening guidelines and diverse stakeholder perspectives

TABLE 11.2
Bioengineering ethics roadmap for BE 2700: bioengineering laboratory principles

Technical Content	Ethics Content
Mechanical testing of animal tissue	Application of ethics principles and regulatory frameworks to animal research
Verification and validation testing of medical devices	Reflection on the adoption of technology, and its intended and unintended use by users; ethical dilemmas in user and human factors validation testing
Wearable health technology design challenge	Stakeholder conflict in the regulatory and economic context of wearable health technology

TABLE 11.3
Bioengineering ethics roadmap for BE 3090: bioengineering modeling, analysis, and design laboratory I

Technical Content	Ethics Content
Kidney dialysis lab	Empathetic engineering as a branch of user-centric design
Limb prostheses design lab	Inclusive design for invisible disabilities using the Universal Design and Empathy Mapping frameworks

TABLE 11.4
Bioengineering ethics roadmap for BE 3100: bioengineering modeling, analysis, and design laboratory II

Technical Content	Ethics Content
Microfluidics and fluid dynamics lab	Accessibility to microfluidic technologies in low-resource settings
Synthetic biology lab: Genetic switches	Responsible release and biocontainment in gene editing technologies
ECG monitoring design lab	Interdisciplinary approaches and regulatory standards for data protection and security in wearable devices
Low-cost diagnostics—spectrophotometer design lab	Institutional Review Boards and protection of human subjects in clinical trials

TABLE 11.5
Bioengineering ethics roadmap for senior design project

Technical Content	Ethics Content
Project proposal development	In-class activity on professional responsibility and ethics
Proof-of-concept presentations	Prepared a document for the senior design instructors with background research on developing course policies for the safe and ethical use of generative AI
Proof-of-concept presentations	Prepared a document with student resources on IP and relevant policies at Penn

The ultimate goal is to have the students understand that all of their professional activities have societal and ethical implications. Two illustrative examples were selected to demonstrate how the ethics content was embedded into the core technical courses and specifically tailored to the format of each course.

11.3.1 Example 1: Ethics Within an Introductory Bioengineering Course

The introductory course selected was BE 1000, a first-year course focused on the areas of concentration in bioengineering taught through eight technical modules, among which we selected the following to accompany with an ethics module: (1) Systems and Synthetic Biology; (2) Neuroengineering; (3) Biomedical Devices; and (4) Biomedical Imaging and Radiation Physics. The Neuroengineering module is described in the following as an example of how the ethics material was matched with the technical material in the introductory course (see Table 11.1).

The Neuroengineering module was divided into two weeks. The first week was focused on the technical material. The students were provided with a series of mini-lectures on the mechanisms of common neurological disorders and various branches of neuroengineering, such as neural electronics and neural tissue engineering.

The second week was devoted to the ethics unit. Each of the four ethics units in BE 1000 consists of an online discussion board response to assigned readings or media, followed by a 45-minute in-class discussion led by the ethics fellows. The resources for the ethics units consist of podcasts, news articles, popular science magazine articles, videos, or other media. Two peer-reviewed journal articles were selected for the module on neuroengineering. The first was a *Neuron* article by Martha Farah, a neuroscientist and Director of the Center for Neuroscience & Society at Penn, selected to provide an introduction to the principles of biomedical ethics and moral philosophy as applicable to bioengineering practice (Farah 2015). The second was an article on the ethical design and development of neuroengineering, assistive, and rehabilitative technologies, which discusses the practical implementation of the principles of user-centered and value-sensitive design for engineers (Ienca et al. 2017).

We designed an in-class group assignment to apply the learnings from the two articles to stakeholder mapping. Students were asked to select an ethical dilemma and present to the class the levels of agency available to the various stakeholders. This activity reinforced the students' understanding of consequentialism, deontological principles, user-based design, and value-sensitive design. The class meetings, which consisted of discussions, small group work, and design challenges, illuminated various facets of bioengineering ethics, as well as the healthcare sector at large, and laid the foundation for the sophomore-, junior-, and senior-level courses.

11.3.2 Example 2: Ethics a Junior-Year Bioengineering Laboratory Courses

The embedded ethics curriculum at the sophomore and junior level has been initiated into three laboratory-based courses (see Tables 11.2–11.4). The technical objectives of all of these courses are achieved through a series of design challenges, each spanning multiple weeks during which students learn and practice the applicable experimental and mathematical modeling techniques. The example used here is associated with a module on cell therapeutics and synthetic biology (see Table 11.4).

For the ethics module, we selected a discussion on responsible decision-making for biocontainment to accompany the technical material. In general, in BE 3090 and 3100, we emphasize specific stakeholder perspectives and sociotechnical concerns for each of the technologies discussed in the course. In this module, the students were provided with the following resources on the release of genetically modified, self-limiting mosquitoes for disease control.

The first assigned readings included a web page on genetically modified mosquitoes and a talk by Natalie Kofler, a microbiologist and founder of the Editing Nature advocacy group for responsible gene editing, as well as an opinion piece published in the *Boston Globe* in which Kofler and Jennifer Kuzma, co-director of the Genetic Engineering and Society Center, discuss the problems with rigor, transparency, and conflicts of interest in the risk assessments preceding the adoption of this technology (Editing Nature 2020; Kofler and Kuzma 2020). The final assigned reading was a web page published on the US Centers for Disease Control and Prevention website, which provides an example of the public educational efforts for this technology (Centers for Disease Control and Prevention).

For seamless integration with the laboratory-based nature of this course, the ethics assignments are embedded into the final lab report for each design challenge. Students were required to reflect in 200 words each on Natalie Kofler's recommendations for effective risk assessment, the thoroughness of the educational material provided by the two parties, and the relevance of the aforementioned resources to their own design challenge.

11.4 CONCLUSION

At the University of Pennsylvania's Department of Bioengineering, we have been able to implement an embedded ethics approach to incorporate sociotechnical training throughout the four-year undergraduate curriculum. The ethics modules were carefully crafted to complement the technical material being taught in a first-year introductory course, three laboratory courses throughout the sophomore and junior years, and senior design.

Reflecting on our experience, as well as themes from the secondary literature, particularly the Harvard Embedded EthiCS publication, we found the following to be instrumental to the success of our initiative and informative for future efforts (Grosz et al. 2019):

- Engaged participation from individual faculty members and course instructors who were committed to partnering with us, making space available for the ethics modules in their coursework, and providing iterative feedback to develop and implement the modules;
- Administrative support from the school and department leadership, including support for the engineering ethics lead and fellows to develop the curriculum;
- An interdisciplinary team bringing diverse areas of expertise;
- Recognition that building the ethics modules is an iterative process requiring adaptability and flexibility;
- Additionally, a genuine interest among the students displayed through thoughtful course discussions, homework submissions, and survey feedback has indicated an engagement with the ethics material.

We have also identified challenges faced with an embedded ethics approach, as well as opportunities for future innovative approaches. This pedagogical approach is difficult to assess in terms of long-term impact. While our current procedures include multiple surveys and analyses of student participation and coursework, there is an opportunity to develop a longitudinal study including alumni. An embedded ethics approach also requires a commitment to continuously update the content and introduce innovative teaching methods, particularly as the regulatory landscape, pedagogical approaches, and the technologies themselves that the students are studying are rapidly changing.

REFERENCES

Bucholz, Elizabeth K., Cameron Kim, Joshua R. Chan, and Christian Ferney. 2024. "The Snail Progression of Ethical Instruction: Nurturing Ethical Mindsets Across the Biomedical Engineering Curriculum." In *ASEE Annual Conference & Exposition Proceedings,* Portland, OR, June 23–26. https://peer.asee.org/48138

Centers for Disease Control and Prevention. n.d. *Genetically Modified Mosquitoes.* Accessed May 29, 2025. https://www.cdc.gov/mosquitoes/mosquito-control/genetically-modified-mosquitoes.html.

Chan, Joshua R., Elizabeth K. Bucholz, and Cameron M. Kim. 2023. "WIP: Integrating Ethics Education Across the Biomedical Engineering Curriculum Increases Student Awareness of Frameworks and Broader Applications to Practice." In *ASEE Annual Conference & Exposition Proceedings,* Baltimore, MD, June 25–28. https://peer.asee.org/42571

Editing Nature. 2020. *GM Mosquitoes.* Accessed May 29, 2025. https://www.editingnature.org/gm-mosquitoes.

Farah, Martha J. 2015. "An Ethics Toolbox for Neurotechnology." *Neuron* 86 (1): 34–7. https://doi.org/10.1016/j.neuron.2015.03.038.

Frow, Emma, Stephen H. Tillery, Jerry Coursen, and James Abbas. 2017. "Building an 'Ethics Spine' into Biomedical Engineering Curriculum at Arizona State University." *Online Ethics Center.* Accessed May 29, 2025. https://onlineethics.org/cases/stem-ethics-projects-2017-present/building-ethics-spine-biomedical-engineering-curriculum.

Grosz, Barbara J., David G. Grant, Kate Vredenburgh, et al. 2019. "Embedded EthiCS: Integrating Ethics Across CS Education." *Communications of the ACM* 62 (8): 54–61. https://doi.org/10.1145/3330794.

Hess, Justin L., and Grant Fore. 2018. "A Systematic Literature Review of US Engineering Ethics Interventions." *Science and Engineering Ethics* 24: 551–83. https://doi.org/10.1007/s11948-017-9910-6.

Hess, Justin L., Elizabeth Sanders, Grant A. Fore, et al. 2024. "Transforming Ethics Education Through a Faculty Learning Community: 'I'm Coming Around to Seeing Ethics as Being Maybe as Important as Calculus.'" *Science and Engineering Ethics* 30: 40. https://doi.org/10.1007/s11948-024-00503-2.

Ienca, Marcello, Reto W. Kressig, Fabrice Jotterand, and Bernice Elger. 2017. "Proactive Ethical Design for Neuroengineering, Assistive and Rehabilitation Technologies: The Cybathlon Lesson." *Journal of NeuroEngineering and Rehabilitation* 14 (1): 115. https://doi.org/10.1186/s12984-017-0325-z.

Kofler, Natalie, and Jennifer Kuzma. 2020. "Before Genetically Modified Mosquitoes Are Released, We Need a Better EPA." *The Boston Globe*, June 22.

Miller, Sharon, Steven Higbee, Joseph M. Wallace, John H. Schild, and Julie Y. Ji. 2020. "WIP: Embedded Ethical Inquiry and Reflection in a Biomedical Engineering Curriculum." In *ASEE Virtual Annual Conference & Exposition Proceedings.* https://doi.org/10.18260/1-2-35536.

Mitcham, Carl, and Elaine E. Englehardt. 2019. "Ethics Across the Curriculum: Prospects for Broader (and Deeper) Teaching and Learning in Research and Engineering Ethics." *Science and Engineering Ethics* 25 (6): 1735–62. https://doi.org/10.1007/s11948-016-9797-7.

National Academy of Engineering. 2016. *Infusing Ethics into the Development of Engineers: Exemplary Education Activities and Programs.* Washington, DC: National Academies Press.

National Academy of Engineering. 2017. *Overcoming Challenges to Infusing Ethics into the Development of Engineers: Proceedings of a Workshop.* Washington, DC: National Academies Press.

Shields, Brit. 2023. "Justice, Equity, Diversity, and Inclusion Curriculum within an Introductory Bioengineering Course." *Biomedical Engineering Education* 3 (1): 39–49. https://doi.org/10.1007/s43683-022-00086-z.

Tang, Xiaofeng, Jeffrey M. Catchmark, Eduardo Mendieta, and Thomas A. Litzinger. 2020. "Infusing Ethics Across the Curriculum in Biological Engineering: Background, Process, and Initial Results." *Advances in Engineering Education* 8 (3). https://advances.asee.org/wp-content/uploads/vol08/issue3/Papers/AEE-NAE-Tang.pdf.

Tonn, Jenna, Brit Shields, Ryan Hearty, and Adelheid Voskuhl. 2025. "Pedagogical Choices for Navigating and Teaching Sociotechnical Landscapes in Engineering Education." In *ASEE Annual Conference & Exposition Proceedings,* Montral, Canada, June 22–25. https://peer.asee.org/57029

12 Developing a Social Disposition in Biomedical Engineers

Curriculum Innovations for Societal Impact

Sharon Aris, Daniela Castro de Jong, and Lauren Kark

12.1 INTRODUCTION

Since its emergence as a formal discipline, engineering has evolved in tandem with societal needs and values. Today, it is widely acknowledged as a sociotechnical profession (Jesiek et al. 2019), shaped by and shaping the social, cultural, political, and economic landscapes in which it operates. Formal consideration of sociotechnical integration in engineering emerged after World War II to describe the necessity to optimize both "technological and social variables" (Bauer and Herder 2009, 601). Prior to this, the expectation was that society would adapt to new technology without considering the interrelationship between the two. The importance of the humanities in engineering education, however, was documented as early as the 1900s, and by the 1930s, it was argued that at least "one-fifth of an engineering curriculum should be devoted to the study of the humanities and social sciences" (Marsh 2025). Nowadays, very few (if any) universities throughout the world could claim that 20% of their engineering curriculum is devoted to the humanities and social sciences (Khalid et al. 2013).

Despite engineering being recognized as a sociotechnical profession, its education remains predominantly technocentric. This technocentric focus may result in graduates who are inadequately prepared for real-world engineering challenges, lacking the capacity to engage with the social dimensions of the profession, essential for responsible practice and long-term career fulfillment (Jesiek et al. 2019). It may also limit recruitment and increase attrition, particularly amongst groups that are underrepresented in the engineering profession (Pleasants et al. 2025). Accrediting bodies have attempted to incorporate more nontechnical training into engineering curricula by explicitly requiring the inclusion of non-technical skills (e.g., ABET, Engineers Australia) However, this approach has drawn criticism as these skills are

DOI: 10.1201/9781003520313-12

often listed separately from technical skills. Some critics argue that this separation depoliticizes non-technical skills in engineering (Cech and Sherick 2015), while others worry about curriculum dilution (Roberts and Lord 2020). Balancing a curriculum to meet professional demands, existing academic capabilities, and societal needs is challenging. Nowhere is this truer than in biomedical engineering.

The disconnect between the sociotechnical nature of engineering and its technocentric education is not new. While the social dimensions of the engineering profession have been debated for over a century, their integration into engineering education remains limited and inconsistent. In their review, Martinez-Marroquin et al. (2024) found that a variety of curricular techniques were used to address the social dimensions of engineering, ranging from standalone core courses and electives to integration into existing courses. The level of sociotechnical integration varied from complete integration to "add-ons" that were independent of the technical aspects of the projects in which students were engaged (Martinez-Marroquin et al. 2024). Currently, there is no consensus on what and how the social aspects of engineering practice should be taught. However, Roberts (in Roberts and Lord (2020, 2)) recently called to action, "that we are now emerging on a next revolution in engineering education, making engineering education sociotechnical."

In this chapter, we aim to contribute to the conversation by proposing an alternative approach to developing biomedical engineers who excel in sociotechnical practices. These engineers are adept at traversing sociocultural and disciplinary boundaries to assemble teams that examine problems through all appropriate lenses, creating the most effective solutions. To achieve this, we propose a conceptual model for fostering a social disposition in biomedical engineering students through deliberate curriculum design, specifically within the context of biomedical engineering. The chapter begins by exploring the social context of biomedical engineering, including a discussion of health and disability as a central influence that shapes both the discipline's knowledge and its practical applications. It then defines the term "social disposition" and explains how it can be developed. We examine current approaches to dispositional development in engineering, followed by a critique of two case studies that have attempted to cultivate a social disposition in biomedical engineering students. The chapter wraps up with a proposed conceptual model for an integrated curriculum to support this development and a call to action for educators and institutions to continue the conversation and share their practices.

12.2 THE SOCIAL CONTEXT OF BIOMEDICAL ENGINEERING

12.2.1 A Multidimensional Understanding of Health and Disability

Biomedical engineering exists across engineering and health. Key to a multidimensional understanding of health is found in the WHO's constitution, which states that it is more about well-being than the absence of a given medical condition (WHO 2020). Health and well-being can be better understood in a social way by exploring the surrounding circumstances to individuals, groups, and communities' lives through the conceptualization of the Social Determinants of Health (SDH) (Marmot et al. 2008):

> The place where you live, the communities you belong to, your education level, ethnicity, race, income and gender, and whether you have a disability, all make a huge difference to how long you can expect to live a healthy life. People in the country with the highest life expectancy will, on average, live for 33 years more than those born in the country with the lowest life expectancy.
>
> (WHO 2025, xii)

Research suggests that health outcomes can be attributed approximately 30% to traditional clinical and therapeutic interventions and 70% to social factors, highlighting the greater impact of social factors on overall health and well-being (Marmot et al. 2010). Regardless of this, traditional clinical and therapeutic interventions prevail, which negatively impacts a more holistic understanding of health in context (Bailey-McHale, Whaley, and Bailey-McHale 2020). The interaction of the different elements within the SDH is complex and cannot be explained in a causal or direct correlation (Braveman 2023; WHO 2025). As Braveman (2023, 12) emphasizes, "health disparities are differences in health among more and less socially advantaged groups of people, which raise concerns about justice." The conceptualization of SDH is helpful for highlighting structural inequalities but also has been criticized for not widely improving the health outcomes for the most disadvantaged communities (Frank et al. 2020).

Just like health, disability is another crucial concept of importance for biomedical engineering. Disability is also a multifaceted construct that has been explored and redefined across history (Koutsoklenis and Adam 2024; Lawson and Beckett 2020). Since 2001, the International Classification of Functioning, Disability and Health (ICF) has offered a globally accepted framework for understanding how health and disability must be seen in context rather than in isolation (WHO 2001). The ICF proposes that disability can be explained through a biopsychosocial model, in which the medical condition must be understood in terms of how it impacts people's engagement in valued activities and participation in society (WHO 2001).

Narratives around disability can use a deficit- or a strength-based approach. A deficit-based approach situates disability as a sole responsibility of the individual and their medical condition(s). On the other hand, the social and human rights models of disability go beyond the ICF and propose a more political approach, explaining how societal barriers cause limited opportunities for those living with a disability (Koutsoklenis and Adam 2024; Lawson and Beckett 2020). The social model of disability is connected to advocacy and empowerment, focusing on how social structures and attitudes can create the conditions for marginalization and disadvantage (Barnes 2019; Lawson and Beckett 2020).

12.2.2 The Intersection of Technology and Health

Given biomedical engineering's role in the development of assistive technology for people living with a disability, it is essential to better understand the growing level of evidence around its impact (Manzoor and Vimarlund 2018). Terminology has evolved over the last two decades, moving from assistive technology in general to more specific ones, such as tele-rehabilitation technology, wearable healthcare technology, ambient intelligent living, or gerontechnology (Manzoor and Vimarlund 2018; WHO and UNICEF 2022). Recently, an expanded call to consider how technology can support quality of life and deal with major societal issues, such as isolation for older people, has emerged (Ravi, Kamalanabhan, and Jawahar 2019). This is in line with WHO's (2022) approach toward the understanding of assistive technology as a means and an end. As a means, it becomes needs-driven as it gives opportunities for people with disabilities to participate as active members of their communities, while, as an end, it is considered a basic human right in terms of ensuring health access (WHO and UNICEF 2022).

While collaboration among biomedical engineering and health professionals, such as physicians, physiotherapists, and occupational therapists, is seen as beneficial for positive health outcomes, some barriers must be acknowledged. These barriers can arise from a lack of mutual understanding due to different professional jargon, as well as a lack of time and opportunities to overcome this issue and build up the collaboration (Mihailidis and Polgar 2016). Therefore, for biomedical engineering, as part of the health management and support personnel group (WHO 2019), it is critical to understand health in a broader manner to support the development of more accessible and affordable assistive technology and medical equipment to reduce such inequities.

12.3 DEVELOPING A SOCIAL DISPOSITION FOR ENGINEERS

Communicating in a language and embracing the required sensibility for this interdisciplinary and user-focused approach require engineers to develop a social disposition to understand how technology is also a human practice with social meaning (Santander Gana and Trejo Fuentes 2006; Williams 2011). This requires an epistemic shift away from technocratic approaches to social ones (Miranda, Goñi, and Sotomayor 2021). Here, thinking tools from sociology, social work, and the social sciences can be usefully adapted to the engineering curriculum (Gilbert et al. 2014; Martinez-Marroquin et al. 2024; Walther, Miller, and Sochacka 2017). These include: social *theories* on how the social world is constructed, who has power to act within this and how this influences individual and collective behavior; developing professional *attributes* such as empathy, critical thinking, imagination, and creativity; and bringing these together in professional *practices* such as critical reflection and co-design to extend established design thinking approaches when working with individuals, groups, and communities to strengthen the effectiveness of a project.

Theoretically, social scientists understand the world as not only physically but also *socially* constructed, consisting of networks of relationships and institutions, cultural norms, and power structures that shape how people live and interact with each other (Giddens and Sutton 2021). These may be formalized into theories on social class, family, cultural and religious values, ideals of power and authority, or expectations as to how individuals should interact or present themselves to the world. These are influenced by people's histories and social context (Durkheim 1982) and shape how individuals unconsciously behave (Bourdieu 1977). Considering some of these variables is the first step to understanding how different groups of people may engage with healthcare systems, what, who, and how they trust, how they communicate their needs or symptoms, or whether they seek any treatment at all.

For biomedical engineers, developing a social disposition means learning to look beyond the technical aspects of innovations in healthcare to also consider how social, cultural, economic, and political factors may be shaping the development and use of medical technologies and how these affect those using these technologies. Specifically, this way of thinking challenges students' taken-for-granted assumptions about health, illness, ability, and disability and technology and provides them with the tools to see and understand unfamiliar social contexts and service or product-users living in these with empathy and critical insight (Berger 1963; Cruz, Nuñez, and Carrell 2024). While there is no firm consensus on what constitutes the social dispositions necessary to engineering practice, most center around a broad conceptualization of empathy and how this can be developed and put to work in practice. This includes having an emotional intelligence about one's own emotions and life experiences and how this shapes one's own perspective, and the commitment to recognize the diverse lived historic, social, and emotional experiences of users and other stakeholders and how this shapes their perspectives (Ruch 2002; Tang 2018). It also encompasses a commitment to social responsibility, an ethic of care and social justice so that designs are human-centered and context-sensitive (Canney and Bielefeldt 2015; Leydens and Lucena 2014).

12.3.1 Teaching for a Social Disposition

While skills and knowledge are often taught through formal instruction and assessed through measurable outcomes, teaching dispositions need to be developed differently. This is most effectively done by fostering integrated and active reflective practice, through mentorship, and exposure to real-world ethical dilemmas (Bogo et al. 2011; Leydens and Lucena 2014). In the following section, two approaches that complement existing design thinking frameworks that guide learners toward this are outlined (Walther, Miller, and Sochacka 2017, 27). These can be adapted for classroom, project-based, and/or work-integrated learning.

Design approaches that focus on the self-defined and contextual needs of the end user to ensure that usability and safety are characterized as human- or user-centered design (Vincent and Blandford 2011). Human-centered design places an emphasis on building empathy with end users to better understand their context and true needs (Rodriguez et al. 2023). This is frequently packaged into a "design thinking" process framework, which broadly consists of a process that begins with seeking an empathic understanding of the needs of the end user, reframing the problem, collecting diverse perspectives, ideating different solutions, and creating and testing prototypes through an ongoing iterative process (IxDF 2016). However, while design thinking has been embedded in biomedical engineering programs, implementation evaluations have demonstrated that qualities including empathy and human-centeredness were not sustained, leading the researchers to conclude that "these concepts are difficult to grasp and retain unless immersed in a setting in which they are valuable" (Davies et al. 2022).

Critical reflection and *co-design* are two social frameworks for approaching clients and communities when developing engineering interventions that can complement design thinking approaches in embedded and meaningful ways that operationalize concepts of empathy and human-centeredness. These bring together *social skills* such as listening and communication, *social theories* focused on understanding the social, historical, and institutional contexts of all participants in a process, and *social practices* for action. Specifically, critical reflection provides a thinking process for engineers to understand their own social expectations and values as well as those of key stakeholders. Co-design provides a model for co-construction with product or end users across a development cycle. Practicing these across a curriculum will greatly help engineering students develop their social disposition.

12.3.1.1 Critical Reflection

Reflection is well established in engineering pedagogy (Cruz, Nuñez, and Carrell 2024). Drawing on Schön's (1983) influential descriptions of "reflection-in-action"—the capacity to think on your feet, and "reflection-on-action"—to learn from experience and plan for future improvement (Boud and Walker 1998), reflection is advanced as a way to enable students to think through past, present, and future actions and to facilitate a professional disposition of "informed self-evaluation" (Mina, Cowan, and Heywood 2015). Reflection also requires the development of skills in listening contextually, identifying structural conditions, acknowledging power to act, increasing opportunities and resources while reducing risks and harm, and enhancing capabilities (Leydens and Lucena 2014).

Critical reflection, borrowed from social work, brings these reflective skills together into a systematic thinking and planning process. This model asks those involved in a project to seek to hear and understand the perspectives of all the stakeholders in a project, particularly checking if some voices are not being heard (Fook and Gardner 2007). It seeks to understand how the influence of social, historic, and institutional values influences a situation, how this shapes the relationship with stakeholders, and how understanding this can inform rethinking of the situation to create practical change (Fook and Gardner 2007; Watts 2018). Adapting Fook and Gardner (2007), the key steps are as follows: (1) describe the key issue and key stakeholders; (2) contextualize understanding of the social, historic, and institutional context of all key stakeholders (including the engineer). This includes noticing the language being used to describe the issue, any assumptions and values being expressed in this also any current adaptions to the issue; (3) use social theories and perspectives to deconstruct or unpack assumptions of the issue and what the stakeholders bring to this; (4) with these new insights, reconstruct understanding of key issue and end-user needs; (5) re-engage with key stakeholders; and (6) continue to plan action incorporating all perspectives. This thus offers practical steps for building empathy, bringing together other social practices noted across the literature as being important including: the principle of always "starting where the client is" (Walther, Miller, and Sochacka 2017, 126); using skills in listening and communication (Leydens and Lucena 2009); and prioritizing social perspective-taking for developing empathy (Hess, Strobel, and Brightman 2017). Ultimately, this process works to ensure that engineers do not make assumptions that can limit their understanding of end users and the strengths and perspectives they may bring, ultimately ensuring the final product developed is fit for purpose and adopted.

In the following case study from the UNSW (Australia), we demonstrate how critical reflection can support the development of social dispositions in undergraduate students tasked with designing a prototype of an assistive technology product for people living with disabilities. For instance, a postural chair that grows with the child or a language-agnostic communication device, both proposed by academic colleagues in the Pacific region. The prototype is developed across the course of a year-long elective course comprising three ten-week terms and a field trip overseas. During terms 1 and 2, students investigate the problem and develop an initial prototype. Between the second and third terms, they travel overseas to engage with key stakeholders in the Pacific region, gather feedback on their design, and explore local manufacturing opportunities. Upon returning to Australia, students spend the final term refining their prototype based on the feedback received during their overseas engagement. This process follows a design-thinking process, deepened by applying critical reflection, as depicted in Table 12.1.

TABLE 12.1
Case study 1: applied critical reflection process for developing assistive technology in low- to middle-income countries

[1] Describe key task	Students research the context in which their prototype will be used and the need it is to address.
[2] Contextualize context	Students examine the country's social context, including its history, current political climate, and the socioeconomic status of its residents. This informs their design proposals and their design and manufacturing choices. While in the country, students participate in historical tours and visit museums to deepen their understanding of its history. Whenever possible, they stay on campus at a partner university where they interact with local students through social activities and meals. If English is not the spoken language, students receive basic language training. Stakeholder engagements may include students presenting their prototypes to people with disability, fellow students, health professionals, teachers, parents, and engineers. To gather effective feedback, students must adapt their communication strategies to the local context.
[3] Deconstruct assumptions	Students frequently describe this experience as eye-opening, testing both their creativity and their sociotechnical assumptions about engineering, seeing potential to positively influence society, which often reaffirms their choice of biomedical engineering and encourages them to use their skills for social good.
[4] Reconstruct the task with new insights	Students use new knowledge and understandings to describe the key problem and technical solution in a new way.
[5] Re-engage with the task from the perspective of users	Students may sometimes feel overwhelmed by the enormity of the problems being faced and may be confused when a problem that seemed solvable through a technical solution cannot be addressed solely with technology. For instance, if there are issues related to resourcing, policy challenges, or societal preconceptions like disability stigma.
[6] Appreciate the task and biomedical engineering as part of a bigger picture	Students become aware of how the needs of the user in their social context. Technical solutions are only effective if they also address the social context. Also, understand that technical solutions can only address some of the wider social needs. Those who grasp this context develop greater resilience, understanding that they are just one piece of a larger puzzle.

12.3.1.2 Co-Design

Complementary to critical reflection is the model of co-design. Co-design is best understood as a research and human-centered design practice that sits on a continuum of research participation (Steen 2008). Participatory research refers to ways of researching that include involvement of, or partnership with, people with lived/living experience, who typically are the subjects or end users of research and design (Bellingham et al. 2023). For engineers, co-design means that their role is not just as "problem solvers" but as facilitators jointly with stakeholders. Early and structured collaboration with the people who will live with, build, and maintain the resulting technology is emphasized (Steen 2013). Co-design is not a one-off activity; rather, it involves cyclical and iterative processes exploring, discussing, acting, and reflecting (Lenette 2022). This too draws on skills and insights from social work and development studies, which emphasize the need to balance power relations between stakeholders through non-authoritarian engagement (Amadei, Sandekian, and Thomas 2009), the importance of active listening (Leydens and Lucena 2009), and recognition and description of existing individual and community strengths, rather than the deficits they lack (Saleebey 2012; Schneider, Leydens, and Lucena 2008).

At a minimum in co-design, there are three iterative phases: (1) co-defining both the key problem or issue and the approach to its solution, with an emphasis on the lived experience of the end user; (2) establishing an ongoing iterative design process and being willing re-visit problem definition and design throughout the duration of engagement; and (3) co-interpretation of findings and design outputs, and transparent reporting (adapted from Bellingham et al. (2023)).

This form of iterative design process with key stakeholders is becoming established as good practice in engineering (De Maria et al. 2022), with evidence emerging that participatory practices strengthen both the technical performance and social applicability and acceptance (Grogan 2021). This is particularly the case in resource-limited social contexts. For instance, Jagtap's (2022) systematic review showed that when engineers co-design with community members—sharing decision-making power and local knowledge—the resulting products are both more culturally appropriate and more highly adopted in the long term.

Studies suggest that engineering students absorb the principles of co-design most effectively when the curriculum itself is imbued with the practice (Mazzurco, Jesiek, and Godwin 2019; Mazzurco and Daniel 2020). This case study, also from the UNSW, illustrates such an approach. It examines the process of pairing student groups with individuals with a disability to collaboratively design and develop customized assistive technologies in a two-term elective course offered to upper-level undergraduate and postgraduate biomedical engineering students. In this course, "Rehabilitation Engineering and Assistive Technology," the primary task is to create a functional prototype that aligns with the managed expectations of the individual with the disability, who actively participates as a co-creator rather than serving as a consultant on their own project.

The course begins by emphasizing non-technical skills essential for the successful delivery of the prototype, including an introduction to disability awareness with activities to develop students' inclusive language and communication skills, identify environmental and attitudinal barriers, and gain an overview of the legislative

TABLE 12.2
Co-design process for developing custom assistive technology

[1] Co-define research design	Students participate in two key activities: (1) a lived experience panel featuring individuals with disabilities, where students are encouraged to ask questions and challenge their assumptions; and (2) an introduction to community-based rehabilitation, helping students understand the context in which they may work as rehabilitation engineers. Scaffolded weekly reflective tasks are used during this phase of the course to help students develop self-awareness and foster both personal and professional growth. After completing these activities, which span the first four weeks of the course, students begin prototyping.
[2] Co-deciding deviations in the design	Students meet with their lived experience consultant on at least three occasions: at the beginning to define the scope, in the middle to give feedback on the proposal, and again at the end to give feedback on the prototype.
[3] Co-interpretation and reporting on design	Final feedback on prototype from lived experience consultant. In the final presentation, students are expected to demonstrate the application of co-design, inclusive design, and universal design in their final prototype presentations.

framework in Australia. Students are introduced to different models of disability, particularly the medical and social models, culminating in the WHO's ICF. Students then move into a co-design cycle for the remainder of the course (summarized in Table 12.2).

12.4 CONCEPTUAL MODEL FOR AN INTEGRATED CURRICULUM

Drawing on the growing body of work on STT as a bridging framework (Rodriguez and Cicek 2024), this section proposes a conceptual model for an integrated curriculum designed to develop social dispositions in biomedical engineering students. To ground this model in current educational practice, we are guided by how STT has been incorporated into engineering curricula. Although pedagogical approaches to STT are still evolving, there is broad agreement that it should not be treated as a standalone topic (Martinez-Marroquin et al. 2024). Instead, the most effective strategy involves repeated and integrated exposure across the curriculum, a view supported by recent literature (Martinez-Marroquin et al. 2024; Rodriguez and Cicek 2024) and consistent with conclusions drawn from our own case studies.

Developing social dispositions in biomedical engineering students requires a framework that integrates sociotechnical dimensions, specifically, the convergence of engineering, health and disability, and social domains. This is conceptualized in Figure 12.1 using a tapered double helix model, where one strand represents critical reflection and the other co-design. These intertwined processes symbolize the reflective and collaborative nature of problem-solving in biomedical contexts. The expanding diameter of the helix signifies the progressive development of students' knowledge and skills over time. Enveloping this structure is a cone of empathy,

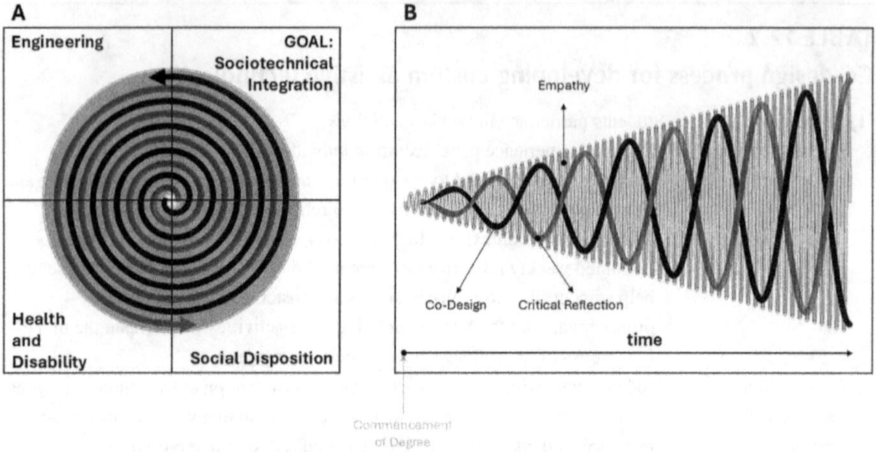

FIGURE 12.1 Conceptual model for an integrated curriculum to develop social dispositions in biomedical engineering students. A and B are orthogonal to one another. A represents the domain through which students must navigate to achieve sociotechnical integration; B represents the student journey throughout (and beyond) their academic studies

which acts as both a guiding principle and a protective sheath. While empathy is often positioned as the initial step in design thinking, we argue for its omnipresence in biomedical engineering practice, so fundamental that it becomes an implicit force guiding every stage, rather than a discrete step to be checked off. This model underscores the imperative that future biomedical engineers not only master technical competencies in engineering and health but also develop social dispositions necessary to design for diverse human experiences and social contexts.

Although Figure 12.1B illustrates critical reflection and co-design with a 90° phase shift, this requirement is not fixed. In practice, both the phase and magnitude of these processes can vary throughout a student's academic journey. The phase shift (i.e., the temporal offset between when each process is emphasized) may expand or contract depending on curricular structure and student needs. Simultaneously, the magnitude of engagement with each of these processes can fluctuate, mirroring the depth and emphasis placed on critical reflection and co-design at different stages. For example, early coursework may emphasize high-magnitude critical reflection to build sociotechnical awareness, while later stages may emphasize high-magnitude co-design in capstone or clinical placements.

Extending the double helix model, the integration of engineering, health and disability, and social domains is further conceptualized through the metaphor of cell membranes—semi-permeable boundaries that regulate the exchange of knowledge, values, and practices between these domains. These membranes are not static; they respond to stimuli such as interdisciplinary learning, critical reflection, and co-design. When stimulated, they open channels that allow for the diffusion of sociotechnical understanding, enabling students to navigate and integrate diverse forms of knowledge. However, in the absence of continued stimulus, such as when learning becomes siloed or reflective practices are neglected, these membranes may close, reducing permeability and reinforcing disciplinary isolation. This dynamic process underscores the need for sustained, intentional curricular interventions to maintain openness and foster integration. As students engage repeatedly with these stimuli at increasing levels of complexity, the membranes become more responsive and adaptive, eventually allowing for near seamless diffusion. The biomedical engineer evolves into a self-diffuse operator—a professional who navigates fluidly across contexts, attuned to their positionality, identity, and the collaborative configurations necessary to address complex health challenges.

While Figure 12.1A depicts the double helix as circular and centered at the geometric origin of the model, this representation is not prescriptive. Educators are encouraged to reconceptualize the helix as elliptical, with its center positioned anywhere within or across the domains of engineering, health and disability, and social knowledge. This flexibility allows for the model to be tailored to the specific entry-level competencies and experiences that students bring to their studies. The orientation and dimensions of the ellipse—defined by the angle of the major axis and the relative length of its axes—can be shaped by the priorities of key stakeholders, including educators, accrediting bodies, industry partners, and government agencies. These parameters can be embedded and assured through intentional curriculum design. Thus, the model accommodates variation in both inputs and outputs, enabling educators to explore and refine the relationships between disciplinary integration and the development of social dispositions in biomedical engineering students.

12.5 CONCLUSION

This chapter proposes a flexible, non-prescriptive conceptual model for developing social dispositions in biomedical engineering students, one that can be meaningfully integrated into diverse curricula through intentional design that prioritizes repeated and sustained engagement with social learning. While critical reflection and co-design are highlighted as foundational practices, the model avoids prescribing specific pedagogies, recognizing that effective teaching must respond to local contexts. Our hope is that it serves as a practical guide and a catalyst for experimentation, adaptation, and collaboration among educators.

REFERENCES

Amadei, Bernard, Robyn Sandekian, and Evan Thomas. 2009. "A Model for Sustainable Humanitarian Engineering Projects." *Sustainability* 1 (4): 1087–105. https://doi.org/10.3390/su1041087.

Bailey-McHale, Rachel, Vanessa Whaley, and John Bailey-McHale. 2020. "Social Determinants of Health." In *Good Health and Well-Being*, edited by Walter L. Filho, Tony Wall, Anabela M. Azul, Luciana Brandli and Pinar G. Özuyar, 647–57. Cham: Springer.

Barnes, Colin. 2019. "Understanding the Social Model of Disability: Past, Present and Future." In *Routledge Handbook of Disability Studies*, edited by Nick Watson, Alan Roulstone and Carol Thomas. London: Routledge.

Bauer, Johannes M., and Paul M. Herder. 2009. "Designing Socio-Technical Systems." In *Philosophy of Technology and Engineering Sciences*, edited by Anthonie Meijers, 601–30. Amsterdam: Elsevier.

Bellingham, Brett, Emily Elder, Bill Foxlewin, Nick Gale, Gail Rose, Kate Sam, Kelly Thorburn, and Jamie River. 2023. *Co-Design Kickstarter.* Sydney: Community Mental Health Drug and Alcohol Research Network. https://mhcc.org.au/wp-content/uploads/2023/06/CMHDARN-Co-design-kickstarter-FINAL.pdf.

Berger, Peter L. 1963. *Invitation to Sociology: A Humanistic Perspective.* New York: Knopf.

Bogo, Marion, Cleo Regehr, Ellen Katz, Carmen Logie, and Maria Mylopoulos. 2011. "Developing a Tool for Assessing Students' Reflections on Their Practice." *Social Work Education* 30 (2): 186–204. https://doi.org/10.1080/02615479.2011.540392.

Boud, David, and David Walker. 1998. "Promoting Reflection in Professional Courses: The Challenge of Context." *Studies in Higher Education* 23 (2): 191–206. https://doi.org/10.1080/03075079812331380384.

Bourdieu, Pierre. 1977. *Outline of a Theory of Practice.* Cambridge: Cambridge University Press.

Braveman, Paula. 2023. "Introduction: What Influences Health? And What Influences the Influences?" In *The Social Determinants of Health and Health Disparities.* Oxford: Oxford University Press.

Canney, Nathan, and Angela Bielefeldt. 2015. "A Framework for the Development of Social Responsibility in Engineers." *International Journal of Engineering Education* 31 (1B): 414–24.

Cech, Erin A., and Heidi M. Sherick. 2015. "Depoliticization and Structure of Engineering Education." In *International Perspectives on Engineering Education*, edited by Steen Christensen, Carl Mitcham, Bernard Newberry, Chris Didier, Andrew Jamison and Michael Meganck, 203–16. Cham: Springer.

Cruz, José, Enrique Nuñez, and Jonathan Carrell. 2024. "Developing Empathetic Dispositions in Engineering Undergraduates Using Humanities-Driven STEM: A Discourse Analysis." *Studies in Engineering Education* 5 (1): 134–56. https://doi.org/10.21061/see.120.

Davies, Thomas C., Jacob Manzin, Melissa Meraw, and Daniel S. Munro. 2022. "Understanding the Development of a Design Thinking Mindset During a Biomedical Engineering Third-Year Course." *Biomedical Engineering Education* 3 (2): 123–32. https://doi.org/10.1007/s43683-022-00093-0.

De Maria, Carmelo, Alejandro D. Lantada, Tuomo Jämsä, Lorenzo Pecchia, and Arti Ahluwalia. 2022. "Biomedical Engineering in Low- and Middle-Income Settings: Analysis of Current State, Challenges and Best Practices." *Health and Technology* 12 (3): 643–53. https://doi.org/10.1007/s12553-022-00657-8.

Durkheim, Emile. 1982. *Rules of Sociological Method.* New York: Simon and Schuster.

Fook, Jan, and Fiona Gardner. 2007. *Practicing Critical Reflection: A Resource Handbook.* Berkshire: Open University Press.

Frank, John, Thomas Abel, Stefano Campostrini, Susan Cook, Vincent K. Lin, and David V. McQueen. 2020. "The Social Determinants of Health: Time to Re-Think?" *International Journal of Environmental Research and Public Health* 17 (16): 5856. https://doi.org/10.3390/ijerph17165856.

Giddens, Anthony, and Philip W. Sutton. 2021. *Sociology.* 9th ed. Hoboken, NJ: Wiley.

Gilbert, Donna J., Mary L. Held, Jennifer L. Ellzey, William T. Bailey, and L. B. Young. 2014. "Teaching 'Community Engagement' in Engineering Education for International Development: Integration of an Interdisciplinary Social Work Curriculum." *European Journal of Engineering Education* 40 (3): 256–66. https://doi.org/10.1080/03043797.2014.944103.

Grogan, Paul T. 2021. "Perception of Complexity in Engineering Design." *Systems Engineering* 24: 221–33. https://doi.org/10.1002/sys.21574.

Hess, Justin L., Johannes Strobel, and Andrew O. Brightman. 2017. "The Development of Empathic Perspective-Taking in an Engineering Ethics Course." *Journal of Engineering Education* 106 (4): 534–63. https://doi.org/10.1002/jee.20175.

Interaction Design Foundation (IxDF). 2016. *What Is Design Thinking (DT)*? https://www.interaction-design.org/literature/topics/design-thinking.

Jagtap, Shirish. 2022. "Codesign in Resource-Limited Societies: Theoretical Perspectives, Inputs, Outputs and Influencing Factors." *Research in Engineering Design* 33: 191–211. https://doi.org/10.1007/s00163-022-00384-1.

Jesiek, Brent K., Nicole T. Buswell, Andrea Mazzurco, and Tia Zephirin. 2019. "Toward a Typology of the Sociotechnical in Engineering Practice." In *Proceedings of the 8th Research in Engineering Education Symposium (REES 2019): Making Connections*, vol. I: 597–606. Cape Town, South Africa, 10–12 July. https://doi.org/10.25916/sut.26251025.v1

Khalid, Ahmed, Christopher A. Chin, Mohammed M. Atiqullah, Jeffrey F. Sweigart, Brian Stutzmann, and Wei Zhou. 2013. "Building a Better Engineering: The Importance of Humanities in Engineering Curriculum." In *Proceedings of the 2013 ASEE Annual Conference & Exposition*. Atlanta, GA. https://doi.org/10.18260/1-2--19270

Koutsoklenis, Andreas, and Sophia Adam. 2024. "The Social Model of Disability." In *The Palgrave Encyclopedia of Disability*, edited by Graham Bennett and Emma Goodall. Cham: Palgrave Macmillan.

Lawson, Anna, and Alison E. Beckett. 2020. "The Social and Human Rights Models of Disability: Towards a Complementarity Thesis." *The International Journal of Human Rights* 25 (2): 348–79. https://doi.org/10.1080/13642987.2020.1783533.

Lenette, Chelsey. 2022. *Participatory Action Research: Ethics and Decolonization*. Oxford: Oxford University Press.

Leydens, Jon A., and Juan C. Lucena. 2009. "Listening as a Missing Dimension in Engineering Education: Implications for Sustainable Community Development Efforts." *IEEE Transactions on Professional Communication* 52 (4): 359–76. https://doi.org/10.1109/TPC.2009.2032383.

Leydens, Jon A., and Juan C. Lucena. 2014. "Social Justice: A Missing, Unelaborated Dimension in Humanitarian Engineering and Learning Through Service." *International Journal for Service Learning in Engineering, Humanitarian Engineering and Social Entrepreneurship* 9 (2): 1–28. https://doi.org/10.24908/ijsle.v9i2.5447.

Manzoor, Muhammad, and Vivian Vimarlund. 2018. "Digital Technologies for Social Inclusion of Individuals with Disabilities." *Health and Technology* 8 (5): 377–90. https://doi.org/10.1007/s12553-018-0239-1.

Marmot, Michael, Jessica Allen, Peter Goldblatt, Tammy Boyce, Dominic McNeish, M. Grady, and I. Geddes. 2010. *Fair Society, Healthy Lives: The Marmot Review*. London: Institute of Health Equity.

Marmot, Michael, Sharon Friel, Ruth Bell, Tanja A. Houweling, and Sebastian Taylor. 2008. "Closing the Gap in a Generation: Health Equity Through Action on the Social Determinants of Health." *The Lancet* 372 (9650): 1661–9. https://doi.org/10.1016/S0140-6736(08)61690-6.

Marsh, Adam. 2025. "Why Engineers Still Need the Humanities." *IEEE Spectrum*, May 5.

Martinez-Marroquin, Enrique, Bahia Senadji, Sally Male, and Lesley Wood. 2024. "Embedding Human and Social Aspects in Engineering Education." *European Journal of Engineering Education* 50 (3): 654–72. https://doi.org/10.1080/03043797.2024.2430532.

Mazzurco, Andrea, and Steven Daniel. 2020. "Socio-Technical Thinking of Students and Practitioners in the Context of Humanitarian Engineering." *Journal of Engineering Education* 109: 243–61. https://doi.org/10.1002/jee.20307.

Mazzurco, Andrea, Brent K. Jesiek, and Allison Godwin. 2019. "Development of Global Engineering Competency Scale: Exploratory and Confirmatory Factor Analysis." *Journal of Civil Engineering Education* 146 (2). https://doi.org/10.1061/(ASCE)EI.2643-9115.0000006.

Mihailidis, Alex, and Jill M. Polgar. 2016. "Occupational Therapy and Engineering." *Canadian Journal of Occupational Therapy* 83 (2): 68–9. https://doi.org/10.1177/0008417416638842.

Mina, M., John Cowan, and John Heywood. 2015. "Case for Reflection in Engineering Education—and an Alternative." In *Proceedings of the IEEE Frontiers in Education Conference (FIE)*, El Paso, TX, pp. 1–6, https://doi.org/10.1109/FIE.2015.7344252

Miranda, Claudia, Javier Goñi, and Tomás Sotomayor. 2021. "Embracing the Social Turn: Epistemic Change in Engineering Students Enrolled in an Anthro-Design Course." *International Journal of Technology and Design Education* 32 (5): 2697–724. https://doi.org/10.1007/s10798-021-09699-x.

Pleasants, Jacob, Ricardo Velasco, Camila Colonnello, Sarah Glenn, Sarah Crapitto, Kelly Raymond, and Benjamin Abbot. 2025. "Promoting Sociotechnical Perspectives of Engineering During a Summer Bridge Program." *Journal of Engineering Education* 114 (1): e20626. https://doi.org/10.1002/jee.20626.

Ravi, Sanjay, T. J. Kamalanabhan, and T. Jawahar. 2019. "Being More Human in the Digital World: Technology to Touch All, Serve All." *Health and Technology* 9 (3): 365–72. https://doi.org/10.1007/s12553-019-00325-4.

Roberts, Catherine, and Sheryl M. Lord. 2020. "Making Engineering Sociotechnical." In *Proceedings of the IEEE Frontiers in Education Conference (FIE)*. Uppsala, Sweden, pp. 1–4. https://doi.org/10.1109/FIE44824.2020.9273957

Rodriguez, Nicole M., Gary Burleson, Jacqueline C. Linnes, and Kathleen H. Sienko. 2023. "Thinking Beyond the Device: An Overview of Human- and Equity-Centered Approaches for Health Technology Design." *Annual Review of Biomedical Engineering* 25 (1): 257–80. https://doi.org/10.1146/annurev-bioeng-081922-024834.

Rodriguez, Raul B., and John S. Cicek. 2024. "A Scoping Literature of Sociotechnical Thinking in Engineering Education." *European Journal of Engineering Education* 49 (5): 807–33. https://doi.org/10.1080/03043797.2024.2346344.

Ruch, Gillian. 2002. "From Triangle to Spiral: Reflective Practice in Social Work Education, Practice and Research." *Social Work Education* 21 (2): 199–216. https://doi.org/10.1080/02615470220126435.

Saleebey, Dennis. 2012. "The Strengths Perspective: Putting Possibility and Hope to Work in Our Practice." In *The Profession of Social Work: Guided by History, Led by Evidence*, edited by Cynthia N. Dulmus and Karen M. Sowers. Hoboken, NJ: Wiley.

Santander Gana, Maria Teresa, and Luis A. Trejo Fuentes. 2006. "Technology as 'a Human Practice with Social Meaning'—A New Scenery for Engineering Education." *European Journal of Engineering Education* 31 (4): 437–47. https://doi.org/10.1080/03043790600676414.

Schneider, Jennifer, Jon A. Leydens, and Juan Lucena. 2008. "Where Is 'Community'?: Engineering Education and Sustainable Community Development." *European Journal of Engineering Education* 33 (3): 307–19. https://doi.org/10.1080/03043790802088640.

Schön, Donald A. 1983. *The Reflective Practitioner.* London: Temple Smith.

Steen, Marc G. D. 2008. *The Fragility of Human-Centered Design.* Amsterdam: IOS Press.

Steen, Marc G. D. 2013. "Co-Design as a Process of Joint Inquiry and Imagination." *Design Issues* 29 (2): 16–28. https://doi.org/10.1162/DESI_a_00207.

Tang, Xiaofei. 2018. "From 'Empathic Design' to 'Empathic Engineering': Toward a Genealogy of Empathy in Engineering Education." In *Proceedings of the 2018 ASEE Annual Conference & Exposition.* Salt Lake City, UT, June 24–27. https://peer.asee.org/from-empathic-design-to-empathic-engineering-toward-a-genealogy-of-empathy-in-engineering-education.pdf

Vincent, Christopher, and Ann Blandford. 2011. "Designing for Safety and Usability: User-Centered Techniques in Medical Device Design Practice." In *Proceedings of the Human Factors and Ergonomics Society Annual Meeting* 55 (1): 793–97.

Walther, Joachim, Sarah E. Miller, and Nicola W. Sochacka. 2017. "A Model of Empathy in Engineering as a Core Skill, Practice Orientation, and Professional Way of Being." *Journal of Engineering Education* 106 (1): 123–48. https://doi.org/10.1002/jee.20159.

Watts, Lynelle. 2018. "Reflective Practice, Reflexivity, and Critical Reflection in Social Work Education in Australia." *Australian Social Work* 72 (1): 8–20. https://doi.org/10.1080/0312407X.2018.1521856.

Williams, P. John. 2011. "Dispositions as Explicit Learning Goals for Engineering and Technology Education." In *Fostering Human Development through Engineering and Technology Education*, edited by Moshe Barak and Marc J. Hacker. Rotterdam: Sense/Brill.

World Health Organization (WHO). 2001. *International Classification of Functioning, Disability and Health (ICF).* Geneva: WHO.

World Health Organization (WHO). 2019. *Improving Health Workforce Data and Evidence.* Geneva: WHO.

World Health Organization (WHO). 2020. *Basic Documents: Forty-Ninth Edition (Including Amendments Adopted Up to 31 May 2019).* Geneva: WHO.

World Health Organization (WHO). 2025. *World Report on Social Determinants of Health Equity.* Geneva: WHO.

World Health Organization (WHO), and UNICEF. 2022. *Global Report on Assistive Technology.* Geneva: WHO and UNICEF.

13 Case Studies and Applications of Prototyping Pedagogy in Biomedical Engineering Education

Katherine Sammy and Matthew Wettergreen

13.1 INTRODUCTION

How can a prototype made from scavenged wood and office supplies outperform a prototype made from custom-machined metal? Moreover, how can BME educators teach students that this is the case?

In BME education, prototyping is more than a hands-on skill; it is a dynamic educational process of iteration, refinement, and discovery. This chapter builds upon the pedagogical strategies introduced in Chapter 5 by analyzing how real student teams move from rough concepts to sophisticated biomedical prototypes. We use detailed case studies to explore how projects evolve across dimensions such as fidelity, function, technical sophistication, and refinement. We also reflect on how prototype types and project durations influence the prototyping process and appropriate tool selection. These real-world examples allow educators to move beyond theory and observe the practical progression of student work.

While Chapter 5 provided a structured framework for understanding fidelity (low, medium, and high) and prototyping intent (e.g., ergonomic and proof-of-concept), this chapter focuses on actual outcomes. We present three extended case studies, from a first-year undergraduate design to a year-long graduate project, to show how real-world factors such as skill knowledge, time constraints, tool access, mentoring, and course structure shape the evolution of student teams' prototypes.

Each case study presents multiple prototypes that are analyzed using two pedagogical tools: (1) photos with a universal prototyping comparison table that tracks fidelity levels, materials, and tools used across prototypes (similar to the excellent depiction of helmet development over time from (Dean 1920, 47); and (2) a set of graphs that map fidelity against functionality, technical sophistication, and refinement. These tools allow us to visualize prototype progression and highlight key design decisions by student teams, showing where projects align with or deviate from idealized trends.

DOI: 10.1201/9781003520313-13

13.2 KEY TERMS AND DEFINITIONS

To analyze prototypes across fidelity levels, we use the following core definitions:

- **Function:** How well a prototype performs its intended task or goal. Functional prototypes meet specified design criteria or user needs. Function typically improves with iteration.
- **Technical Sophistication:** The depth of knowledge and skill reflected in the design and fabrication of a prototype. This incorporates factors such as appropriate tool use, integration of multidisciplinary knowledge, detailed implementation, and design elegance. For instance, a perf board circuit with intentional component selection reflects higher sophistication than a loose breadboard setup.
- **Refinement:** The finish quality, precision, elegance, and aesthetic resolution of a prototype. This could include smooth edges, functional assembly, or a visual clarity in the prototype that resembles a manufactured object.

13.3 IDEALIZED MODEL FOR PROTOTYPING PROGRESSION

Using these definitions, we introduce an *idealized model* for prototype development in BME education to serve as a benchmark and a teaching tool. In this *idealized model*, students begin with a low-fidelity prototype, such as a sketch or a 30-minute prototype, intended to explore design blocks, communicate initial ideas, and rapidly test assumptions. These early efforts should use basic materials like cardboard or foam and prioritize communication of design intention. Function may be minimal or non-existent at this stage, and technical sophistication is also absent. However, these early prototypes are essential in revealing abstract ideas in a tangible form.

As students gain insight into their problem space, their prototypes evolve into medium fidelity. These designs begin to incorporate actual functionality using accessible fabrication tools such as 3D printing, laser cutting, or breadboarding. At this stage, complexity (as seen through total part count) often increases as students add design features. At the same time, technical sophistication begins to emerge as decisions are now informed by a deeper understanding of the design blocks. Functionality improves, even if aesthetic refinement remains ignored.

The final set of high-fidelity prototypes, as made by teams, reflects the convergence of their ideas, the collective prototyping skill, aggregate mentorship, and execution. These models may integrate mechanical, electrical, and digital systems; employ advanced fabrication techniques such as CNC machining or custom electronics; and reflect a high degree of visual refinement and clean part organization. At this stage, technical sophistication peaks as students leverage their combined skills and the mentorship networks they are leveraging. The total number of parts typically reduces in these prototypes as the final prototypes are highly integrated and refined.

Figure 13.1 visualizes this ideal trajectory in the three graphs comparing fidelity versus functionality, fidelity versus technical sophistication, and fidelity versus refinement. In all three cases, an idealized prototyping path should move from the bottom left to the top right. While real student work often deviates from these paths,

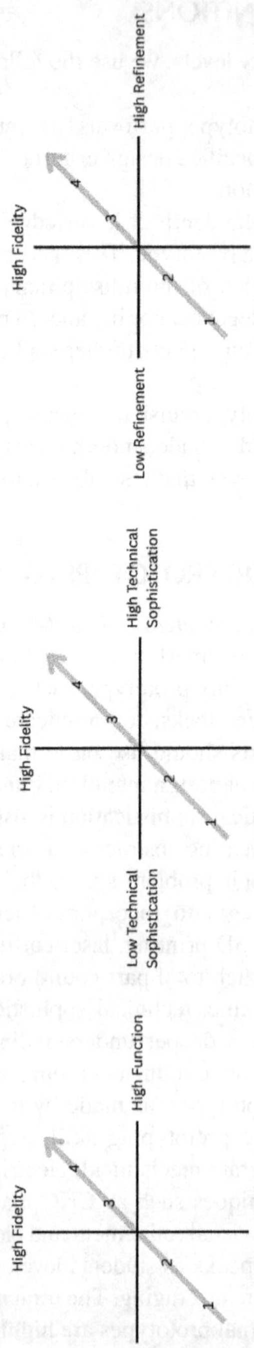

FIGURE 13.1 Prototype 1–4 progression (low to high fidelity) across three dimensions (function, technical sophistication, and refinement) with idealized trendlines

this visual model offers a shared vocabulary for diagnosing progress, setting milestones, and providing structured feedback throughout the prototyping process.

In this chapter, we review three student projects:

1) A first-year undergraduate project that developed a training mannequin for dislocated elbow reduction;
2) A multi-year undergraduate project to create an ergonomic soap grater;
3) A graduate-level, year-long project to develop a low-cost tele-retinal camera for diabetic retinopathy (DR) screening.

These projects were selected because they span a range of fidelity levels, tools, and learning environments. Each example includes photos, analysis of prototyping decisions, materials and tools list, and the comparative assessment using the fidelity versus function/sophistication/refinement graph introduced earlier.

By tracing these prototypes from sketch to near-product, this chapter offers educators a roadmap for recognizing effective prototyping progress, diagnosing roadblocks in team prototypes, and scaffolding project-based prototyping for biomedical engineers at every academic level. It is intended that BME educators understand the idealized versions of a prototype progression and how this happens in practice, so they can guide students in producing prototypes that balance functionality with technical sophistication and refinement, no matter their starting skill level.

Following the case studies, which highlight prototypes from a fidelity perspective, we present two additional frameworks to understand prototyping in the BME curriculum better. Section 13.4 re-categorizes projects according to the type of prototype they produced, independent of fidelity. Section 13.5 examines how project duration (e.g., a two-hour sprint versus a two-semester capstone) influences the number of iterations, tools employed, and overall prototype quality. These comparative frameworks give BME educators a multidimensional view of how biomedical engineering students engage in iterative design and how course structure and support systems can guide more effective prototyping practice.

13.3.1 Case Study 1: Training Mannequin for Nursemaid's Elbow

Our first case study highlights a one-semester project titled "Training Mannequin for Dislocated Elbow," developed by a first-year team at Rice University's OEDK in the ENGI 120: Introduction to Engineering Design course. Despite having no prior fabrication experience, the team iterated through five major prototypes, producing a functioning device that simulated the relocation technique for a common pediatric injury, Nursemaid's Elbow. The project description and resulting outcome are as follows:

> Many children under five experience Nursemaid's elbow, a dislocation of the radial bone caused by a sharp upward pull on the arm. Despite its clinical frequency, there were no existing tools to train physicians in the proper relocation technique at the time. This project developed a mannequin arm that simulates the relocation process, allowing physicians to practice before treating patients and seeking to reduce associated

> pain and stress. The design includes three plastic bones and a spring-loaded metal pin in the radial head. When the correct motion is performed, rotating the forearm palm-up and bending it toward the shoulder, the pin snaps into place, providing visual and tactile feedback. The radial bone can be reset for repeated use. This low-cost tool aims to improve physician effectiveness and patient care for Nursemaid's elbow.
>
> (Danckers 2014, 1)

We selected this first case study because it shows that by using simple materials and tools, the function can be achieved and iterated over successive prototypes in order to achieve a level of refinement necessary for a project solution. We show photos of the successive prototypes and a table that discusses the different materials in the comparison graphs; these can be found in Figures 13.2 and 13.3 and Table 13.1.

Over the semester, the team produced five successive prototypes. These are shown in Figure 13.2, which visually traces the evolution from initial concept sketch to a high-fidelity anatomically based prototype. Table 13.1 shows how the materials and construction methods evolved across all five versions. The team's first prototype was a hand-drawn sketch that clearly mapped out the desired motion and included arrow-labeled annotations to describe the intended internal mechanism. This early design was notable for its completeness and clarity; it served to communicate an idea and as a roadmap for the functional system the team would build.

The second prototype was constructed from low-cost, readily available materials. There was a wide range of these materials: pine wood, dowels, wire, rubber bands, and tape, totaling 27 individual parts, assembled with both hand and power tools. This low-fidelity prototype was unexpectedly functional, an unusual success for a first-year team with no prior fabrication training. Despite its low fidelity and lack

TABLE 13.1
Elbow Mannequin: materials and construction methods across prototypes 1–5

Prototypes	1	2	3	4	5
Materials	Paper, pencil	Wooden dowels, wire, wooden peg, plywood, PVC, plastic sheet, metal hinge, screws, tape	Pine wood, dowels, nail, metal hinge, screws, rubber bands, staple, tape	Pine wood, plywood, wire, dowel, screws, rubber bands, staples, metal hinge	Plastic humerus, plastic radius, plastic ulna, screws, spring, metal washer, metal hinge, rubber band, acrylic sheet
Number of unique materials	2	9	8	8	9
Number of parts	1	27	18	18	12
Tools used	Sketching	Hand tools, power tools	Hand tools, power tools	Hand tools, power tools	Hand tools, power tools

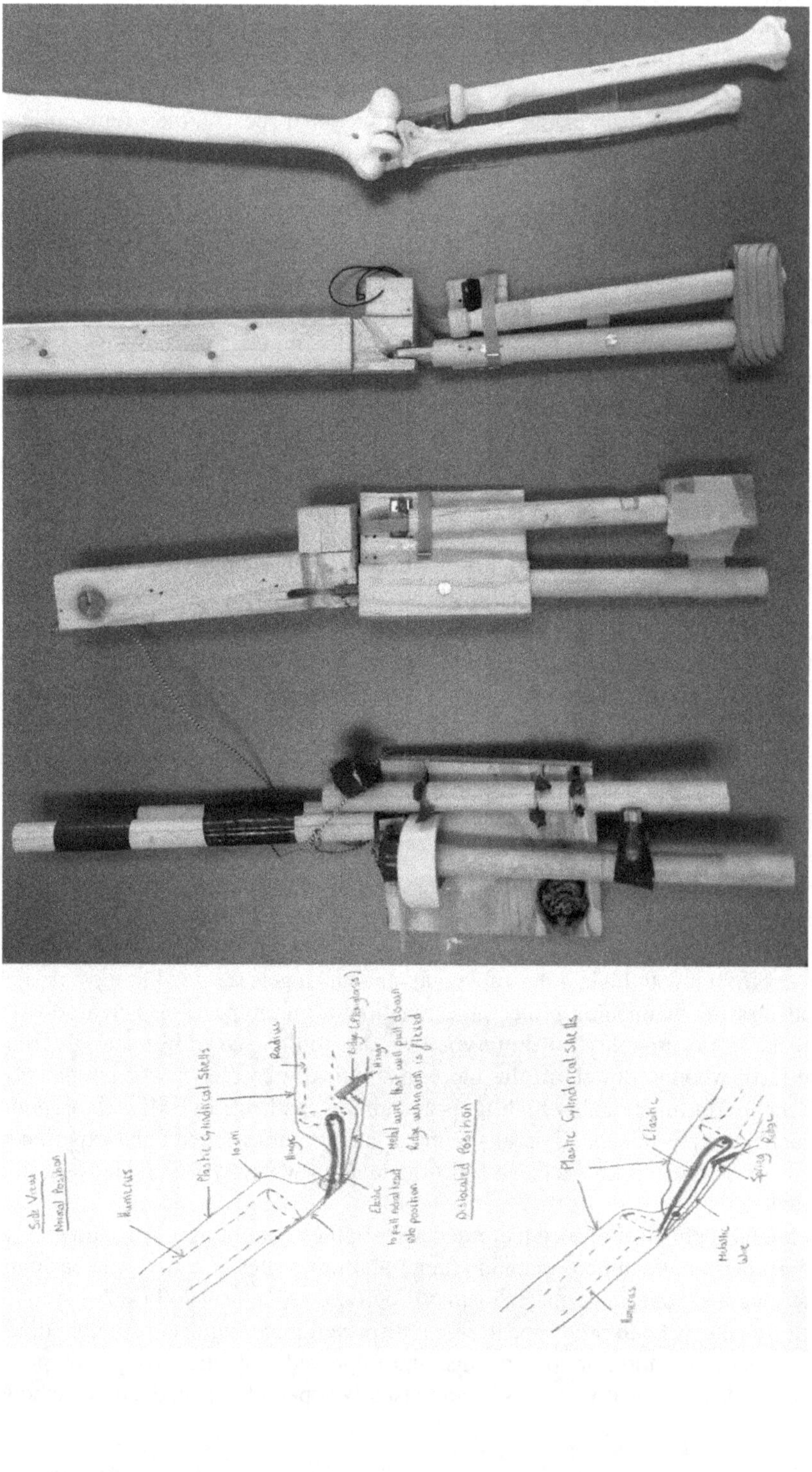

FIGURE 13.2 Elbow Mannequin prototypes 1–5, showing progression from concept sketch to high(medium)-fidelity anatomical model

of refinement, the mechanism effectively simulated the locking and release action of the elbow relocation. The elbow joint could be "reset" and reused, and the entire device demonstrated an intuitive and physical response when manipulated correctly. It is rare for a first prototype at this academic level and skill to achieve such precise functionality, especially using mostly rigid materials, which are hard to shape and work with. Since the team experienced early functional success, their future prototypes iterated toward greater refinement of the existing materials and a reduction of the total number of parts.

In later prototypes (three and four), the team kept the overall layout of the wooden platform but began refining the bone structures and the mechanics. Although the type of material remained relatively constant, the number of parts dropped to 18 for both prototypes. Tape as a fixation device was replaced with fasteners; wood components were sanded and shaped. The "bones," initially improvised from dowels, were whittled to mimic anatomical proportions better and enhance rotational alignment. Prototypes three and four prioritized maintaining function as they refined individual elements.

Prototype 5 departed from the evolutionary exploration of prototypes 2–4 and sought to maintain function while achieving greater anatomical realism for training purposes. The team substituted the dowels for the commercially available Sawbones representations of the humerus, radius, and ulna. Rubber bands were still used to provide the necessary resistance and snap-in functionality, and clear acrylic was substituted for the plywood base to hold everything in place. While more visually compelling and containing the fewest parts (12), this prototype performed functionally worse than the previous wooden versions. The Sawbones models' irregular geometries and awkward connection surfaces introduced significant challenges for joint assembly and reliable motion. Functionality suffered, demonstrating that increased fidelity in prototypes does not always mean that a prototype is more successful; in fact, it can represent a step backward in prototyping.

Figure 13.3 compares the prototypes analyzing fidelity against function, technical sophistication, and refinement. While these graphs have inherent limitations: they are representational, not quantitative; they are intended to highlight the progression and tradeoffs inherent in iterative prototyping. Across all five prototypes, fidelity increased from low to high, a desirable outcome and a general trend in most design projects. For the mannequin project, the function of prototypes 1–4 increased with a decrease in functionality for prototype five, due to the change in materials from the uniform wooden dowels to the more anatomically correct Sawbones models. This decrease in functionality highlights a common challenge in BME prototyping: do students use physiologically realistic materials to prototype with and experience struggle, or do they seek to achieve full functionality with physical analogs (in this case, dowels)?

Technical sophistication also increased across all five prototypes: the team moved from improvised attachment methods (tape) and raw material cuts to increasingly precise cuts and repeatable mechanisms. Prototype refinement followed a similar upward trajectory. Each prototype iteration displayed more uniform assembly quality, a cleaner integration of components, and improved aesthetics. By prototype 4, the model was functionally successful and visually apparent as a model of the elbow,

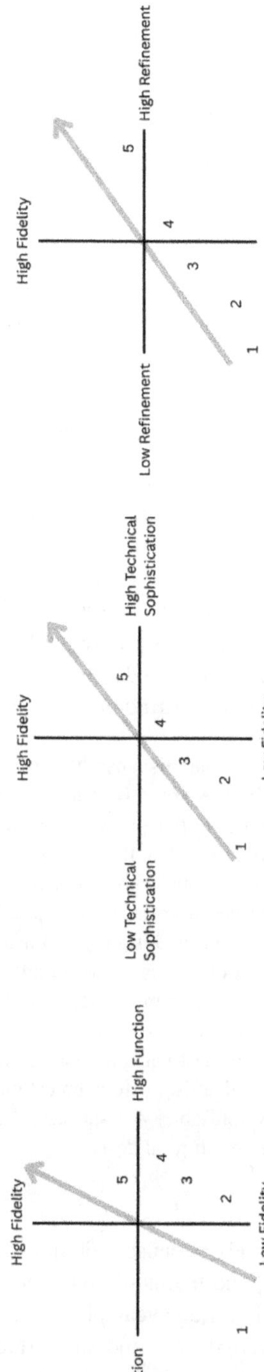

FIGURE 13.3 Elbow Mannequin prototype comparison graphs (fidelity, function, technical sophistication, and refinement)

containing the three bones. This refinement continued through prototype 5, the most visually impressive due to its anatomical realism.

This case study highlights several important insights. First, this study demonstrates that individuals without prior fabrication experience can produce functional prototypes in a setting with proper tools, instruction, mentorship, and support. Second, students can develop a deep insight into engineering mechanisms even with simple materials, such as wood, rubber bands, and wire. Third, full functionality can be achieved even with low- or medium-fidelity prototypes. This is especially important as this team's final prototype, prototype 5, a high-fidelity prototype, was less functional than earlier versions; this serves as a valuable example that higher fidelity and higher levels of refinement do not necessarily yield improvements in other dimensions, especially in functionality.

13.3.2 Case Study 2: Hand-Powered Soap Dispenser for Bar Soap

Our second case study highlights a multi-year undergraduate project titled "Safe Soap," also known by its earlier name "Fork Yeah." Initially launched by a first-year team in the ENGI 120: Introduction to Engineering Design course at Rice University's OEDK, this project evolved over six semesters and culminated in a high-fidelity, technically sophisticated prototype. Over time, the team iterated through six major versions of a soap dispenser that incorporated culinary elements to align with the branding of The Pass and Provisions, a James Beard-nominated restaurant in Houston. The project description and resulting outcome are as follows:

> Team Fork Yeah's goal is to design a soap dispenser that integrates kitchen equipment to grate bar soap for a restaurant in downtown Houston, the Pass and Provisions. The owners of the Pass and Provisions want all aspects of their restaurant to be innovative and reflect their kitchen theme. To accomplish this goal and fit the restaurant's overall uniqueness, a normal liquid soap dispenser is not adequate. A bar soap dispenser that utilizes a commercially available cheese grater will help enhance the overall dining experience and contribute to the restaurant's success. Our design meets several constraints outlined at the beginning of our project, including: 1) our device must match the design and décor of the bathroom, 2) it must mount to the already installed bathroom mirrors, 3) it must dispense standard bar soap and mimic the idea of a kitchen environment in the final design. In order to accomplish our design objectives, the following are our design criteria: intuitive use, safety, entertaining/unique, durable, low cost, easily replicable, and easily refillable. All successful and necessary prototype features have been implemented into our final design.
>
> (Grace et al. 2013, 1)

We selected this second case study because it demonstrates that long-term prototyping success is not often linear, and teams often experience setbacks or pauses in forward progress. Additionally, this multi-year project demonstrates what students can learn and accomplish in a well-staffed and supported makerspace, starting as underclassmen. Photos of the successive prototypes and a table that discusses the different materials in the comparison graphs can be found in Figures 13.4 and 13.5 and Table 13.2.

TABLE 13.2
Safesoap: materials and construction methods across prototypes 1–6

Prototype	1	2	3	4	5	6
Materials	Springs, acrylic, metal bracket, screws, balsa wood, pine wood, rubber bands, metal washer, hot glue, grater, soap, sharpie	Butcher block wood, microplane grater, acrylic, springs, plastic frame, soap	Hair tie, soap, acrylic, plastic frame, springs, butcher block wood, microplane grater	80/20 aluminum framing, soap, sheet metal, angle brackets, machine screws, metal washers, metal "U" channels, microplane grater, springs	Butcher block wood, acrylic, sheet metal, steel block, machine screws, plastic grater case, microplane grater, springs, soap	Sheet metal, steel block, butcher block, metal U channels, springs, soap, microplane grater, screws
Number of unique materials	8	6	6	9	9	7
Number of individual parts	50	15	14	29	17	27
Tools used	Hand tools, power tools, drill press	Hand tools, power tools, laser cutter, mill	Hand tools, power tools, laser cutter, CAD, CNC	Hand tools, CAD, CNC, sheet metal bender	Laser cutter, CAD, CNC, machining, sheet metal bender, hand tools	Machining, CAD, CNC, sheet metal bending, hand tools

Abbreviations: CAD, Computer-Aided Design; CNC, Computer Numerical Control

This playful yet technically demanding concept, a cheese-grater-style bar soap dispenser, challenged students to iterate across materials, mechanisms, and tools, while preserving core functional requirements and responding to actual client needs, as shown in Figure 13.4. The final device grates soap onto the user's hand using a mechanical handle that mimics the motion of grating material in the kitchen. Throughout the project, the team conserved key design elements (such as vertical soap orientation and integrated frame geometry) while steadily increasing technical sophistication and refinement.

Over six semesters, the team advanced from a low-fidelity, hand-assembled prototype to a fully machined, CNC-cut, sheet metal-bent final product. The earliest prototype (prototype 1) was the most component-dense, containing over 50 parts sourced from readily available materials in the OEDK, such as springs, acrylic, pine, and balsa wood, all assembled using basic tools such as hand tools, a drill press, and basic fasteners. This prototype demonstrated the basic concept, a palm-activated mechanical soap dispenser, although it lacked refinement and technical sophistication. In prototype 2, the students streamlined their design, significantly reducing the total part count to 15. They incorporated some elements that would continue through to all of the prototypes: butcher block wood, a spring-loaded mechanism, and a vertical orientation for the bar of soap. Prototype 2 exhibited higher functionality due to the use of channels cut into the wooden block, which stabilized the movement of the grater. This prototype also marked the team's first use of digital fabrication tools, including a laser cutter to cut the acrylic and a manual mill to drill holes.

Prototype 3, completed after one year of working on the project, reflects that the team had self-trained to use CAD and CNC machining to produce the channels in the wooden housing, which guide the motion of the cheese grater. Functionality further improved in this prototype, and the design began to resemble the final form while maintaining the relatively same number (18) of parts as the previous prototype (19). The students also introduced a new method of providing compressive force between the bar of soap and the grater, in this case, a hair tie, which provided a compressive force.

Prototype 4 marked a deliberate departure: built from 80/20 aluminum extrusion, it was intended not as a refined solution but as a learning platform. This prototype version was constructed quickly, but by using 80/20, the students ended up with a prototype that worked uniformly, allowing them to explore and test out a range of physical models produced with CAD, CNC machining, metal cutting, and sheet metal bending. While prototype 4 had lower fidelity, functionality, and refinement, it offered a critical opportunity for skills acquisition and tool experimentation.

In the later prototypes, the skills acquired in prototype 4 incorporated CNC metal cutting and sheet metal bending. In prototype 4, the team returned to their refined butcher block frame but incorporated these new machined metal elements, including a metal soap holder chamber made from bent CNC machined metal, and U-channel guides that secured the grater in a sled. Prototype 6, the team's final prototype, was the most technically sophisticated, highest fidelity, most refined, and most functional of all of the prototypes. The soap enclosure had been modified to incorporate a new understanding of the user base, low-resource settings, where bar soap was a target

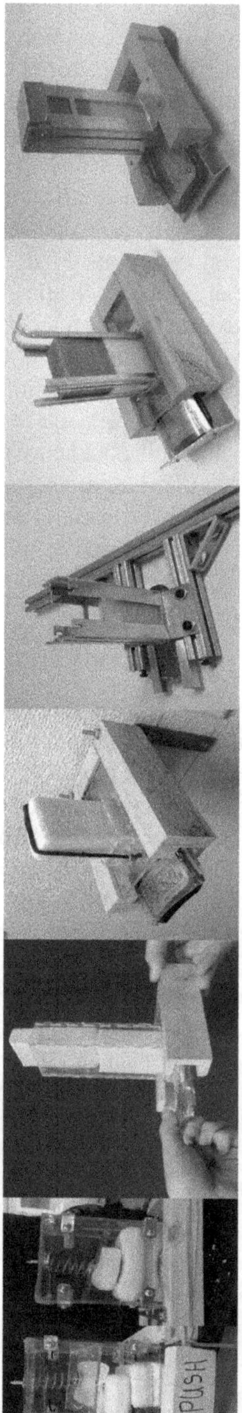

FIGURE 13.4 Safesoap prototypes 1–6, showing progression from low- to high-fidelity models, left to right

for theft. Though this final version had more parts than previous versions (27), this was due to the number of fasteners required to assemble the precision components.

Figure 13.5 compares the prototypes along axes of fidelity, functionality, refinement, and technical sophistication. The trend for fidelity, functionality, technical sophistication, and refinement generally reflects an increase between prototypes 1 and 6. However, these figures show that the team's progression to a final solution was not strictly linear. Prototype 4 stands out as an anomaly to these positive trends, reflecting a strategic pit stop used for skills development.

This case study reinforces several key points. First, successful prototyping is not merely about linear progress; it can include tactical setbacks that set up long-term successes. Prototype 4 is a prime example where a less functional but highly instructive tool unlocked future advancements. The setback that the team experienced in case study one is similar to the use of the 80/20 in prototype 4, as it reduced the prototype's functionality, but the team learned a valuable lesson that they then built upon in the future. Perhaps the elbow mannequin could have taken what was learned from prototype 5 and applied it to successful future prototypes if they had had more time in their project. Another outcome is that the team retained the core design elements across iterations, for example, the vertical soap chamber, palm-actuated handle, or the grater mount. This action provided a stable foundation for experimentation.

13.3.3 Case Study 3: Low-Cost DR Camera for Telemedicine

Our third case study features a year-long graduate project, "Innoscope," developed by students in the Global Medical Innovation Master of Bioengineering program at Rice University. This professional master's program prepares students for careers in the medical device industry by combining rigorous coursework with industry-sponsored design experiences. Innoscope was developed in partnership with the University of Texas School of Public Health in the Rio Grande Valley, targeting a specific unmet clinical need: screening for DR in low-resource settings. Over one academic year, the team developed and refined a portable tele-retinal camera capable of capturing retinal images in primary care or community health settings. The project's objective and resulting outcome are described as follows:

> Diabetic retinopathy (DR) is a complication that leads to irreversible blindness. While preventable through early eye screenings, DR remains underdiagnosed in low-resource settings due to inaccessibility to ophthalmologists and the prohibitive cost of traditional retinal cameras (~$20,000). Innoscope offers a low-cost, portable retinal imaging system that enables primary care nurses to screen for DR in community-based or home settings. The device includes a handheld housing with custom optics, a Raspberry Pi microprocessor, a pellicle beam splitter, LED illumination, and an integrated LCD screen. The estimated unit cost is $400 at high-scale production, substantially lower than current commercial devices. Initial usability testing showed significantly improved user scores compared to an existing clinical comparator.
>
> (Chen et al. 2023, 3)

This case was selected because it highlights the technical challenges and design considerations unique to biomedical devices with complex technical requirements,

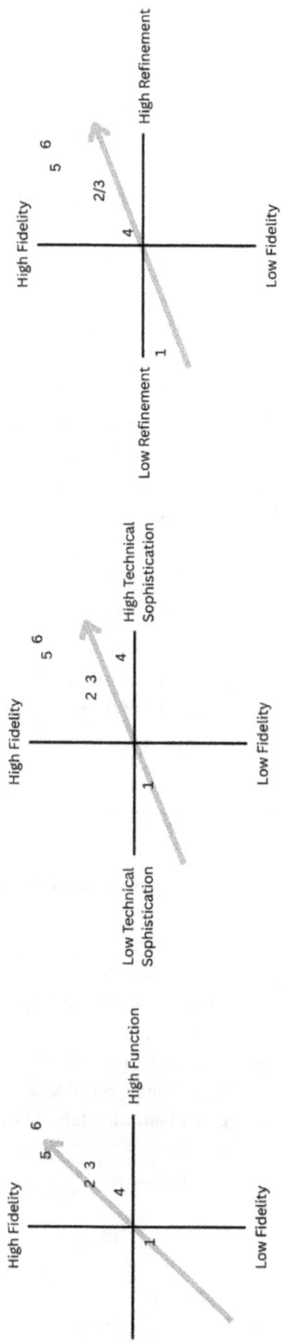

FIGURE 13.5 Safesoap prototype comparison graphs (fidelity, function, technical sophistication, and refinement)

such as optical or electronic components. It also demonstrates how a project can evolve in a one-year design team experience, from a detailed sketch to a fully functional, near-deployable prototype over two semesters, leveraging advanced fabrication tools, expert mentorship, and structured iteration.

Photos of the successive prototypes and a table that discusses the different materials in the comparison graphs can be found in Figures 13.6 and 13.7 and Table 13.3. These illustrate how the team produced low-fidelity prototypes that communicated a refined vision of the device, but then, when technical function was addressed, required the team to start with an unrefined, technologically complex prototype and iterate up to a refined and functional prototype.

The team produced four major prototypes, as shown in Figure 13.6. The first prototype was a detailed sketch that included labeled drawings of intended components such as the camera, an LED ring light, a battery, a microprocessor, and a potential solar charging panel. This annotated drawing served as a visual aid and a systems-level concept map, clearly communicating functional design blocks, hardware needs, and spatial organization. For a sketch, the level of specificity was high, giving the team a direction to prototype for their first physical prototype, and demonstrating that the team had an idea of engineering requirements for the project's demands.

The second prototype was a low-fidelity physical model made primarily of just five materials: cardboard, hot glue, foam, paper, and popsicle sticks. This prototype builds off the team's ideas from the detailed sketch, and similarities between these two are apparent. The prototype communicates how the user might interact with this device, hold it, and receive visual feedback. Despite lacking any function,

TABLE 13.3
Innoscope: materials and construction methods across prototypes 1–4

Prototype	1	2	3	4
Materials	Paper, pencil	Cardboard, popsicle stick, foam, paper, hot glue	Computer monitor, peripheral cords, desktop computer, mouse, keyboard, Raspberry Pi, breadboard, optical lens, pink foam, wire, tape, bolts, wood, optical equipment	Optical equipment, optical lens, Raspberry Pi camera sensor, breadboard, DSI screen, wire, rocker switch, toggle switch, hose clamp, 3D printed case, micro SD card, battery bank, charging port, USB terminal blocks, flashlight
Number of unique materials	2	5	14	16
Number of parts	1	14	>30	<30
Tools used	Sketching	Hand tools	Hand tools, CAD, 3D printing, coding, electronics	CAD, 3D printing, coding, electronics

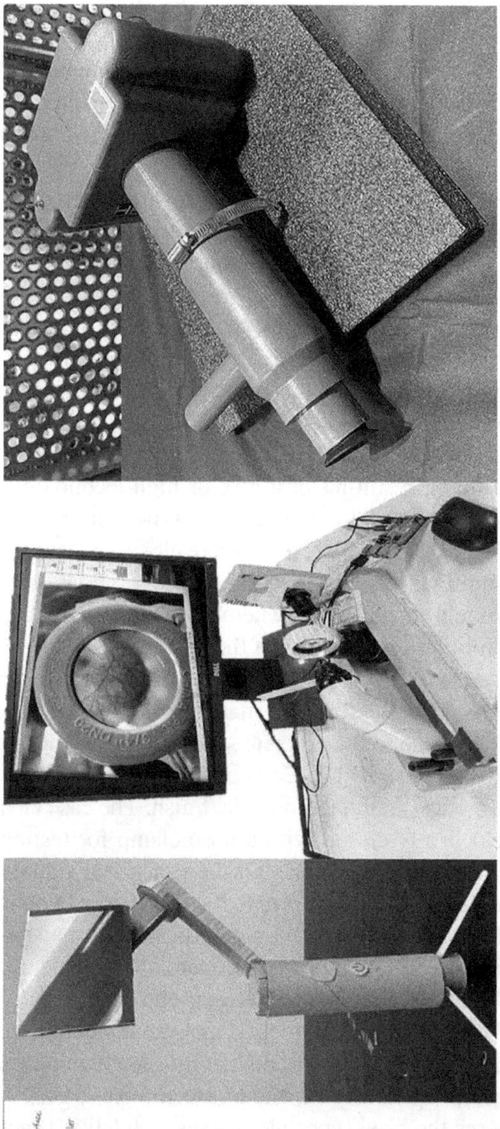

FIGURE 13.6 Innoscope prototypes 1–4, showing progression from concept sketch to high-fidelity functional model

it successfully mapped the design blocks from the sketch into a physical space, facilitating meaningful feedback during a design review. Low-fidelity prototypes like this are especially valuable for BME educators in medical device development, as they allow instructors and stakeholders to challenge assumptions and help students prioritize system elements before investing in more complicated technical development.

Prototypes 3 and 4 were developed during the spring semester of the course, and they represent a prioritization of function and integration. Prototype 3 was a semi-functional prototype incorporating over 14 unique materials with more than 30 total parts. The prototype included elements of low, medium, and high fidelity, such as tape and foam, breadboards, Raspberry Pi, and optical equipment such as pellicle beam splitters and aspheric lenses. The device could capture images, though not yet at the clinically relevant resolution or magnification. The device was also not portable and required an external computer interface. The device did not yet include any housing and was loosely assembled using basic mounts and available lab hardware, like wood, tape, and foam, resulting in a mix of high-technology electronics and low-fidelity structural elements. This type of prototype, common in early technical prototypes, reflects a blend of fidelity levels, where electronic subsystems are robust, but form factors are improvised. This mix of fidelities should be encouraged: it does not matter what the mount looks like or whether it is functional at this point, since the technical underpinnings are the focus of the prototype.

Prototype 4 was the team's final, high-fidelity prototype. This prototype maintained around the same number of unique materials as the prior prototype, but the total part count decreased due to the efficient space management offered by the custom 3D printed enclosure, designed in CAD and post-processed using wet sanding and paint to create a smooth, manufactured-like finish. The case closed with snap-fit elements and was held firmly closed with a hose clamp for testing. The case was designed to perfectly and elegantly house all the functional subsystems: the optics technology block, the flashlight, the USB hub, the Raspberry Pi board, and the LCD screen. Power, control switches, and a charging port were embedded in the housing, providing a user experience comparable to commercial handheld devices. This fully functional prototype allowed users at the final year-end design showcase to take retinal images on-site. The functionality, fidelity, and refinement reflected not just the students' technical growth but also the product of the mentorship they received: from their course instructor, an optics expert, and an electronics expert.

Figure 13.7 compares the prototypes along axes of fidelity, functionality, refinement, and technical sophistication. For this project, fidelity, functionality, and technical sophistication increased across all prototypes moving from the sketch to the high fidelity version. Refinement offers an interesting lesson in prioritizing design outcomes; prototypes 1 and 2 were refined, expressing specific design intentions, but prototype 3 prioritized function and technical operation, and thus refinement temporarily dropped. This is similar to case study 2, where the team paused on integrated evolution to prioritize another design need temporarily. Unlike the earlier undergraduate case studies, the graduate team's trajectory reflects conceptual low-fidelity prototypes before successive technically driven solutions, rather than using a low-fidelity model and evolving function on that model.

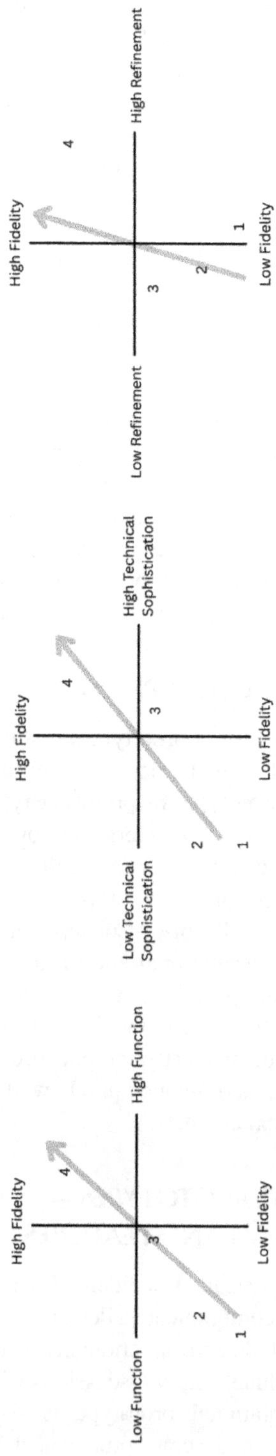

FIGURE 13.7 Innoscope prototype comparison graphs (fidelity, function, technical sophistication, and refinement)

This case study offers an interesting discussion around the dramatic difference between the low-fidelity prototypes (1 and 2) and the medium-/high-fidelity prototypes (3 and 4). This team spent time making a detailed sketch and a detailed low-fidelity prototype from that sketch, only to need to then focus on the function of the device, which sent the final prototype in a completely different direction. A concern for BME educators may be that the team lost time or work by not developing upon the low-fidelity prototype. Nevertheless, this progression is typical for design teams. Getting teams to develop early prototypes can simply be about helping them to gain momentum. After they get started and take team ownership of the prototype, they can sustain that momentum, as this team did, moving from the idea of their low-fidelity prototype into the desktop version of their technical functioning prototype.

This case study underscores several important points about advanced BME prototyping. First, teams working on highly technical systems, such as optics, electronics, or diagnostics, benefit from using low-fidelity prototypes not to demonstrate function, but to scope design elements and manage complexity strategically. Second, scaffolding from instructors and subject-matter mentors played a critical role in bridging the gap between vision and execution, thanks to the instructor connecting the team with the right experts to maintain momentum (optics expert and electronics expert). In conclusion, fully functional systems can be built by student teams when they are given time, structure, mentorship, and access to appropriate fabrication tools.

13.4 CASE STUDIES BY PROTOTYPE TYPE

While fidelity is one way to evaluate a prototype's maturity and how well it meets design goals, another valuable lens is the design intent, or prototype purpose. This section re-categorizes selected prototypes by prototype type rather than fidelity. This new lens gives BME educators a way to understand how different prototypes serve different goals, even if they share similar levels of refinement or fidelity.

As described in Chapter 5, prototype types fall into several categories: Representational, Mockup/Visual, Proof-of-Concept, Ergonomic, and Functional. For simplicity, we combine representational and visual mockup prototypes in this section, as they serve overlapping purposes in the early design stages. Each prototype that a team creates contributes value to the design process. BME Instructors can use these categories to help students clarify the purpose of their prototype, choose appropriate evaluation criteria, and understand how different phases of design require different kinds of physical artifacts.

13.5 REPRESENTATIONAL PROTOTYPES—"SYMBOLIZES DESIGN AND FEATURES"

Representational prototypes are typically low-fidelity sketches, drawings, mockups, or physical prototypes intended to communicate a designer's internal ideas in the physical realm. They most likely include zero functionality, but help visualize form, size, or features, and can facilitate valuable early discussions with users or stakeholders.

An example of a representational prototype is shown in the drawings in Figure 13.8, where a student designed a conceptual wheelchair for a pediatric patient.

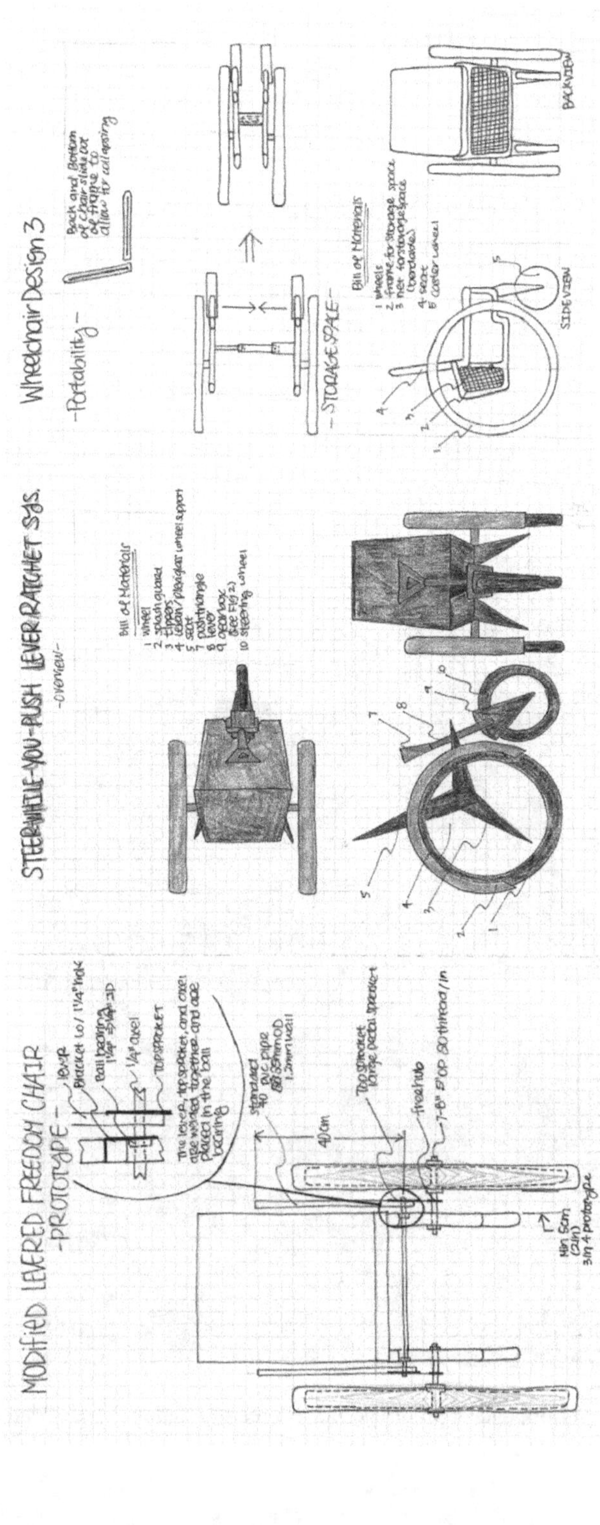

FIGURE 13.8 Early representational sketches of a custom wheelchair, used to communicate design and features

The design includes multiple annotated views highlighting the planned features, such as accessory locations or functional components, before any building has begun. Representational prototypes are particularly useful during stakeholder engagement and early design planning, as drawings like this can be brought to the instructor and mentors to seek direct feedback before resources are invested in building.

13.6 PROOF-OF-CONCEPT PROTOTYPES—"WORKS LIKE"

Proof-of-concept prototypes aim to demonstrate that at least one critical function or design element is feasible, proving the design team's ideas about solving a design problem. These prototypes sacrifice refinement, aesthetics, or even usability to validate a core technical principle, which can be shown to a client or instructor as evidence of a feasible solution. These prototypes are essential for making binary decisions. Will they work, or won't they?

Figure 13.9 presents an early version of a forearm rotation measurement device. Constructed from basic materials, the prototype was not intended for patient use,

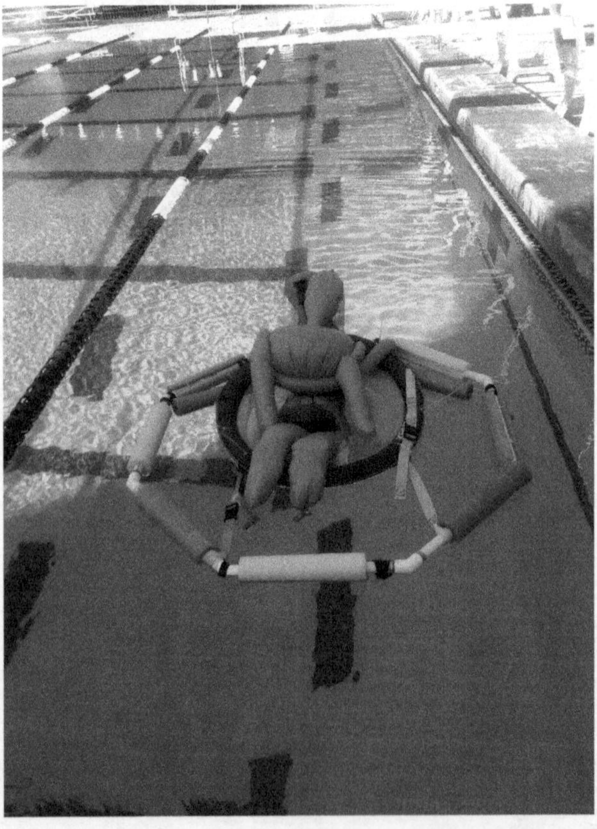

FIGURE 13.9 Proof-of-concept prototypes for a forearm rotation device, used to test core functions

but it successfully demonstrated the team's approach to capturing forearm rotational angle. This proof-of-concept enabled the team to move forward confidently and was a communication tool for instructors and advisors.

13.7 ERGONOMIC PROTOTYPE—"FEELS LIKE"

Ergonomic prototypes simulate or represent how a user interacts with a device. These prototypes prioritize size, form factor, feel, and physical interactions over proper functionality or technical sophistication. These prototypes are especially useful for uncovering usability, comfort, and safety concerns that might not arise until functional testing.

Figure 13.10 shows an ergonomic prototype for a flotation device intended for a patient with ataxia who enjoys water-based activities. While not functional (or safe!), the prototype was fabricated at full scale using floatable materials and realistic straps to simulate how the user would wear the device in the water. Ergonomic prototypes

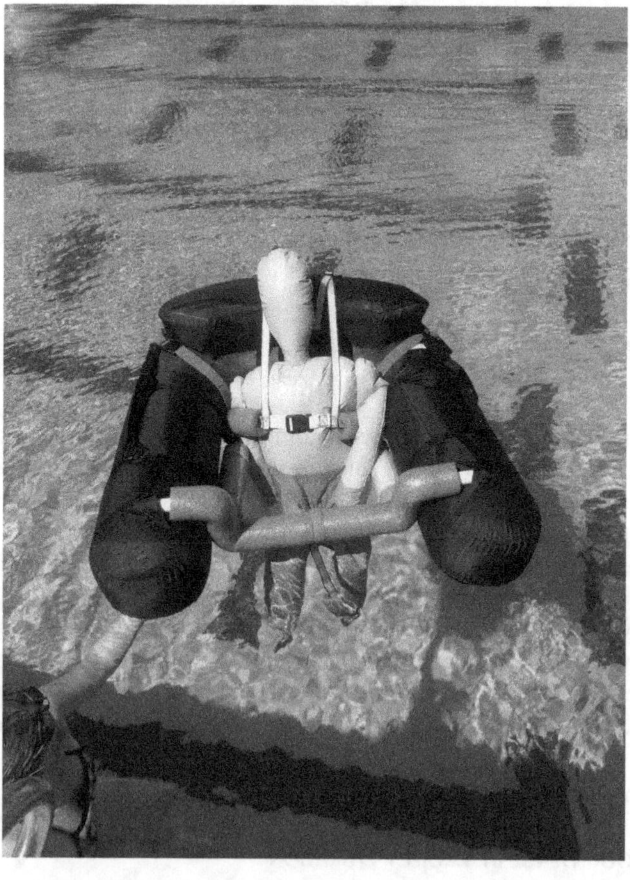

FIGURE 13.10 Ergonomic prototypes for a patient-specific flotation device, tested and refined for user comfort and safety

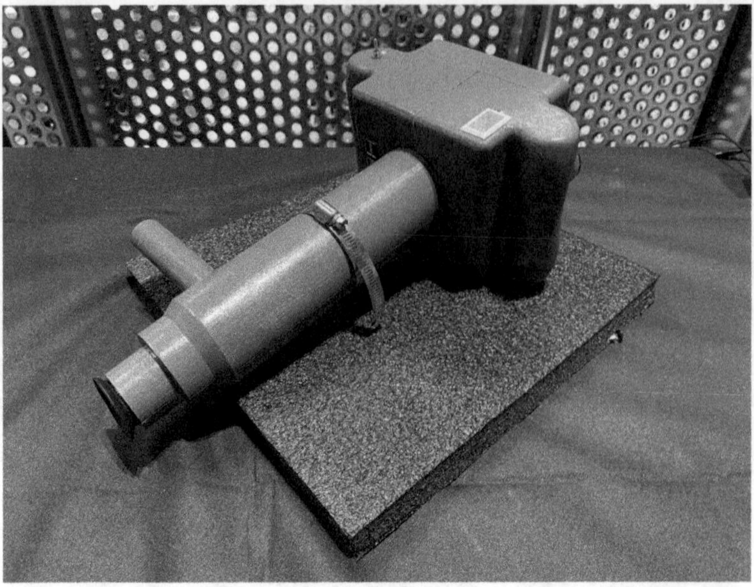

FIGURE 13.11 Functional prototypes for innoscope, which integrate mechanical, electronic, and software components

like this one help teams identify design improvements related to user interaction and offer an important opportunity for early user feedback.

13.8 FUNCTIONAL PROTOTYPES—"LOOKS LIKE, FEELS LIKE, AND WORKS LIKE"

Functional prototypes are the most evolved form of student prototypes, fully integrating the features, achieving full functionality of the design goals, being refined, and being technically sophisticated. These are often the final deliverables of long-term projects, capstone or graduate-level projects, and can ideally serve as an alpha prototype or be adopted by a client. In Figure 13.11, we present the final prototype from the Innoscope team, their low-cost tele-retinal camera for DR screening. Their final prototype integrates optical, electronic, and mechanical systems into a device that performs all the intended device's core functions while demonstrating a high degree of refinement. Functional prototypes showcase the entire arc of iterative prototyping and reflect deep student engagement with design goals and user needs.

13.9 CASE STUDIES BY PROJECT DURATION

13.9.1 Tool Usage by Project Duration

Figure 13.12 suggests that the percentage of time each tool could be used across four project lengths: two-hour prototype, hackathon, one-semester, and two-semester

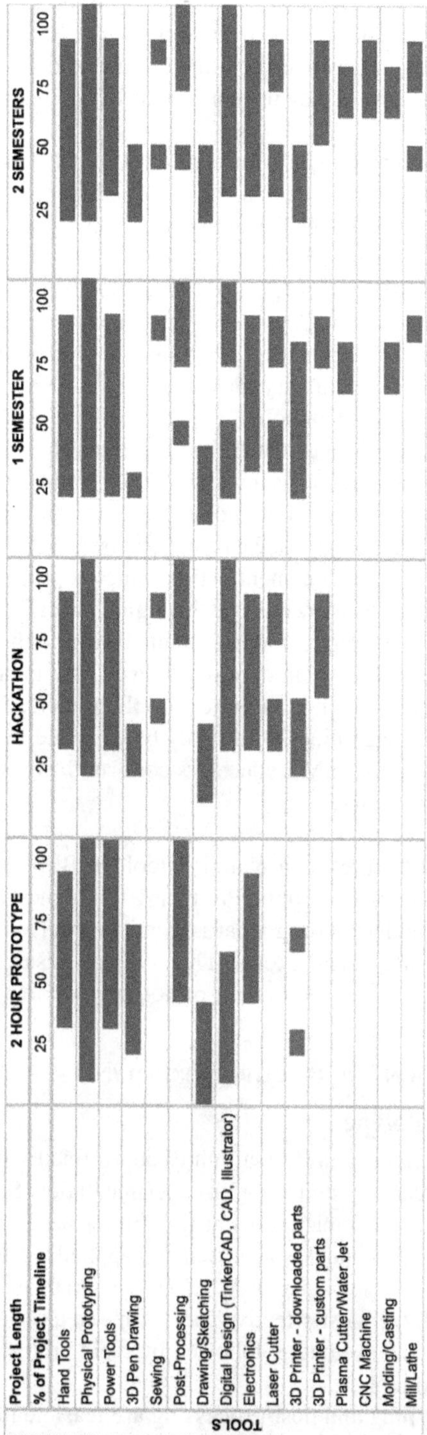

FIGURE 13.12 Tool usage mapped across different project durations (two hour, hackathon, one semester, two semesters), showing when specific design tools are typically used

projects. Each bar illustrates when a given tool is likely to be used during the project timeline. Tools are grouped by type, from simple sketching and hand tools to advanced fabrication techniques such as molding, casting, and CNC machining.

This visualization offers several key insights for BME educators:

- **Tool selection must match the timeline:** Only rapid, low-barrier tools, such as sketching, 3D pens, or hand tools, are advised in short-duration projects. Complex tools like CNC machining or custom casting are impractical due to setup and learning time.
- **Iteration is timeline-dependent:** Projects shorter than a weekend often leave little time for iteration. Conversely, one- and two-semester projects allow for structured prototyping design–build–test cycles, where students can develop multiple evolutionary prototypes, while increasing fidelity through increasingly advanced tools.
- **Advanced tools require longer timelines:** For tools such as laser cutters, custom 3D printing, and electronics integration, successful use often depends on projects extending over a minimum of multiple weeks. High-complexity tools (CNC machining, molding, and casting) can be used for initial fabrication and iterative prototype refinement in two-semester projects.
- **Scaffolding matters:** Educators can use this figure to scaffold tool instruction appropriately. For example, students should be explicitly encouraged to utilize digital design tools early in semester-long courses in order to support potential later fabrication with laser cutters or 3D printers. Similarly, milling, casting, or CNC machining should only be expected in later stages of long projects, ensuring that BME educators confirm the existence of or set up training where necessary.

Ultimately, Figure 13.12 serves as a planning tool for BME educators to align design expectations with time constraints. Producing the highest-fidelity prototype for each project requires understanding what is possible in given time frames and what is reasonable based on academic level. This tool can ensure that students are both challenged and set up for success in their prototyping efforts.

13.9.2 Project Duration and Resulting Prototype

13.9.2.1 Two-Hour Prototype

A two-hour prototyping challenge offers a tightly constrained window that fosters quick decision-making, creativity, and low-risk experimentation. Students should not be expected to iterate or use complex tools at this timescale. Instead, they should rely heavily on tools that can be quickly accessed and applied, such as sketching, 3D pen drawing, simple digital design software (e.g., TinkerCAD), and basic hand tools. As shown in Figure 13.12, the most effective use of time in a two-hour prototype is spent up front in ideation and sketching, followed by rapid prototyping using easily manipulable materials and tools.

While physical prototyping and post-processing are feasible in this time frame, tools such as CNC machines, molding/casting, or even advanced electronics should be avoided. Students may occasionally incorporate downloaded, pre-made 3D parts or off-the-shelf electronics (like Arduino shields and downloadable project files), but it should be expected that these would be integrated without any time for iteration. Achieving functionality in a two-hour prototype is unrealistic, but when it exists, it is rudimentary. The most valuable outcomes of two-hour prototypes are the communication of design goals and a visualization of core intended functionality.

A recurring less than two-hour design challenge that has been held at the OEDK challenges students to design a spoon that can be used by individuals with arthrogryposis multiplex congenita, a condition marked by joint contractures and limited upper limb mobility. Students begin by rapidly sketching and prototyping their concepts using low-fidelity materials. Despite the limited timeframe and owing to the simplicity of the challenge, students routinely generate clever, expressive solutions, many of which can tell a compelling story about how the device would work in a higher-fidelity version. Figure 13.13 shows several spoon prototypes generated over the years, all constructed using low-fidelity, low-cost material.

13.9.2.2 Hackathon

Hackathons provide slightly longer timelines (typically a weekend) that open up the possibility for more advanced tool usage and the potential for limited iteration in the prototypes. Students can move beyond quick sketches to refine their ideas and even translate them to a higher level of CAD (such as SolidWorks). The ability for the students to spend more time developing their initial ideas means that they can plan for the incorporation of tools such as breadboards, laser cutters, downloaded or custom 3D printed parts, and even simple electronics or coding platforms. However, it is worth reflecting on Figure 13.12 to observe that while more tools become available, in a weekend-long hackathon, their usage remains concentrated late in the timeline, and getting more than a couple of iterations is unlikely.

Digital design, sewing, laser cutting, 3D printing, and kit-based electronics are often prioritized during hackathons due to their relatively fast turnaround and medium-fidelity outputs. Custom 3D printed parts or laser-cut enclosures can be rapidly produced, allowing final prototypes to be visibly refined, even if technical sophistication is low. More complex tools (e.g., CNC, molding, and casting) should be avoided and only be introduced if pre-setup and staff support are available.

At the OEDK's three-day Medical Device Design-a-thon, teams prototyped solutions to real-world design for disability challenges. Three final prototypes are shown in Figure 13.14, ranging from low fidelity to high fidelity, and two of these have low levels of refinement. However, the winning team created a syringe locking mechanism to prevent accidental reuse of syringes. This team spent the majority of their working hackathon time doing early design work and then applied that design to the production of CAD files, which they sent off to the 3D printer (and then the team went home early!). The three outcomes reflect that a hackathon can support a range of outcomes for novice designers and that the best designers can produce a high-fidelity prototype in the time allotted, given a highly selective use of tools.

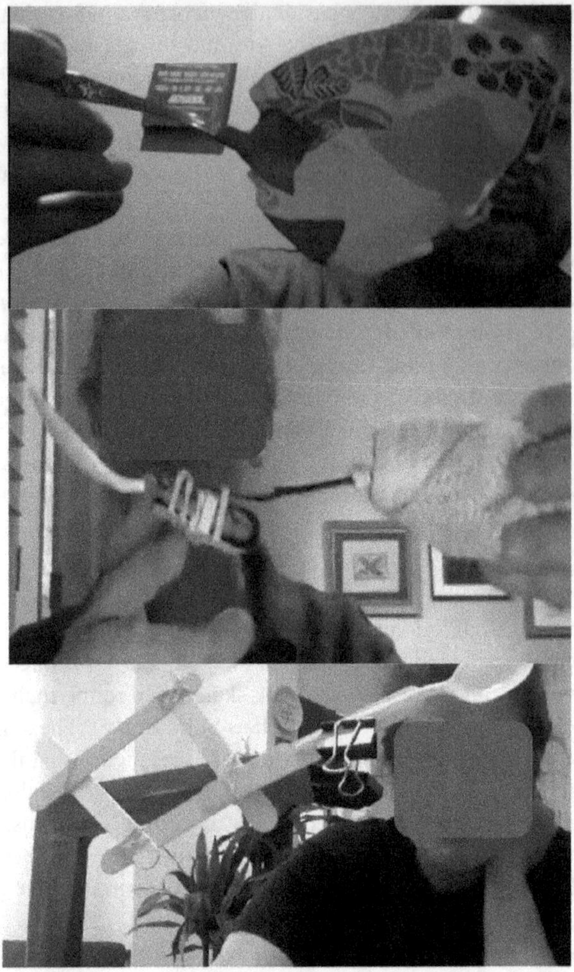

FIGURE 13.13 Prototypes from the Arthrogryposis Project, a design challenge to create an adaptive spoon for promoting independent eating in individuals with joint contractures

13.9.2.3 One-Semester Project

Semester-long courses, particularly first-year and sophomore-level design classes, allow students to engage in iteration and prototyping refinement and include the possibility of scaffolding tool use. Reflecting on Figure 13.12, students can use nearly every tool category in these courses, though the most complex machines (e.g., CNC, plasma cutter, and molding/casting) should be limited to instructor- or technician-facilitated fabrication or for one-off parts that will not be iterated upon. Tools with a low or lower barrier to entry, such as hand tools, power tools, TinkerCAD, laser cutters, simple electronics, and simple 3D printing, can be incorporated into the student's prototyping process with ample time for iteration of the tool to drive increased functionality of the prototype.

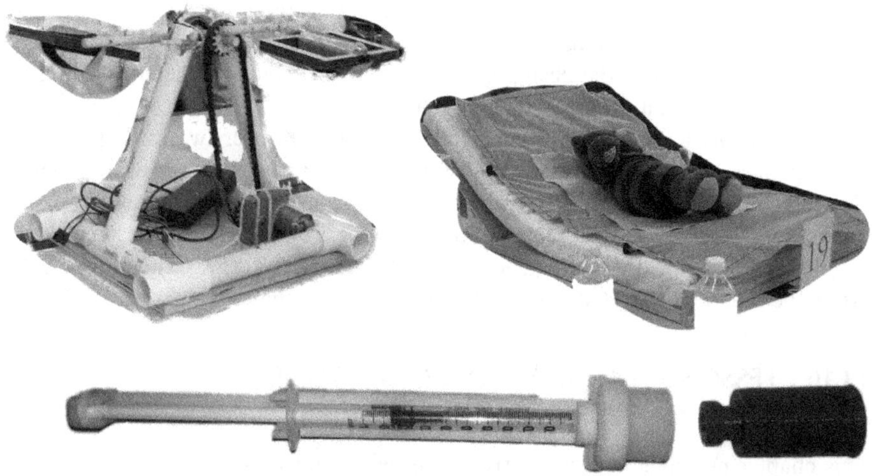

FIGURE 13.14 Sample prototypes from the OEDK design-a-thon, illustrating that iteration is possible even with low- to medium-fidelity prototypes, and highly trained students can create custom 3d printed solutions with the appropriate available tools in an accelerated experience

The beginning weeks of the project should prioritize early design process steps, and it is acceptable to begin to ideate through digital design tools and sketching (by hand, by 3D pen) in these early weeks. In a one-semester project, physical prototyping should start no later than halfway through the academic term. In a project of this length, educators have ample time to have conversations with each team and coach them through transitioning prototypes to higher fidelity, higher function, and attempting to achieve technical sophistication.

The Safe Soap team developed their first low-fidelity prototype, shown in Figure 13.4, over the span of their one-semester design class. This prototype was constructed using only hand and power tools and a drill press to make holes, which an OEDK lab technician facilitated. While neither refined nor possessing technical sophistication, the team's low-fidelity prototype demonstrated function, included some aspects of a medium-fidelity prototype, and informed future iterations by the team.

13.9.2.4 Two-Semester Project

Capstone or graduate-level courses often span two semesters, offering students the opportunity to pursue full iterative design–build–test cycles and produce high-fidelity, near-product prototypes. Figure 13.12 shows that nearly every tool becomes available over time, including (as needed) CNC machines, custom PCB fabrication, milling, molding/casting, or complex electronics. These longer timelines allow the curriculum to support functionality, technical sophistication, refinement, and multiple cycles of functional testing.

Two-semester projects should emphasize full engagement with the iterative design–build–test process, including structured design reviews, prototype evaluations, and the expectation for targeted improvements to the prototypes. Students should be expected to transition through all fidelity levels and finish with an integrated prototype that meets all of the design goals in a refined prototype, demonstrating the potential for clinical usability and client handover.

The graduate team that developed Innoscope worked over two semesters, moving from sketches to an integrated, high-fidelity prototype containing custom optics, electronics, and a custom-designed and printed 3D housing. As shown in Figure 13.6, this prototype has all the hallmarks of a successful prototype after two semesters: it is functional, technically sophisticated, and refined. The result was a near-deployable prototype that demonstrated clinical potential for their client.

13.10 LESSONS LEARNED FROM CASE STUDIES AND CONCLUSION

This chapter presented a comparative analysis of student-built prototypes through multiple lenses: fidelity progression, prototype goal, and project duration. We traced how real-world constraints and instructional contexts shape student design decisions over time by examining three extended case studies: the Elbow Mannequin, SafeSoap, and Innoscope. Across these projects, we analyzed trends in functionality, technical sophistication, refinement, material, and tool usage. Additional case studies explored how design goals such as ergonomics or proof-of-concept prioritize prototyping strategies while de-emphasizing others. We also examined how project length, from a two-hour sprint to a two-semester capstone, impacts which tools should be used, how much iteration should be advocated, and what students might be able to achieve.

Throughout this chapter, a set of common themes and recommendations was made for BME educators:

13.10.1 Common Challenges and Solutions in Biomedical Prototyping Projects

Across the case studies, students faced several challenges routinely. Prototypes often lost functionality when the teams attempting to refine their prototypes began using more advanced tools or materials, as seen in the Elbow Mannequin project. Not highlighted in these case studies, but endemic globally, is limited access to specialized fabrication tools or parts, which can present a barrier to producing higher-fidelity prototypes. Available project time was a critical decider on how much teams could accomplish, especially in short- and medium-length projects. To address these challenges, we recommend that educators positively encourage the use of low-fidelity prototyping to define critical design blocks and identify potential high-risk functions early. Additionally, BME educators should offer real-time feedback and troubleshooting support to help students sustain momentum through inevitable prototyping setbacks. Finally, we encourage BME educators to set realistic guardrails on tool use and project scope based on course duration and student readiness.

13.10.2 The Role of Mentorship, Faculty Guidance, and Peer Review in Student Success

Mentorship is among the most significant mediators of final prototype and student team success. A web of mentors: faculty, peers, technical staff, and clinicians, helps students acquire critical prototyping skills, especially when navigating unfamiliar tools or design challenges, such as in one-semester or longer-term projects. We encourage BME educators to calibrate expectations for SOs based on available mentorship. Inside classes, foster a culture of peer review to shift student mindsets toward improvement, not perfection, and develop their capacity to "hear" feedback as a process, not a personal comment. Where possible, actively structure mentoring interactions with available networks to support teams' technical, process, and communication skill growth.

13.10.3 Reflection on Iterative Design

Iteration is a critical factor mediating student team prototyping success. Projects that embraced rapid low-fidelity prototyping at early stages typically progressed further and demonstrated greater refinement in later stages. Teams that engaged in iteration, especially after failure, tended to produce more sophisticated, higher-functioning final prototypes. Students should be taught that failure is not an endpoint but a tool for uncovering weak assumptions, flawed design blocks, or a key milestone along the journey to accomplishment. BME educators should look out for the effect that strategic exploration of new techniques may produce temporary setbacks for teams, but this can yield stronger prototype outcomes over time. Educators should seek to help student teams gain momentum from early wins (e.g., proof-of-concept prototypes), which can support confidence and help them move faster in future prototype development.

13.10.4 Scalability While Prototyping

Translating student prototypes into clinically relevant or commercially viable solutions requires more than technical sophistication and functionality. Functional prototypes must eventually meet regulatory, safety, and manufacturability standards. While these constraints may not be actionable in lower-fidelity prototypes, they should be introduced conceptually as students begin producing medium- or high-fidelity prototypes. Students benefit when educators consistently emphasize manufacturability and documentation during the prototyping process in a way that does not interrupt student progress. Topics such as materials selection, safety concerns, and testing strategies should be discussion items during design reviews, not just protocols turned in as assignments. BME educators can encourage teams to think about their prototypes on a long-term scale, even as they focus on producing low-fidelity models; this can build awareness of the entire prototyping timeline for the final outcome.

13.11 FINAL THOUGHTS ON THE SCAFFOLDING OF PROTOTYPING THROUGHOUT THE BME CURRICULUM

Prototyping remains one of the most essential skills for BME education and for preparing future biomedical engineers. Prototyping draws from a range of engineering disciplines, mechanical, electrical, computational, and biological, and allows students to marry their conceptual knowledge with hands-on execution. When scaffolded effectively across the curriculum, prototyping enables students to build, test, iterate, and ultimately design solutions that are technically feasible, user-centered, and impactful.

Students must be equipped to prototype at all levels of fidelity. Early-stage experiences should focus on rough mockups, analog materials, and sketches to rapidly explore ideas. Mid-level courses should use digital tools, standard components, and structured iteration to encourage developing functional design blocks. By the time students reach capstone, they should be capable of delivering integrated, high-fidelity prototypes that meet clinical or technical specifications, with supporting documentation for performance, usability, and manufacturability.

Crucially, impactful prototyping does not require a high-end lab. As shown throughout this chapter, meaningful prototypes can emerge from modest settings using cardboard, tape, 3D pens, and practical ingenuity. Prototyping can, and must, happen anywhere. What matters most is a mindset of exploration, iteration, and thoughtful execution.

As educators, we are responsible for cultivating environments that support this mindset. We must teach students that failure is part of the process, that low-tech solutions can solve high-stakes problems, and that design grows through continuous iteration and learning. By embedding prototyping deeply and intentionally into the BME curriculum, we equip students with the skills and resilience to create solutions that matter, regardless of context, tools, or constraints.

ACKNOWLEDGMENTS

This work was completed at the OEDK and spans many courses in the design curriculum over the previous 15 years. We thank Paige Rennie for the copyediting and suggestions for improving this chapter. Photos from this chapter have been collected through the course of normal educational experience, where, at the beginning of the semester, students acknowledge their approval for the future usage of these materials anonymously, based on the course syllabus.

REFERENCES

Chen, Laurel, Asma Farooqui, Anjitha Saji, and Haruto Sasajima. 2023. *Innoscope: An Affordable, Portable Retinal Camera for Remote Diabetic Retinopathy Screening in Low-Resource Settings*. Unpublished manuscript.

Danckers, Ericka. 2014. *Training Mannequin for Dislocated Elbow*. Unpublished manuscript.

Dean, Bashford. 1920. *Helmets and Body Armor in Modern Warfare*. New Haven, CT: Yale University Press. https://lccn.loc.gov/20017513.

Grace, Josiah, Sarah Hernandez, Marie Hoeger, and Kayla McCarty. 2013. *Executive Summary for Kitchen-Themed Soap Dispenser*. Unpublished manuscript.

14 Biodesign Innovation at the University of Meldine—A Case Study in Multidisciplinary Medtech Education

David B. Grayden

14.1 INTRODUCTION

As described in Chapter 6, Biodesign Innovation has emerged as a highly successful program to equip students and fellows with the skills necessary to identify unmet clinical needs, develop innovative solutions, create business plans, and take their concepts through to commercialization. With the goal of bringing together engineering, business, and clinical perspectives to training in medical technology (medtech) innovation, the University of Melbourne, Australia, developed a Biodesign Innovation program in 2016 that is jointly taught as electives within the Master of Biomedical Engineering and MBA degrees and in close association with the university's teaching hospitals. Specifically, students undertaking the relevant degrees enroll in the subjects BMEN90030 Biodesign Innovation[1] and MGMT90231 Biodesign Innovation[2] that are taught by the Department of Biomedical Engineering and the Melbourne Business School, respectively. The handbook entries were informed by a similar program set up a few years before at the Hebrew University of Jerusalem,[3] Israel, and the curriculum is based closely on the textbooks, *Biodesign: The Process of Innovating Medical Technologies* (Yock 2015) and *Disciplined Entrepreneurship: 24 Steps to a Successful Startup* (Aulet 2013).

The University of Melbourne Biodesign Innovation program was awarded the University of Melbourne 2021 Norman Curry Award for Innovation and Excellence in Educational Programs, and was shortlisted for the Engagement Australia 2020 Excellence Awards and the Universities Australia 2024 Shaping Australia Awards. The following sections describe the structure, pedagogical approaches, outcomes, and lessons learned from the program, providing insights for those seeking to implement similar initiatives in medtech innovation education.

DOI: 10.1201/9781003520313-14

14.2 PROGRAM STRUCTURE AND CURRICULUM

The University of Melbourne's Biodesign Innovation program is structured over two semesters (from March to November), allowing for a deep dive into the Biodesign process and for students to learn and experience the whole process from initial need identification to development of prototypes and business models. Crucially, the two-semester period allows the subject to replace the typical Capstone Project or Research Project subject that engineering students must undertake in their final year of study. For the MBA students, the subject counts as three electives in the MBA degree program. The program runs with 12 weekly evening classes of three hours duration in each of the semesters. The classes include didactic lectures, guest lectures, in-class exercises, and breakouts for team-based activities.

The program is closely aligned with the Stanford University Biodesign Innovation process (Yock 2015). The first semester focuses on needs finding, including clinical immersion and needs validation and specification, and then the initial stages of concept generation. The second semester builds on this foundation, transitioning to prototype development, business modeling, and preparation for potential commercialization.

The integration of students undertaking engineering and business administration is a distinguishing feature of the program. The first three to four weeks of the program include exercises and activities that enable the cohort to get to know each other for the purpose of team formation. The students are free to form their own teams, subject to the requirement that each team must include at least two students from each discipline. In recent years, the teams have comprised three engineering students and two or three MBA students, depending on the number of students enrolled. The teams are encouraged to develop a team mission that matches the priorities of the individuals and the team. This involves analyzing the strengths and weaknesses of the team and developing a set of acceptance criteria that would make a project attractive to the team.

14.2.1 Needs Finding

The curriculum is structured around the three core components that mirror the key stages of medtech innovation. The first aspect, needs finding, is one of the most important aspects of the curriculum. Students may enter the course with preconceived ideas of how they would like to use some interesting type of technology or AI approach within the course. However, the course emphasizes that first finding a need to solve is of far greater value than trying to squeeze a solution into a need. Classes teach the process of needs finding, largely following the Biodesign textbook (Yock 2015). Once teams are formed, students engage in clinical observations, stakeholder interviews, and background research to identify unmet needs in different clinical settings.

The needs finding process commences with each team nominating their top two to four areas of clinical interest. The instructors then endeavor to make introductions to clinicians within the teaching hospitals of the university and other sources so that the team can make contact, arrange interviews, and, if possible, obtain access to observe clinical practice in the clinical environment. The students sometimes already have some clinical contacts in different areas through pre-existing networks, which they are encouraged to tap into, and they often cold-call clinicians across the city, country, and around the world to expand their needs finding scope.

Each team typically compiles a list of 30–200 needs, which they must narrow down to a short list of needs that they wish to consider pursuing. They do this with reference to their acceptance criteria and team mission. Usually, the teams conduct a voting process to rank the needs and obtain the top three to five needs. They then create need statements that specify the problem, population, and outcome, refining and validating these specifications through further background research, interviews, and observations.

At the mid-semester point, the students are required to submit their first assignment. This written assignment includes three aspects:

1. A brief statement and description of the team and its strategic focus, including descriptions of the criteria established by the team for deciding which clinical areas to pursue, the team's mission, the strengths and weaknesses of the team, and the acceptance criteria.
2. A brief description of the methodology that the team followed to conduct the needs exploration, including descriptions of background research, observations, and interviews.
3. A detailed presentation and explanation of one need statement, including supporting background information needed to understand the need statement. The students must describe and justify the problem, population, and outcome aspects of the need statement, and how these relate to the team's acceptance criteria, building upon insights from their background research, observations, and interviews.

14.2.2 Concept Generation

The second stage is concept generation, when students are now encouraged to develop solutions to unmet needs. Building on their identified needs, the teams brainstorm and develop potential solutions. In classes, the students are introduced to training in ideation techniques, including brainstorming, initial concept selection, concept exploration, and testing. They are also trained at this stage in business models and stakeholder analysis, including market entry and beachhead strategy and entrepreneurial strategy, as well as IP considerations.

The teams now spend considerable amounts of time in their brainstorming and concept development activities. They revisit their clinical contacts for validation of their ideas, and they continue to expand their list of contacts and deep dive into potential technologies.

At the end of the first semester, the students are required to submit their second assignment. This written assignment includes three deliverables:

1. The first section is a short update on the team and the medical need that they plan to address. This is an opportunity to provide an update if the need to be pursued is different from the one described in the first assignment.

2. A detailed description of two or three concept ideas. In this section, they are expected to describe the processes used to develop the concepts, provide a concept map, provide clear explanations of the background, rationale, and solutions of their chosen concepts, and provide clear descriptions of the extent to which the concepts address the need statement and the team's acceptance criteria.
3. A description of one preliminary business model. In this section, the expectation is for a business model that would guide the commercialization of the preferred device concept, including a BMC focusing mainly on customer segments, value propositions, revenue streams, and channels to market.

14.2.3 Prototyping and Business Modeling

The third stage is Prototyping and Business Modeling, when students now start to implement their solutions. The second semester commences with the third assignment: an oral presentation of a plan to build a medical device. This assignment is an opportunity to present what was written in the second assignment to an expert panel, obtaining feedback that can help guide testing and prototyping productively during the second semester. The presentation must include detailed descriptions of the following:

- An unmet clinical need and a related need statement;
- A broad market review, including customer analysis, beachhead segment and attractiveness, and the value proposition to serve that market;
- Engineering concepts for up to three solutions, indicating the team's preferred solution;
- Business model and commercialization approach;
- IP challenges and opportunities.

The second semester classes cover more details of the medtech commercialization process, with guest lectures provided by experts in pitching, accelerators and incubators, funding, reimbursement, clinical trials, regulations, IP strategy, design and fabrication, quality management systems, and others.

The teams create and iterate on prototypes of their proposed solutions. Since it is nearly impossible for a device to be completed within the three months of the semester, the students are encouraged to focus on the aspects of their prototyping that will mitigate the risks of their devices. They rank the key assumptions of their device concept and then test these through benchtop experiments, conversations with clinicians and other key stakeholders, tissue testing, and, when possible, evaluation with human volunteers. Access is provided to design-and-build facilities, research laboratories, and other facilities that can enable the prototyping work to proceed as far as possible.

The teams develop comprehensive business plans for their innovations, considering market analysis, regulatory pathways, IP strategies, and financial projections. In this case, the students are also encouraged to test their assumptions through background research, interviews with key stakeholders, and modeling. Outside of classes, the instructors meet with the teams separately each week to discuss progress and address needs and concerns in each of the device prototyping and business plan development.

At the end of the second semester, the students are required to submit their fourth and final assignment, which comprises three components: a layperson oral presentation, a detailed oral presentation, and a professional project report.

14.2.3.1 Layperson Oral Presentation

This is a public presentation at an exhibition of final year engineering projects, conducted alongside students enrolled in engineering disciplines. The students deliver a 90-second pitch, as if to potential investors or business partners, followed by a question-and-answer session. They are also expected to have an exhibit of their project along with a poster.

14.2.3.2 Detailed Oral Presentation

This is a detailed description of the technical aspects of the final product and business plan. The presentation includes the following aspects and should include technical analyses, including methodology, data, calculations, and results:

- The formulation of the problem and need, background material, and a brief survey of previous work;
- The solution concept, including device prototype design, development, implementation, and testing outcome(s);
- The business approach, including value proposition, business model validation, target customer(s) and market overview, proposed approach for market entry and competing/collaborating in the market, regulation, reimbursement, and IP strategies, traction, team, and next steps.

14.2.3.3 Professional Project Report

This major report described the final prototype device and business plan. The report should contain the following:

- Design, implementation, and testing of the device: background on disease state fundamentals and existing solutions (identify), description of the concept design (invent), and detailed description of the device prototyping process, evaluation methods, and results (implement).
- Business approach: value proposition, business model, and results of validation, target customer(s) and market overview, proposed approach for market entry and competing/collaborating in the market, reimbursement strategies.
- Next steps, including future product development and regulation and IP strategies.
- Each student should include a final page with reflections, recommendations, and conclusions about their project and key learnings from their team's efforts.

14.3 PEDAGOGICAL APPROACHES AND METHODOLOGIES

There are several key aspects of how the program is taught that have led to its success, and these are highlighted in the following sections.

14.3.1 Multidisciplinary Teams

A strength of the program is that it trains students enrolled in Engineering and Business coursework programs as part of the requirements for their master's degrees. Internationally, the most similar program is that of the Hebrew University of Jerusalem, which engages engineering PhD students and MBA coursework students. The program creates teams of typically mid-career MBA students, keen to apply the lessons from their workplace and other courses (marketing, strategy, negotiations, and finance), with typically younger engineering master's students, eager to explore new technological pathways as they obtain their engineering qualifications. The flipside, however, is that the program faces the challenge of needing to work alongside other coursework requirements (especially for engineering students) and employment (especially for the MBA students). These challenges were successfully surmounted by scheduling evening classes and facilitating the initial clinical immersion to enable out-of-hours access to clinicians.

14.3.2 Clinical Observations and Engagement With Local Hospitals

The generous support of clinicians, hospitals, and medtech experts in the program provides an excellent learning experience for the students, reinforced by the academic team. The University of Melbourne has many teaching hospitals, which are important partners in the program, providing access to clinicians and to clinical immersion, including St Vincent's Hospital, Melbourne Health, Austin Health, Royal Women's Hospital, Royal Victorian Eye and Ear Hospital, Western Health, and Northern Health. Furthermore, other hospitals have provided strong support, including Eastern Health, Alfred Health, and many smaller public and private hospitals. The clinicians and hospitals have very quickly understood the value of Biodesign Innovation and are keen to participate because it provides an opportunity to articulate unmet clinical needs and for potential solutions to become available to them.

14.3.3 Diverse Clinical Domain Exposure

The most important partners in Biodesign Innovation are the clinicians, who are critical as they provide the background information, expert insights, and clinical access required for optimal needs finding and concept development. The minimum requirement is the clinicians' time to meet with the students for interviews and to facilitate clinical observations. However, most of the clinicians are keen to contribute through ongoing discussions, brainstorming, and, for some, essentially becoming part of the team.

The primary clinical partners come from a broad range of clinical areas, including neonatal intensive care, neurology, orthopedics, cardiology, respiratory medicine, aged care, dentistry, general practice, optometry, ophthalmology, anesthesia, psychiatry, intensive care, nephrology, women's health, and vascular surgery. This wealth of opportunity has allowed the teams to select initial areas of medicine in which they have a strong interest, and greatly increases the scope of needs that can be sourced. There have also been around ten times as many experts accessed as secondary partners. This includes those introduced by primary partners or engaged through direct contact made by the students who have sought to expand the base of expertise to pursue their needs validation and concept development. These have mainly been clinicians, nurses, hospital administrators, paramedics, and others. Some teams have engaged with other regions of Australia and overseas contacts.

14.3.4 Industry Expert and Alumni Guest Lectures

Our other partners are guest speakers, advisors, and mentors. While some guest lectures have been delivered by people internal to the University of Melbourne, many external guests from the teaching team's own personal networks have been engaged to cover topics including IP, commercialization, moving beyond the prototype, regulations, quality management, and reimbursement. The insights from professionals working actively in different areas or developing their own start-up have been extremely valuable to the students. Likewise, the guests are keen to meet the students as they view them as potential future employees or start-up investment targets. Importantly, the growing alumni of the program have been an incredible resource, especially in joining in most of the first semester classes to share about their own experiences in the needs finding and concept development processes.

Guests have also included patent attorneys, angel investors, start-up founders, medtech company executives, and accelerator coordinators. They have provided students with skills that are highly transferable for seeking a career in established medtech companies or founding their own start-up. As a result, the program has successfully contributed to the growing entrepreneurial ecosystem within Melbourne and Australia. The teams have developed shovel-ready prototypes and business plans that are well-positioned to leverage the growing national appetite for MedTech start-ups.

14.3.5 TBL and Peer Review

There is substantial peer-to-peer learning in the program: MBA students learn about engineering prototyping and regulations, while engineering students learn about business models and marketing. This uniquely positions them for entrepreneurial or professional careers.

The online tool CATME SMARTER Teamwork[4] is used with each assignment to survey the team members on their interactions and levels of contributions to the work of the assignments. The evaluations provided by the tool, based on the student responses and comments, are used by the instructors to look for any difficulties that the teams may be having and to intervene, if necessary, to facilitate better team cohesion and effectiveness; these interactions are seen as important learning opportunities for the students. The assignment marks may also be adjusted based on the peer-assessed contributions to the work, although, in each instance, this is discussed extensively between the instructors.

14.3.5.1 Milestone Assessments

The training in BioDesign Innovation is highly interactive, including assessment and feedback processes. The assignments throughout the course are aimed at ensuring that the teams are achieving the intended learning outcomes. The milestone assessments also ensure that progress is made consistently throughout the course. The needs finding assignment ensures that the students describe an unmet clinical need as a need statement and can fully justify the validity of this need by describing the background, disease fundamentals, anatomy and physiology, problem, population, and outcome. The concept development assignment ensures that the teams can describe their concepts, including clear descriptions of the background and rationale for their concepts and their preliminary business models. The prototype development oral presentation ensures that the teams are prepared for the difficult job ahead of developing their solutions and business models. Finally, the final assignment components not only require the students to describe their outcomes across different formats but also meet the requirements for accreditation of the engineering degree.

Throughout these assessment items, the students are guided and advised along the way, but since their projects are sourced by them and are specific to each team, they must do most of the work independently as a team. This is a huge step for many of the students, but the approach encourages them to think in a holistic, integrative manner and to make new connections in clinical, academic, and industry environments. Crucially, extensive feedback is provided to the teams after marking the reports and oral presentations. For the oral presentations, experienced guests from across the University and the commercialization ecosystem are invited, and they also provide useful feedback to the teams. The feedback is provided in written form and also in the weekly discussions that the instructors have with the teams.

The instructors interact with the teams and individuals often through online resources and weekly meetings with the teams after the lectures. Furthermore, separate meetings with the engineering teams are held weekly in the second semester to guide and advise them in the prototyping processes. However, in all cases, the students are the leaders within their own projects, and the instructors act as mentors and guides.

14.4 PROGRAM OUTCOMES AND IMPACTS

14.4.1 Start-Ups

From the start of the University of Melbourne Biodesign Innovation program, there have been a remarkable number of teams that have chosen to pursue the subsequent commercialization of their devices. Of the five teams that participated in the first year, 2016, three teams participated in Medtech's Got Talent 2016, Australia's premier medtech pitching competition, with two of the teams reaching the final and receiving funding. Four of the teams subsequently attempted to commercialize their devices, entering accelerator programs in Australia and the United States.

While three of these have subsequently folded, one is still ongoing, Navi Medical Technologies, which received FDA clearance for their Class II device for neonatal care in 2025.

In the following years, at least one team from each cohort made a serious attempt to commercialize their devices. On average, roughly half of the teams across the cohort between 2016 and 2024 incorporated, with many participating in pitching competitions and accelerator programs, such as the Medtech Actuator, Melbourne Accelerator Program, Translating Research at Melbourne, and others. As expected of start-ups, most have folded, but some are ongoing, and we are keen to see the future impact that they will have across different areas of need.

14.4.2 Student Feedback and Satisfaction

Student feedback has been very favorable for the program. The program has scored highly in the University of Melbourne's Student Experience Survey formal feedback process that seeks student responses to questions such as "This subject was intellectually engaging and stimulating," "I received useful feedback on my progress," and "Overall, I had a very good learning experience in this subject."

Some student comments about the course include the following:

- "Participating in the Biodesign Innovation program has undoubtedly been the highlight of my studies. The program's unique approach to real-world innovation, bringing together Master of Business Administration and Master of Biomedical Engineering students in multidisciplinary teams, has equipped me with invaluable skills that extend far beyond the classroom setting."—Engineering Alumnus
- "The Biodesign Innovation program is a truly unique experience, made possible with the generous and enthusiastic support of fantastic subject leaders, clinicians, mentors and alumni from the startup community."—MBA Alumnus
- "Participating in the program transcended academic learning and reshaped my professional journey. Far from being a conventional curriculum, this program was an incubator for inventive thinking and a practical arena for applying diverse skills in a concerted effort."—MBA Alumnus
- "What sets the Biodesign Innovation program apart is its real-world experience and highly collaborative approach. Learning from industry experts and expanding our professional network, we developed essential skills in problem solving, prototyping, business opportunity assessment, teamwork and communication."—Engineering Alumnus.

14.4.3 Development of Industry-Ready Skills and Knowledge

The program's focus on practical, hands-on learning ensures that graduates develop a set of industry-ready skills highly valued in the medtech sector and other industry sectors that go beyond typical engineering and business courses. A key aspect is needs assessment. The ability to identify and validate unmet needs through observation and stakeholder interviews is a skill that translates across many domains. The students also develop their interdisciplinary collaboration by working in diverse teams and bridging the gap between technical and business perspectives. Finally, experience and training in pitching and presentation help to develop the ability to communicate complex ideas to diverse audiences, from clinicians to investors

14.5 CHALLENGES AND SOLUTIONS

14.5.1 Balancing Diverse Student Backgrounds and Skill Sets

The multidisciplinary nature of the program, while a strength, presents challenges in ensuring that all students can contribute effectively regardless of their background. The focus initially upon get-to-know-you exercises, working toward team formation, helps to allay concerns by the students about the disparate backgrounds across the cohort. The requirement to develop the team mission and team acceptance criteria, along with analyses of the team's strengths and weaknesses, brings to the forefront the strengths that come from diversity in the team. It is also important to emphasize peer-to-peer learning within the teams to leverage individuals' strengths. Finally, the design of the assignments that require input from both the technical and business perspectives encourages collaboration.

14.5.2 Maintaining Clinical Partnerships and Access

Securing and maintaining partnerships with clinicians and healthcare institutions for clinical interviews, observations, and validation activities can be complex and time-consuming. This is mitigated to some extent by cultivating a network of clinical champions for the program within the institutions. For example, in one hospital, a close relationship with the Chair of Medicine has maintained a strong connection with that hospital. In another hospital, a working relationship with a team of entrepreneurial anesthetists has facilitated many opportunities for clinical connections. However, there have been instances where some clinicians have invested their time in the needs finding exercise, but no team has pursued a need in their area, and so they have withdrawn from engaging with the program. Therefore, there is a continuing need to cultivate the network of clinical contacts to maintain the program.

14.6 CONCLUSION

The University of Melbourne's Biodesign Innovation program demonstrates the powerful impact of a well-structured, multidisciplinary approach to training in medtech innovation. Such programs will be instrumental in equipping future innovators with the skills, knowledge, and mindset needed to drive meaningful advancements in medical technology and patient care. By embracing these principles and learning from successful models like the University of Melbourne's program, institutions can play a pivotal role in nurturing the next generation of medtech innovators and contributing to advancements in global healthcare.

NOTES

1 https://handbook.unimelb.edu.au/subjects/bmen90030
2 https://handbook.unimelb.edu.au/subjects/mgmt90231
3 https://bioengineering.huji.ac.il/biodesign
4 https://www.catme.org

REFERENCES

Aulet, Bill. 2013. *Disciplined Entrepreneurship: 24 Steps to a Successful Startup.* Hoboken, NJ: John Wiley & Sons.

Yock, Paul G., ed. 2015. *Biodesign: The Process of Innovating Medical Technologies.* 2nd ed. Cambridge: Cambridge University Press.

15 A Design Continuum That Mimics Workplace Organizational Structure

Jennifer R. Amos, Joe A. Bradley, and Holly McIlwee Golecki

15.1 OVERVIEW OF DEPARTMENT STRUCTURE AND CAPSTONE PROGRAMS

The Bioengineering Department at the University of Illinois Urbana-Champaign participates in several levels of design across programs, from our undergraduate senior capstone design in the Bioengineering Bachelor's program, the Professional Capstone in the Master of Engineering (M.Eng.) in Bioengineering, and the Capstone Course in the Carle-Illinois College of Medicine. Having multiple disconnected levels of design presents numerous challenges, such as sourcing projects, structuring the scope of projects, and sharing physical and personnel-related resources. We chose to address these challenges by creating a design continuum of biomedical-focused project teams that mimic workplace organizational structure (Golecki et al. 2023).

15.1.1 Bachelor's Program

The Bioengineering program at the University of Illinois Urbana-Champaign provides a comprehensive engineering education that prepares graduates to attain positions in industry, pursue graduate education, or professional healthcare training. Undergraduates take four semester credit hours of Senior Design in their final year of the program. In this course, they are tasked with demonstrating knowledge and skills gained in prerequisite courses in a team-based and client-driven design project. The course learning outcomes for BIOE400 are listed in Table 15.1.

15.1.2 Master Program

The M.Eng. in Bioengineering is a one-year professional master's program tailored to the needs of industry (Gray et al. 2024; Stukes et al. 2023). The program admits students with a variety of engineering backgrounds as well as science backgrounds. This program comprises 32 credit hours of graduate credit, including six semester credit hours of capstone split across the fall and spring terms of an academic year, BIOE 575. During their enrollment in the program, the students also take

 DOI: 10.1201/9781003520313-15

TABLE 15.1
Learning outcomes for each course

BS in Bioengineering Program—BIOE 400	M.Eng. in Bioengineering Program—BIOE 575	College of Medicine Program—BSE 685
1. Identify, formulate, and analyze complex engineering problems by applying principles of engineering.	1. Acquire and apply skills and knowledge in customer discovery.	1. Identify a problem or deficiency in the delivery of healthcare that can be improved or solved with an engineering approach.
2. Apply engineering design to produce solutions that meet specified needs with consideration of public health, safety, and welfare, as well as global, cultural, social, environmental, and economic factors.	2. Apply engineering design to develop solutions for complex engineering challenges.	2. Identify and form a team of interdisciplinary collaborators across campus and Clinical Partners to solve a clinical problem that has been identified.
3. Create documentation and presentations to communicate effectively with a range of audiences.	3. Acquire and apply skills and knowledge in engineering management and business operations.	3. Communicate the importance of the problem and the technical solution to a group of engineering, clinical, and business professionals.
4. Apply ethical and professional responsibilities in engineering and make informed judgments, with regard for global, economic, environmental, and social contexts.	4. Gain the knowledge and skills required to take an engineering project from problem discovery to appropriate deliverables.	4. Guide a team that will conduct a full design review process outlining the proposed solution, technical details, timeline, cost to produce, requirements and verifications, and safety and ethical considerations through a collaborative team-based approach.
5. Function effectively on a team whose members together provide leadership, create a collaborative and inclusive environment, establish goals, plan tasks, and meet objectives.	5. Acquire and apply skills and knowledge on client relationship building and client management during project execution.	5. Design a technology-based solution to a challenging contemporary healthcare delivery and clinical problem, within realistic constraints and utilizing appropriate standards.
6. Create and apply appropriate experimentation, analysis, and interpretation of data using engineering judgment to draw conclusions.	6. Acquire and apply knowledge of effective practices in teamwork and effective project management.	6. Demonstrate a working device or technical innovation through quantifiable metrics for gauging a successful outcome.
7. Understand and apply new knowledge as needed, using appropriate learning strategies.		7. Assemble financial, physical, and intellectual resources in order to develop a team-based Capstone project.

technical courses and business courses that are tailored to the bioengineering industry. Through business-focused courses, M.Eng. students gain skills in design, product and project management, and product innovation processes. Given the nature of the M.Eng. training and the fact that students are enrolled in both semesters of capstone, M.Eng. students are ideal for taking on a managerial role in the capstone projects. The course learning outcomes for BIOE 575 are listed in Table 15.1.

15.1.3 Medical School Program

Carle Illinois College of Medicine, the world's first accredited engineering-based medical school, represents a new concept in the field of healthcare education. Innovation is the cornerstone of the curriculum, with emphasis on human factors, design thinking, medical technologies, and entrepreneurship. Unlike traditional medical education, Carle Illinois' curriculum immerses students early in clinical, case-driven, problem-based active learning intended to instill passion and creativity for discovering innovative solutions to the world's most difficult healthcare challenges.

The medical students are enrolled in a one-year-long capstone, BSE 685, during the last year of medical school. The relevant learning outcomes for the BSE 685 capstone course are listed in Table 15.1.

15.2 INTERVIEW AND LITERATURE REVIEW OF THE BENEFITS OF CROSS-DISCIPLINARY TEAMS

15.2.1 Interview Findings From Program Participants for Each Program

At the beginning of the integrated capstone course development, we interviewed former students who had participated in our capstone course prior to the combined capstone formation. These interviews provided us with critical feedback regarding which activities were helpful to the students' learning and what was important in preparing them for their first role postgraduation. Feedback suggests that the students found the validation and verification activities very useful and relevant in their current careers. The students appreciated practicing in the biodesign process, but would like to explore additional prototyping methods. The students expressed some concerns about how the course materials were sequenced. For example, some of the didactic sessions on the BMC and customer discovery process would be more helpful if discussed closer to the start of the course.

15.2.2 Literature Findings on Cross-Disciplinary Teams

Interprofessional teams bring together individuals from different disciplines. The synergy created by these diverse perspectives fosters creative problem-solving and holistic thinking (Kimpton and Maynard 2025). The integration of different professional perspectives is especially critical in human-centered design, where understanding the end-user needs requires empathy and insights beyond traditional engineering parameters. Interprofessional collaboration enhances not only the robustness of solutions but also their usability and social relevance. For successful team dynamics and execution within interprofessional teams, it is important to understand the potential differences in communication styles, problem-solving approaches, and professional cultures. Implementation in the classroom may require a structured collaboration process, reflective practices, and maybe formal didactic or active learning training activities.

Interdisciplinary learning environments can provide students with the training and tools to tackle complex routine and non-routine challenges (Boyd et al. 2025). This environment provides an opportunity to address problems that cannot be solved by a single disciplinary perspective. The interdisciplinary capstone provides our students with an opportunity to practice their learning and apply that knowledge to a real-world problem (Ashby and Exter 2019).

15.2.3 User Profiles for Motivation and Learning Needs

The interdisciplinary capstone project course has collaboration amongst undergraduate bioengineering students, graduate bioengineering students, and medical students, who also collaborate with business students (MBA). For each of the courses, we constructed a persona to represent each of the student groups, as shown in Figure 15.1. The persona that represents a student in undergraduate bioengineering is excited about applying the skills gained over the last four years to building something. Additionally, the undergraduate student is not completely sure of post-graduation plans. For M.Eng. graduate students, they would like to level up their skills and move into management. They are interested in aspects of the integrated capstone that will enhance managerial skills, for example, project management. For the medical student, they would like to work with a team to bring ideas that they document from their clinical experience into a solution that will be successfully adopted. These students do not have as much time to dedicate to the problem, but can provide clinical feedback and, in some cases, engineering expertise.

15.2.4 Competencies and Deliverables for Each Program

In developing this integrated capstone, we reviewed the syllabi for each course with a primary focus on course objectives, session objectives, and assessment criteria. We identified nine competencies that we would like to observe and measure. These competencies are as follows: Need Identification, Project Management, Prototyping, Design Verification, Design Validation, Client Interaction and Management, and Leadership. We reviewed these competencies in relation to how important (*not important* to *very important*) they are to the goals for each of the three student cohorts, separately. The result of the ratings exercise is shown in Figure 15.2.

15.3 THE DESIGN OF THE COMBINED CAPSTONE EXPERIENCES

15.3.1 Course Structure Alignment—Lecture Schedule, Due Dates, and Handoff/Transition

The development of the cross-program design capstone at the University of Illinois Urbana-Champaign is executed over a multi-year curricular process. Here, medical

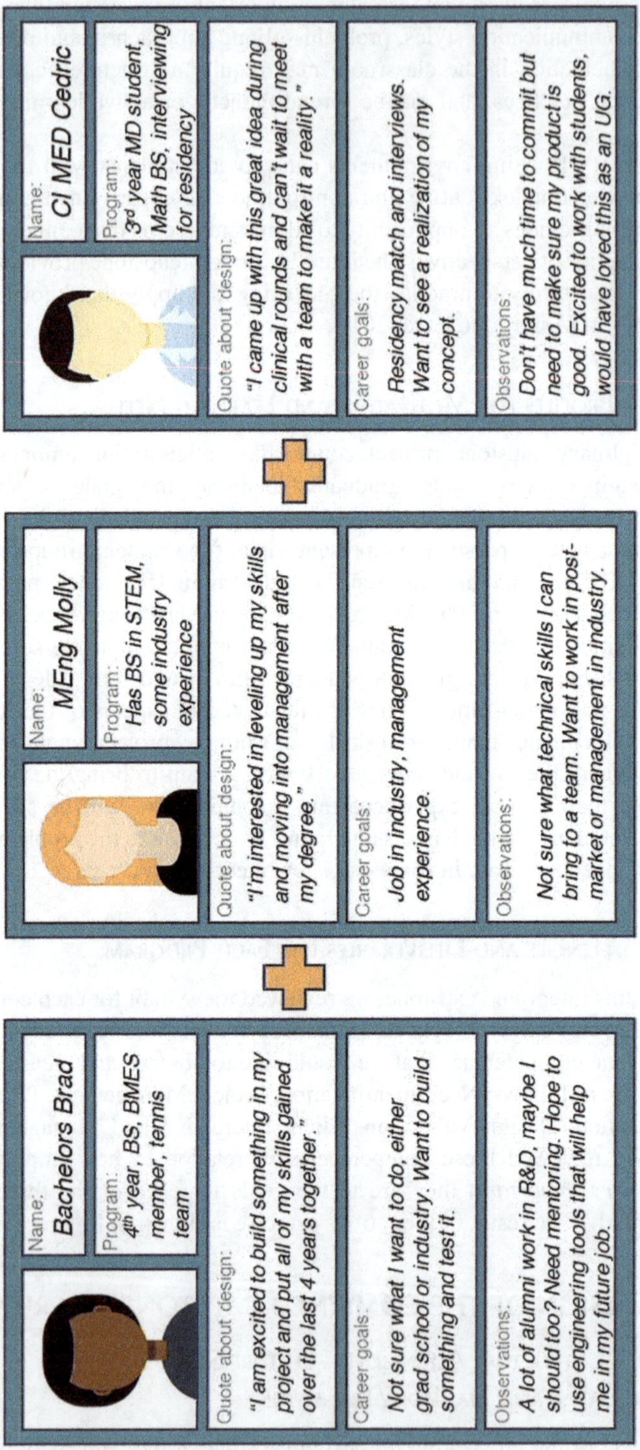

FIGURE 15.1 User personas showing the attitudes and values of each involved student group.

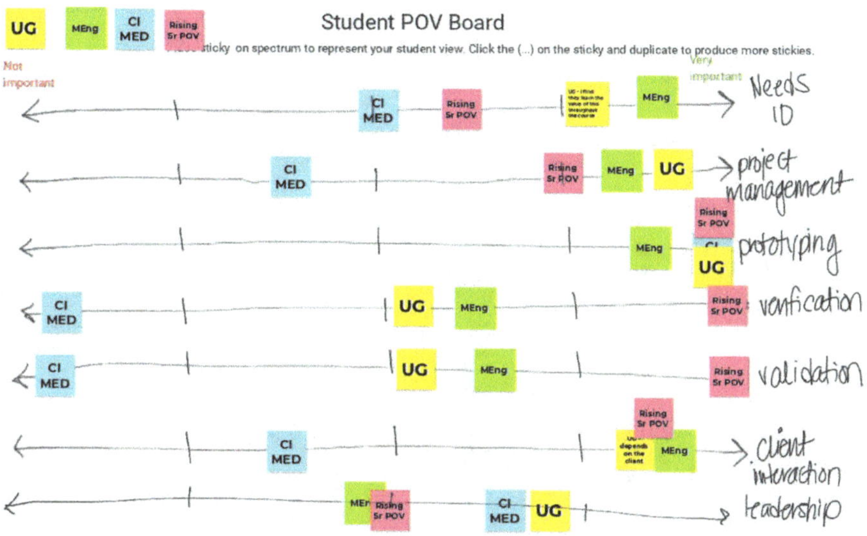

FIGURE 15.2 Student point of view board showing the student values of each of the competencies.

students serve as clients for engineering capstone projects; M.Eng. students serve as project managers; and undergraduate students serve as technical leads. The engineering course also accepts projects from industry, academia, and community sponsors. This case study chapter focused on projects that are sponsored by medical student teams. Project concepts are first initiated during the Carle Illinois Engineering sequence and further developed through multiple cycles of design in the Bioengineering design courses. Figure 15.3 illustrates the overall timeline of the capstone sequence.

Two courses at the medical school lead up to the presentation of design projects to engineering students. Innovation, Design, Engineering, and Analysis (BSE680) is an engineering design course in which medical students conduct needs identification in seven clerkship rotations in their M3 year. From these seven ideas, students form teams and choose or develop a new idea for a capstone project at the start of the M4 year. In BSE685, capstone medical students conduct rigorous needs finding, stakeholder interviews, and initial solution concepts. After this, medical students pitch the projects for engineering students to develop during the fall of the M4 medical school year. From here, medical students assume the role of project clients, similar to those projects sponsored by industry, academic, or community partners.

In the first week of the BIOE Capstone class, the medical students present short project pitches to the class. Pitches provide an overview of the project background, the identified need, and practical details about the type of design and prototype the client seeks. Students use this information to vote for projects. After voting, course instructors assemble teams composed of two to three medical students as clients with one to two M.Eng. students and three to five UGs, depending on project needs, enrollment, and interest. Once teams are formed, the BIOE Capstone course commences.

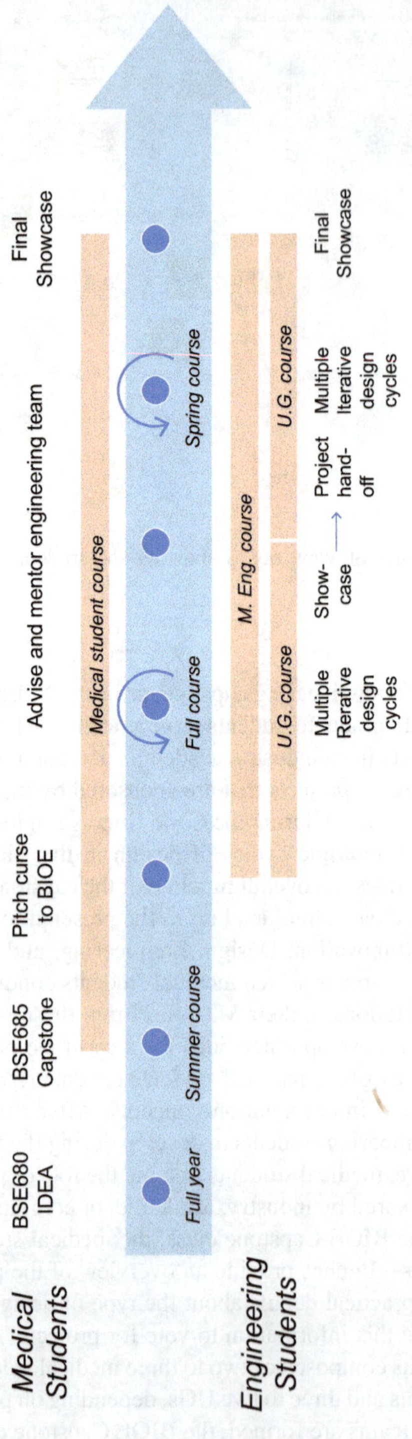

FIGURE 15.3 Timeline for each student cohort involved in the design continuum.

The Illinois BIOE Capstone classes (UG and M.Eng.) meet twice a week for 80 minutes together (referred to as "lecture"). Lecture times include not only didactic content delivery but also workshops, student presentations, and scaffolded team activities (Bethke, Ansari, Amos et al. 2024). Teams meet individually with course staff to present and discuss project-specific updates (referred to as "team meetings"). Students also work outside of class (approximately ten hours per week) with clients and their teams.

During the lecture, students experience instructor presentations on design topics, guest speakers with particular design expertise, presentations, and structured teamwork time. The M.Eng. and UG capstone courses meet together to facilitate teamwork during open lab times and reflection on lecture topics. Topics covered in the BIOE capstone course are detailed in Table 15.2.

These topics are primarily new to all undergraduates within the context of capstone design. For example, undergraduates learn ethics in a first-year course through project-based work (Miller et al. 2022), but it is focused broadly on the field of bioengineering, while in this course, the focus is on engineering design and specific challenges they may face in their project and teams (H. Golecki and Bradley 2024). M.Eng. students may have taken courses in these topics at their undergraduate institution if they majored in engineering. M.Eng. students attend lectures in the fall semester and can reinforce topics when they are delivered in the second semester to the new team of UGs.

From this point, both M.Eng. and UG students use skills previously learned in their respective curricula and a series of modules taught in this course to confirm the project need through stakeholder interviews, prior art investigation, and development of design criteria in collaboration with clients. M.Eng. students are concurrently enrolled in a business/project management course. The management course includes principles of design, management, and improvement of business operations

TABLE 15.2
Topics covered in BIOE575 and 400 Capstone design

Topics covered in BIOE575 and 400 Capstone Design
• Teamwork
• Project management
• Biodesign framework
• Technical writing
• Technical communication
• Library resources
• Patents
• Technical standards
• Regulatory processes
• Engineering ethics
• Technology translation
• *Prototyping workshops*: soft material molding, microcontrollers, CAD, additive manufacturing

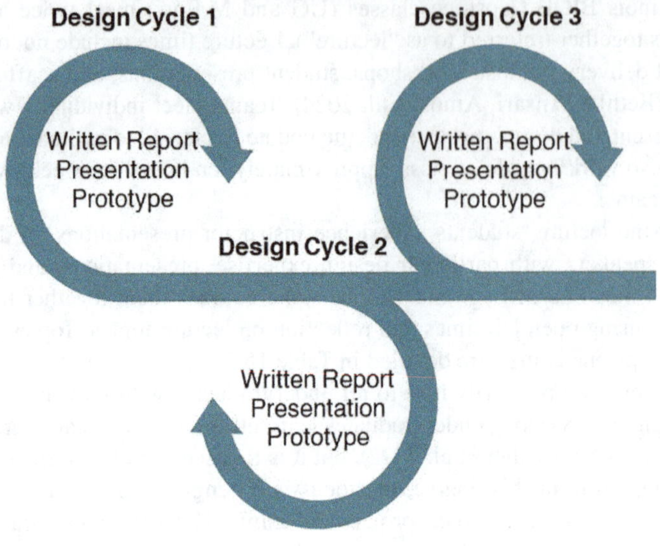

FIGURE 15.4 Design timeline showing iterative writing and prototyping cycles.

and product innovations. Strategies and techniques for managing processes, projects, process improvement, and new product development are emphasized in these courses. Additionally, students learn how to define and analyze strategic problems stemming from innovation and technological change and identify sources of competitive advantage. Project management skill development was evaluated and assessed by M.Eng. instructors. Throughout the semester, students engage in three design cycles, each with associated assignments.

As shown earlier in Figure 15.3, students in BIOE Capstone work through multiple iterative design cycles each semester. Each cycle is documented through a series of assignments as shown in Figure 15.4. Students complete a written report that is modeled after the US Food and Drug Administration Design History File documentation (Fargen and others 2013). Undergraduates take the lead on written documentation as they also earn advanced composition credit, a university-wide writing-intensive course requirement, in the Senior Design course. Undergraduates submit drafts to M.Eng. project managers for review. Student teams create a presentation to share with the class on project updates. M.Eng. students take the lead in organizing these presentations. Finally, students present a prototype iteration in each design cycle, starting with a conceptual design and progressing to a testable prototype. Prototyping is led by undergraduates, but M.Eng. and medical students often participate in this hands-on work.

15.3.2 Assessment Design

Similar to assignments, student assessment in the course is iterative and collaborative. Students complete report drafts and revisions for each section of the written report. Instructors provide both inline comments and analytical rubrics for formative feedback throughout the semester. Analytical rubrics were developed for undergraduates and M.Eng students for presentations. Summative feedback is provided to students after the final demonstration day presentation of the poster and prototype, and completion of the final report. Instructors also assign a Professionalism grade that is based on attendance and participation in class and meetings, regular email communication with clients, and lab maintenance. The objective is for students to have real-time feedback on course performance and opportunities for growth and improvement. There are at least three opportunities for clients to provide informal feedback to instructors and one opportunity for formal feedback that informs final Professionalism grades.

In addition to receiving feedback from course staff and clients, learning to provide peer feedback is an important part of the BIOE Capstone. At the start of the semester, students develop team contracts to set expectations across the team. After this, at multiple points in the semester, teammates provide feedback on each other's performance in the project and adherence to the team contract (Bethke, Ansari, Bradley et al. 2024). Teams, led by M.Eng. project managers, draft contribution statements to accompany each design cycle. Students provide informal feedback to instructors through discussions and meetings, but are also guided by formalized feedback tools.

15.3.3 Feedback Mechanisms

It is critical to train the next generation of engineers for effective and efficient collaboration in their careers (Galbraith and Webb 2013). Team communication facilitates collaboration and continuous improvement processes (Raappana and Horila 2019). To evaluate team dynamics, the Comprehensive Assessment of Team Member Effectiveness (CATME) was originally developed from an assembly of teamwork survey items from the literature (Layton et al. 2007). After survey validation, 87 items were assembled to measure 29 features of team member contributions in an online tool referred to as CATME (Beigpourian et al. 2019). M.Eng. and undergraduate students reflect on their own project performance as well as their peers. CATME provides multiple dimensions for students to rate each other on that includes feedback training and opportunities to share responses with team members or only with instructors. CATME responses are factored into final Professionalism grades as they provide a broad overview of team performance, despite the lack of project management-focused items.

Project management training is crucial for students undertaking a combined bachelor's and master's capstone experience in biomedical engineering. This training equips students with essential skills to effectively plan, execute, and manage complex projects, ensuring they meet deadlines and stay within budget. It fosters teamwork and communication, enabling students to collaborate efficiently with peers and mentors. Additionally, project management training helps students develop problem-solving abilities and adaptability, which are vital in the dynamic field of biomedical engineering (Stukes et al. 2023). By mastering these skills, students are better prepared to tackle real-world challenges, innovate solutions, and contribute meaningfully to advancements in healthcare technology. The course instructors decided on the following skills as key to success for the projects: planning and scheduling, communication, leadership, risk management, budgeting, problem-solving, time management, and quality control.

Some of the skills were already assessed using the CATME tool, but others needed to be assessed separately. We wanted to keep the same 360° review structure as the CATME survey, so we created a feedback tool to collect student feedback and self-assessments of project management skills. A detailed rubric was created with an accompanying Qualtrics questionnaire to collect the self-ratings and team member ratings for each M.Eng. student.

15.3.4 Assessment of Learning Outcomes and Student Experiences in Cross-Disciplinary Teams

Deciding how to grade the students in a combined class with different learning outcomes was a challenge. As outlined in Section 15.1, the course outcomes have some overlap but not complete overlap, so the classes have some common assessments and some unique assessments to fully assess the learning outcomes for each cohort.

15.3.4.1 Project Reports

To reflect the disparity in emphasis on writing skills and mimic workflow in an industry workplace, the undergraduates are tasked with writing the reports. They then turn the reports in ahead of the due date to their M.Eng. members for editing and revision suggestions, as one might turn a report in to a manager before submitting to an upper-level administrator in a company. The group then submits the report to the instructional team. All students on the team receive the same grade for the report. This division of responsibilities allows for each cohort to have a clear role in the quality of the report and a stake in the grade of the report.

15.3.4.2 Project Presentations

Both programs have a focus on communication; therefore, all students have the responsibility to prepare and present presentations. All students in the team receive the same grade for each presentation.

15.3.4.3 Team Assessments

All students are asked to perform a self-evaluation and a peer evaluation of the behavioral aspects of teamwork needed for success in their project. A summary of common themes in both positive and negative feedback is provided in Table 15.3.

15.3.4.4 Project Manager Assessments

All students are asked to perform a peer evaluation of the project management skills needed for success in their project. M.Eng. students are also asked to submit a self-evaluation of their skills. This is performed twice each semester to provide a mid-point formative evaluation before the summative assessment. The PM grade

TABLE 15.3
Positive and negative traits for team performance

Positive Traits for Team Success	Negative Traits For Teammates
• Effective communication and responsiveness to the team and the client	• Sporadic communication and poor attendance at team meetings.
• Contributing technical skills to the team, such as CAD, coding, and prototyping skills	• Procrastination, which leads to last-minute work and increased stress for the team
• Displaying a high level of commitment to the project helped the team get through challenges	• Creating tension or conflict within the team, thereby affecting collaboration and morale
• Consistently meeting deadlines and producing high-quality work	

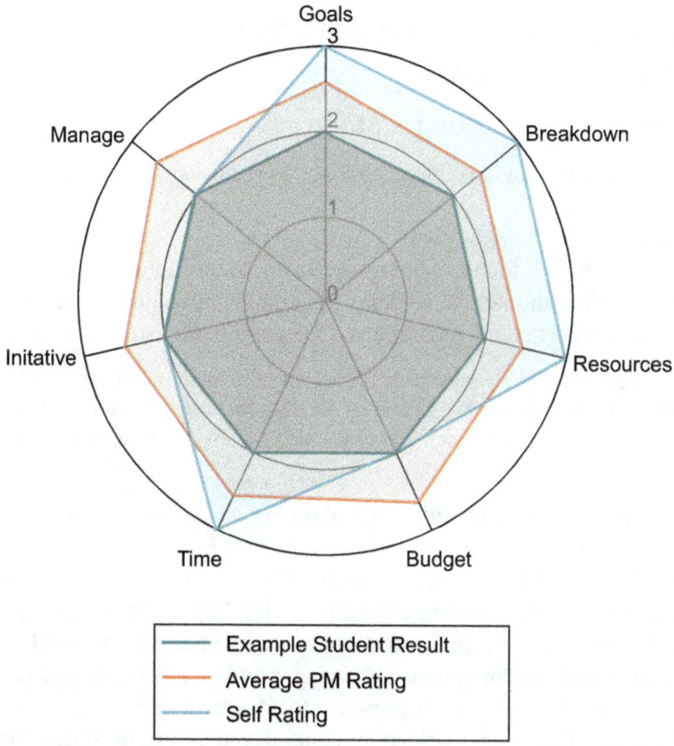

FIGURE 15.5 Spider plot showing sample performance feedback of the PM competencies

is equally weighted with the participation and professionalism grade for the UGs. Figure 15.5 shows an example of the PM feedback, including the student's self-rating, peer rating, and average rating for the cohort. A summary of common themes in both positive and negative feedback is provided in Table 15.4.

TABLE 15.4
Positive and negative traits for project manager performance

Positive Traits for Project Managers	Negative Traits for Project Managers
• Responding to UG questions and client communications in a timely manner • Helping to review and revise coursework for BIOE 400 students, especially design history file reports • Taking a proactive role in managing tasks and enhancing team communication • Running efficient meetings	• Not attending meetings or participating in team discussions or a lack of overall interaction with the team • Lack of initiative and involvement in project-related tasks • Not keeping up to date on BIOE 400 deadlines or not being proactive in reviewing materials before submission

15.4 BEST PRACTICES IN MANAGING CROSS-DISCIPLINARY TEAMS

15.4.1 Student Feedback on the Model

Students are asked to provide course feedback to the instructor about this model and suggest improvements.

Clinical Clients. We found that engineering students appreciate the opportunity to work with medical students to complement their engineering training or to support career aspirations. One engineering student stated,

> This project is definitely my top choice because I'm interested in being able to work directly with real gynecologists and medical students who can give insight into the doctor/patient perspective, something you don't often get as an engineer designing a product.

And another student expressed, "I am planning on applying to medical school soon, so I am interested in working with CIMED students on this project."

Real-World Team Structure. Many students found the course engaging, rewarding, and a valuable learning experience. They felt that the course provided practical insights into real-world applications and industry-level projects. Students cited the continuous check-ins, professional input, and guest lectures as aspects of instructor presence that were valued.

Skill Building. The course helped students develop various skills, including project management, communication, teamwork, and technical skills. Students expressed that they felt more confident in their abilities to work in teams and manage time effectively. Furthermore, the experience of working with clients and managing real projects was highlighted as a significant positive aspect.

Emphasis on Writing. Some students felt that there was too much emphasis on writing the design history file and not enough on prototyping. Suggestions were made to increase the focus on hands-on prototyping activities.

Assigned Team Roles. A few students struggled with understanding their roles and responsibilities within the team. They suggest clearer role definitions and more guidance from M.Eng students and instructors.

15.4.2 Instructor Perspectives of Benefits and Challenges

The consolidation of capstone cohorts represents a strategic initiative aimed at enhancing the efficiency, quality, and impact of experiential learning within our academic programs. By streamlining the project recruitment process, this approach significantly reduces administrative burden while ensuring that all projects are clinically vetted to address authentic, high-priority needs in the field. This vetting process not only enhances the relevance of student work but also strengthens the translational potential of project outcomes. The collaborative structure allows for increased oversight and iterative feedback, as multiple faculty members and staff contribute to project evaluation and student mentorship. Furthermore, the inclusion of project managers as embedded instructional support provides an additional layer of guidance, functioning similarly to TAs to ensure team accountability and progress.

However, this model also introduces several operational challenges that require careful planning and resource allocation. The most challenging are the complexities of coordinating instructional roles and responsibilities across multiple faculty members, particularly when pedagogical objectives and assessment standards vary. Furthermore, the management of the course website and LMS becomes increasingly intricate due to the diversity of assignments and instructional approaches. Additionally, maintaining consistency and equity in grading across cohorts necessitates the development of robust evaluation frameworks and shared rubrics. Emphasizing design through UG curricula will also enhance the hands-on prototyping aspects of the senior design course (Cvetkovic et al. 2024; Golecki et al. 2024). Addressing these challenges is essential to fully realizing the benefits of this integrated model and ensuring a high-quality, equitable learning experience for all students.

15.4.3 Guidelines for Adopting This Approach

To ensure the success of the integrated capstone model, it is essential that the instructional team operates with a shared set of goals and a unified pedagogical vision. Establishing a collaborative working relationship among faculty and staff fosters consistency in instruction and enhances the overall learning experience for students.

Given the large size of student teams and the complexity of their roles and responsibilities, it is also critical to implement effective systems for tracking individual and group contributions. Without such mechanisms, managing workflow and ensuring accountability within teams becomes increasingly challenging, potentially impacting both project outcomes and student development.

15.5 CONCLUSION

The integrated capstone model described in this chapter represents a transformative approach to experiential learning in biomedical engineering education. By aligning the educational goals of undergraduate, graduate, and medical students within a shared design continuum, the program fosters authentic collaboration that mirrors real-world organizational structures.

This model not only addresses logistical and instructional challenges inherent in multi-cohort design education but also enhances student learning. The inclusion of medical students as clients, M.Eng. students as project managers, and undergraduates as technical leads creates a dynamic learning environment that prepares students for the complexities of modern healthcare innovation.

Despite operational complexities in coordinating diverse instructional goals and maintaining equitable assessment frameworks, the benefits of this approach are many. Students gain exposure to interdisciplinary collaboration, develop critical technical and professional competencies, and engage in meaningful problem-solving grounded in clinical relevance. As institutions seek to prepare students for collaborative, interdisciplinary careers, the practices and insights shared in this case study offer a blueprint for capstone design reform.

REFERENCES

Ashby, L., and M. Exter. 2019. "Designing for Interdisciplinarity in Higher Education Considerations for Instructional Designers." *TechTrends* 63 (November): 202–8.

Beigpourian, B., D. M. Ferguson, F. C. Berry, M. W. Ohland, and S. Wei. 2019. "Using CATME to Document and Improve the Effectiveness of Teamwork in Capstone Courses." In *2019 ASEE Annual Conference & Exposition*. Tampa, FL. https://doi.org/10.18260/1-2-33497.

Bethke, Eliot, Ali Ansari, Jennifer Amos, Joe Bradley, Ruth Ochia, and Holly Golecki. 2024. "Bridging Extracurricular Skill Needs in Bioengineering Capstone Design with Just-in-Time Workshops." In *2024 ASEE Annual Conference & Exposition Proceedings* (Portland, Oregon), 48410. https://doi.org/10.18260/1-2-48410.

Bethke, Eliot, Ali Ansari, Joe Bradley, Jennifer Amos, and Holly Golecki. 2024. "An Adaptive Scaffolding Approach Based on Team Dynamics in an Integrated Masters and Undergraduate Bioengineering Capstone Design Course." In *2024 ASEE Annual Conference & Exposition Proceedings* (Portland, Oregon), 46542. https://doi.org/10.18260/1-2-46542.

Boyd, L., J. Bradley, M. Gray, and others. 2025. "Enhancing Biomedical Engineering Education Through Curricular Innovation: Developing Industry-Ready Engineers." *Biomedical Engineering Education*, ahead of print. https://doi.org/10.1007/s43683-025-00171-z.

Cvetkovic, Caroline, Sarah Lindley, Holly Golecki, and Robert Krencik. 2024. "Biofabrication of Neural Organoids: An Experiential Learning Approach for Instructional Laboratories." *Biomedical Engineering Education* 4 (2): 409–19. https://doi.org/10.1007/s43683-024-00145-7.

Fargen, K. M., and others. 2013. "The FDA Approval Process for Medical Devices: An Inherently Flawed System or a Valuable Pathway for Innovation?" *The Journal of NeuroInterventional Surgery* 5 (4): 269–75. https://doi.org/10.1136/neurintsurg-2012-010400.

Galbraith, Diane D., and Fred L. Webb. 2013. "Teams That Work: Preparing Student Teams for the Workplace." *American Journal of Business Education (Online)* 6 (2): 223-n/a. https://doi.org/10.19030/ajbe.v6i2.7687.

Golecki, Holly, Jennifer Amos, and Joe Bradley. 2023. "Designing Capstone Experiences for Interdisciplinarity in Biomedical Engineering Education." In *2023 ASEE Annual Conference & Exposition Proceedings*, June, 42977. https://doi.org/10.18260/1-2-42977.

Golecki, Holly, and J. Bradley. 2024. "Experiential Learning: Exploring Nuances When Making Ethical Decisions in a Capstone Design Course." *Biomedical Engineering Education* 4: 163–70. https://doi.org/10.1007/s43683-023-00126-2.

Golecki, Holly, Jason Robinson, Caroline Cvetkovic, and Conor Walsh. 2024. "Empowering Students in Medical Device Design: An Interdisciplinary Soft Robotics Course." *Biomedical Engineering Education*, ahead of print, April. https://doi.org/10.1007/s43683-024-00143-9.

Gray, M., J. R. Amos, S. Bailey, and others. 2024. "BME Master's Programs: Who Are They for and What Can They Offer?" *Biomedical Engineering Education* 4: 175–83. https://doi.org/10.1007/s43683-024-00141-x.

Kimpton, C., and N. Maynard. 2025. "Factors Shaping Teamwork Skills Development in Tertiary Engineering Education." *European Journal of Engineering Education* 50 (2). https://doi.org/10.1080/03043797.2024.2357343.

Layton, R., M. Ohland, and H. R. Pomeranz. 2007. "Software for Student Team Formation and Peer Evaluation: Catme Incorporates Team Maker." In *2007 Annual Conference & Exposition* (Honolulu, Hawaii). https://doi.org/10.18260/1-2-2355.

Miller, I., S. Lamer, A. Brougham-Cook, and others. 2022. "Development and Implementation of a Biometrics Device Design Project in an Introductory BME Course to Support Student Wellness." *Biomedical Engineering Education* 2: 75–82. https://doi.org/10.1007/s43683-021-00060-1.

Raappana, Mitra, and Tessa Horila. 2019. "Team Communication in the Workplace." *Workplace Communication*: 28–40. https://doi.org/10.4324/9780429196881-3.

Stukes, S., E. Bethke, M. J. O'Donnell, and others. 2023. "Biomedical Specialized Masters Programs: What Are They and How Do They Meet the Needs of Employers?" *Biomed Eng Education* 3: 291–301. https://doi.org/10.1007/s43683-023-00115-5.

16 Engaging Biomedical Engineering Students in the United Nations Sustainable Development Goals

Joseph Tranquillo

16.1 INTRODUCTION

Engineering programs and instructors struggle to prepare graduates for an impactful and fulfilling 40+ year career. As the world changes, the competencies an engineer needs to remain relevant change, too. A grounding in applied science and math may have sustained the engineers of the past throughout their careers. However, graduates today must integrate traditional engineering skills with topics that include ethics, sustainability, entrepreneurship and innovation, business and regulatory processes, intellectual property, and industry standards, all in a global context. To be effective, they should be creative designers, good communicators, contributors to multidisciplinary teams, and competent managers of complex projects. To sustain a career, especially in biomedical engineering, graduates must stay up-to-date with the latest knowledge, tools, and techniques in the biological and medical sciences, breakthroughs in technology, and the ever-evolving healthcare ecosystem (regulatory, finance, marketing, policy, and clinical care).

Our graduates should be simultaneously workforce-ready and attractive to graduate and professional programs. The challenge to programs is that all of this must happen in four (or perhaps five) years in a way that does not silo technical and non-technical abilities. As stated, this seems to be an impossible task.

If we examine most of our curricula (that of the author's as well), it is similar to going to the gym. We isolate specific topics (muscles) and then assess growth (how much they can lift). Just as a lifter may have a "leg day" and an "arm day," we teach Thermodynamics on a Monday and Statics on a Tuesday. There is nothing wrong with this approach, but it tends to silo learning and can easily lead to assumptions that include the following:

- Students accepted to an engineering program are motivated and enter with the technical skills needed to successfully navigate a rigorous engineering curriculum.

 DOI: 10.1201/9781003520313-16

- Practicing scientific and technical skills will be enough to get students hired, and they will learn the rest on the job or in graduate school.
- There is no room in the curriculum to add more content.
- It is the position of this chapter that the secret sauce of an engineering education, one that addresses the impossible tasks above, is engaging students in complex and challenging projects. To continue with the fitness analogy, these experiences are intellectual cross-training. Just as a cross-trainer will engage in non-linear exercises to more holistically strengthen their bodies, we can engage learners in the integration of their skills and knowledge through authentic challenges.

This chapter will detail the author's exploration of immersive design experiences based on the United Nations Sustainable Development Goals (SDGs). The pedagogy, however, is applicable to a broader range of complex design challenges. An overview of the UN SDGs is provided along with a four-part sustainable educational framework. The general outline of an experience with the SDGs is shared with learning objectives, assignments, and assessment ideas. Several variations, both in and out of the classroom, are shared along with pedagogical techniques and a summary of program assessment.

16.2 THE UN SDGS

This section reviews the intersection of engineering and sustainability, the origin of the UN SDGs, and a rationale for introducing the SDGs to biomedical engineering students.

16.2.1 Sustainability and Engineering

The current definition of sustainability emerged from the environmental movement that acknowledged the human impact on the natural world (Gibson 2006; Gibson & Venkateswar 2015). The Brundtland Commission of 1987 broadened the definition to include social, economic, and environmental sustainability. These three dimensions are interwoven and counterbalancing in such a way that business and policy decisions should consider the impact on all three. Although alternative frameworks exist (e.g., Gibson's seven principle approach, Gibson, Hassan, and Tansey 2013), the Triple Bottom Line (TBL) is widely used in both industry and higher education. The TBL sometimes goes by other names such as The Three Pillars, The Three Legged Stool, The Three E's (Environment, Ecosystem, and Economy), and The Three P's (Planet, People, and Profit).

Engineering, both industry and education, was an early adopter of sustainable thinking. Product developers design for Life Cycle Assessment (LCA), using terms such as "Cradle to Grave" and "Cradle to Grave to Cradle," as a way to assess the holistic impact of a product on the world.

Likewise, Environmental Impact Assessment has expanded to include Life Cycle Sustainability Assessment, Life Cycle Costing, and Societal LCA. Within engineering education, the ABET Criteria 3(2) reads "an ability to apply engineering design to produce solutions that meet specified needs with consideration of public health, safety, and welfare, as well as global, cultural, social, environmental, and economic factors." Criteria 3(4) reads "an ability to recognize ethical and professional responsibilities in engineering situations and make informed judgments, which must consider the impact of engineering solutions in global, economic, environmental, and societal contexts" (ABET 2024). In addition, several engineering professional societies, including ASCE, ASME, ASEE, AICHE, and IEEE, have subsections on the importance of sustainable design. Many undergraduate institutions have chapters of these organizations that encourage sustainable thinking. Although the Biomedical Engineering Society does not have a specific sustainability subsection, many different biomedical engineering programs build sustainability into their curricula (Tranquillo n.d.).

16.2.2 The UN SDGs

At the turn of the millennium, an international taskforce developed eight challenges for the 192 members of the United Nations (http://www.un.org/millenniumgoals/). The eight goals, with accompanying metrics, were meant to stimulate efforts to meet the needs of the most disadvantaged people on the planet. An ambitious target date of 2015 was set to meet all of the metrics. In 2015, a report was issued outlining the state of progress. While some metrics were met, many were not. This prompted a reframing and restatement of 17 SDGs (Figure 16.1), approved by the United Nations on September 25, 2015, that will be in effect until 2030. The purpose is to provide sub-goals and measurable outcomes that will focus the allocation of resources toward solving the world's most pressing problems. The website (sustainabledevelopment.un.org) is well organized and contains information on several hundred sub-goals.

16.2.3 Properties of Wicked (and Super Wicked) Problems

The SDGs are "Wicked Problems," a term coined in 1967 by C. West Churchman, but more formally defined in 1973 by Rittel and Webber. Wicked problems affect many stakeholders yet seem impossible to solve because of incomplete, changing, and contradictory constraints that emerge from the complex interplay between socio-cultural, economic, technological, geo-political, and legal dynamics. Any sustainable solution will necessarily involve large-scale collaboration, coordination, and compromise. Because there is no optimal solution, it is often not clear what to measure, if progress is being made, or even when the problem has been solved. Every wicked problem is wicked in its own way, so there are no silver bullets, general frameworks, or formulas for solving them. Furthermore, the unintended consequences of interventions are difficult to predict because most wicked problems are intertwined with other wicked problems.

In 2012, a further set of complexities (Levin et al. 2012) was articulated that turn a wicked problem into a super wicked problem:

- There is a deadline on finding a solution, beyond which severe and irreversible consequences will affect all stakeholders.

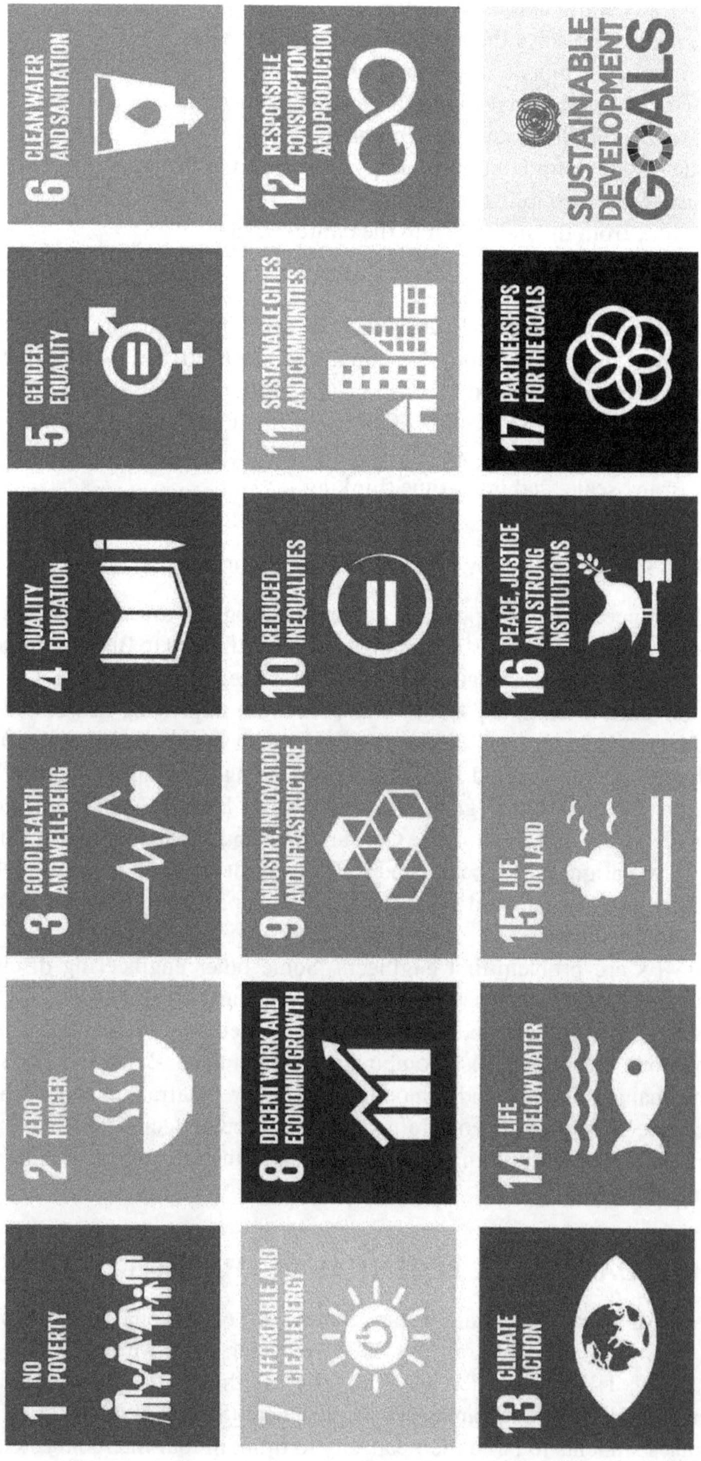
1 NO POVERTY
2 ZERO HUNGER
3 GOOD HEALTH AND WELL-BEING
4 QUALITY EDUCATION
5 GENDER EQUALITY
6 CLEAN WATER AND SANITATION
7 AFFORDABLE AND CLEAN ENERGY
8 DECENT WORK AND ECONOMIC GROWTH
9 INDUSTRY, INNOVATION AND INFRASTRUCTURE
10 REDUCED INEQUALITIES
11 SUSTAINABLE CITIES AND COMMUNITIES
12 RESPONSIBLE CONSUMPTION AND PRODUCTION
13 CLIMATE ACTION
14 LIFE BELOW WATER
15 LIFE ON LAND
16 PEACE, JUSTICE AND STRONG INSTITUTIONS
17 PARTNERSHIPS FOR THE GOALS
SUSTAINABLE DEVELOPMENT GOALS

FIGURE 16.1 Summary of the UN SDGs

- There is no central authority responsible for finding a solution.
- Those seeking to solve the problem are also causing it.
- Certain policies impede future progress.
- Declaring a problem to be wicked is a strategy that aims to.
- Call broad attention to an urgent problem.
- Provide direction for attention, energy, effort, and resources.
- Encourage interdisciplinary collaborations.
- Scale work from the individual to the entire world.
- Suggest metrics that point to signs of progress.

There are lists of wicked (and super wicked) problems (Omenn 2006), such as the NAE Grand Challenges (Mote, Dowling, and Zhou 2016) (e.g., Enhance VR and Secure Cyberspace), Google Moonshots (e.g., Programming Plants to be more Resilient and Sustainable), and UNESCO Engineering Challenges (2010). However, the UN SDGs are the ultimate super wicked problems in that they require trans-disciplinary, trans-scale, and trans-time thinking.

16.2.4 The SDGs Are Ready Made for BME Students

Biomedical engineers are well-positioned to make progress toward addressing the SDGs for several reasons. First, students are typically attracted to BME because they want to be in a technical field that is inherently about helping people.

Second, our interdisciplinary training and focus on improving health and well-being (Azlina et al. 2013) is in direct alignment with many of the goals, including Zero Hunger (Goal 2), Good Health and Well Being (Goal 3), and Clean Water and Sanitation (Goal 6). Other goals, such as Gender Equality (Goal 5), Reduced Inequalities (Goal 10), and Responsible Consumption and Production (Goal 12), have sub-goals that are aligned with health and well-being. Because all of these problems are interwoven, progress toward one often has an impact on the others (Goal 17, Partnerships for the Goals).

Third, BMEs are problem-first engineers. Some other engineering disciplines start with a sub-domain of physics, chemistry, or math and only later look for applications. BMEs, on the other hand, start with the problem and then broadly explore possible solutions that might be a combination of technical skills and knowledge (e.g., fluid mechanics, circuits, and computing). BMEs are unafraid to choose the best solution because they are not constrained by a particular technical domain. The SDGs require this kind of thinking, and BME students thrive in environments where the problem comes first.

16.3 THE PEDAGOGICAL POTENTIAL OF THE SDGS

The SDGs have great potential in the context of educational programs (UN Education, Scientific and Cultural Org 2004; Wheeler 2014; Murphy et al. 2009; Sipos et al. 2008; Tillbury 2011; Wiek et al. 2011). In this section, we expand upon the Sustainability Education Framework for Teachers (SEFT) (Warren et al. 2014) that encourages students to build their capacity to think in four interconnected ways (systems, values, strategies, and future). It is holding all of these ways of thinking together in one's mind, often in tension, that induces cognitive stretching and the ability to navigate a wicked problem (Stibbe and Luna 2009; National Research Council 2000; Caine 2009; Bybee 2002; Byrne et al. 2010; Huntzinger et al. 2007). In the following, each of the ways of thinking is reviewed (modified from the SEFT) and paired with a pedagogical movement within engineering education.

16.3.1 Systems Thinking and Wicked Problems

Systems Thinking emerged from logic, mathematics, and the scientific method but has been adopted by many other fields, including anthropology, art, politics, and economics. An abbreviated list of systems thinking abilities is as follows:

- Seeing network effects, inertia, positive and negative feedback loops, system delays, path dependencies, bottlenecks, flows, and cascading effects (Tranquillo 2019b);
- Recognizing patterns and underlying relationships across different bodies of knowledge and processes (from man-made to natural), places (from local to global), and times (from geo-evolutionary history to the future);
- Making sense of a complex system by extracting the dimensions that matter most (Casti and Karlqvist 1986), so that one can intentionally make incremental interventions that will change the future trajectory of the system;
- Distinguishing between observed symptoms/signals and underlying interconnected system dynamics (Meadows 2008);
- Dissecting how past decisions led us to the problems of today;
- Viewing a particular problem/solution as only one of a constellation of interconnected problems/solutions that could exist (Grunwald 2004);
- Seeking sustainable solutions by considering a wide range of stakeholders, including policymakers, innovators, and citizens.

There are educational movements that are closely aligned with Systems Thinking. For example, the Liberal Arts challenges students to view the world through multiple perspectives. Games, simulations, role-playing, and toy models are excellent ways to teach systems thinking (Bodnar et al. 2016; Tranquillo 2008, 2014) and have been used in disciplines ranging from physics and management to anthropology and psychology. Likewise, a well-orchestrated discussion or debate can help students actively explore unexpected connections that lie beyond the information in a primary or secondary source. Among engineering educators, there has also been an emphasis on the T-shape (Tranquillo 2017a) and Entrepreneurship and Arts combined with STEM.

Engineering educators have adopted several pedagogical approaches that support systems thinking, including PBL and PjBL (Blumenfeld et al. 1991; Prince 2004; Prince and Felder 2007; Bell 2010). In PjBL, student teams are presented with a problem that is ambiguous and/or has incomplete information or constraints. Often, the problem inherits multiple constraints from different natural and man-made systems that may be in conflict with one another. Solutions are not prescribed or predetermined ahead of time, and students are given autonomy over design decisions. The outcome may be a functional (physical) artifact (PjBL) or an on-paper solution concept (PBL).

16.3.2 Values Thinking and Live Case Studies

Values thinking derives from the ethical dimensions of over-consumption and the inequitable distribution of resources, but extends beyond these considerations (Veugelers 2000). An abbreviated list of elements of value thinking is as follows:

- Considering how various views, values, and cultures have been constructed from past choices and preconceived value-based beliefs (Rawls 1985);
- Recognizing major human conflicts as arising from clashing worldviews, unequal resource allocation, and historical biases (Ostrom 1990);
- Positioning value-based tensions between stakeholders in ethical terms;
- Finding ways to be more inclusive and equitable across stakeholders to reduce bias in the status quo;
- Determining the justice, equity, and social-ecological impact of proposed solutions (Holifield et al. 2010);
- Ensuring broad-based consensus and transparency in decision-making (Fischer 1993; Corburn 2007; Bäckstrand 2003).

Values thinking helps students seek out and understand different points of view, as well as develop (and perhaps question) their own personal point of view. Engagement with values thinking can be emotional and can therefore lead to "sticky" learning environments (Caine 2009). Active listening/participation, role-playing, debates, Structured Academic Controversy, and case studies have all been shown to be effective techniques in the classroom. Out of the classroom, several high-impact practices (Kuh 2008) build value thinking, such as community-based learning, service learning, and diversity/global learning. Engagement in these practices has many overlaps with self-determination theory (Gagné and Deci 2005), most specifically the need to see a wider purpose in one's actions.

Live case studies are a particularly powerful pedagogical technique that can highlight the elements of value-based thinking (Beaury et al. 2010). Traditional case studies, especially those from engineering and business, are retrospective—a story is told of a problem and decision-making pathway that resulted in a particular solution, followed by an analysis and take-away message that can be applied in other situations. The learner in these types of case studies is often passive and is not asked to contribute to a solution. A live case study, on the other hand, places the learner in the problem, encouraging active exploration and engaging in value creation. Most live cases are presented as a current problem that, if solved, would provide measurable value to one or more stakeholders.

Each of the SDGs is a live case study that naturally encourages values thinking. The rise in student outreach clubs, study abroad, service learning, and community-based learning all demonstrate that current students are more aware of their privileged place in the world and are looking to make a difference. Biomedical engineering programs have been early adopters of values thinking, most especially through Devices for the Disabled (Enderle 1999), EWH (www.ewh.org), e-NABLE (enablingthefuture.org), and the proliferation of programs that specifically consider design for the developing world.

16.3.3 Strategic Thinking and Design Challenges

Strategic Thinking emerged from the business literature and includes engineering project management and, more recently, Design Thinking (dschool.stanford.edu). Elements of strategic thinking include the following:

- Seeing inefficiencies, tensions, and stakeholder pains as opportunities for a new or improved value proposition;
- Identifying stakeholders and users, uncovering the history of a problem, researching previous attempts to solve the problem, and listing constraints coming from a wide range of disciplines;
- Developing an inspirational vision and strategy that brings people and resources together;
- Exercising creativity in developing potential solutions that take into account needs and constraints (Costanza 2012; Gibson 2006; Lawrence 1999);
- Demonstrating sound decision-making in selecting a particular solution that will best balance the competing needs and demands of stakeholders;
- Developing tactics that will make the most of the available resources and skill sets of individuals and groups;
- Finding quick wins that will build further consensus and collaboration so that the solution will propagate outward to meet the problem everywhere that it may be;
- Considering how a solution will scale across time and space for various stakeholders (Loorbach 2007) so as to ameliorate negative unintended consequences.

Strategic thinking often feels natural to engineers and is woven into the design process. The general idea of strategic thinking, however, can be applied broadly beyond the development of products to include the generation of new policies, institutional frameworks, and governance. From a pedagogical perspective, learning is greatly facilitated by real situations and contexts where the strategies employed are the decision of the students (e.g., there is no "right" path laid out ahead of time). From self-determination theory, this is the ability to have autonomy in the face of ambiguity (Gagné and Deci 2005). As the UN SDGs are layered, nested, and far too large for any particular group to make significant progress, they require all of the elements of strategic thinking to be engaged.

A movement that has taken place over the past few decades is to issue students design challenges, both inside and outside the classroom, usually lasting a day to a few weeks. As such, they are immersive, moving from start to finish quickly, putting disparate concepts close to one another in time in such a way that they can potentially form a cognitive bond (discussed in Section 16.6.1). They are sometimes referred to as Innovation Challenges (Condoor and Keogh 2012), Design Sprints, Hack-a-thons, Start-up Challenges, and Pitch Competitions. The topics can range from trivial (e.g., design a lunch box for school children and logic puzzles) to very grand (e.g., exploring a world-changing entrepreneurial venture). Biomedical engineering was an early adopter of such challenges in required classes (Tranquillo and Cavanagh 2009; Gimm et al. 2011; Kelly 2013; Dolan 2013). Advice on running design challenges can be found in the online article by Tranquillo (2012).

16.3.4 Future Thinking and the Entrepreneurial Mindset

Future thinking, also known as anticipatory thinking, foresight, or trans-generational thinking (Rockström et al. 2009), emerged from social justice, community organization, and the environmental movement. It includes the following elements:

- Recognizing how decisions, actions, and inactions made by others in the past affect our options, constraints, and problems today, and likewise how our decisions, actions, and inactions today will impact others in the future (Brundtland and Khalid 1987);
- Viewing current driving forces and emerging trends as guides to possible future trajectories (Robinson et al. 2011; Kuhlmann 2001);
- Envisioning possible futures (e.g., utopian, dystopian, plausible, desirable, and likely) (Selin 2007) and contrast them with the present status quo as a means of building forward-thinking strategies or "backcasting" (Robinson et al. 2011);
- Considering intergenerational perspectives, including interventions, ideas, and/or solutions that might create cascading effects that become tomorrow's problems (Gibson 2006);
- Using both causal and effectual thinking (Sarasvathy 2001) to actively bias history toward a safer, happier, and healthier future for all (Newman and Jennings 2008).

The UN SDGs are perhaps the most ambitious acknowledgement that the world is not as it should (or could) be. The engagement with a future that is larger than oneself can prompt deeper thought into how one might impact the world, today and in the future.

Entrepreneurship and sustainability often seem to be at odds with one another because one is pitched as being about making money as quickly as possible, while the other is about saving the world and society. Yet Tranquillo (2017b) has argued that both require systems, value, strategic, and future thinking. Although entrepreneurship typically focuses on short-term value (often localized to particular stakeholders), while sustainability focuses on long-term value (often regionally or globally), there is much overlap. Programs such as social entrepreneurship in engineering schools and sustainable finance programs inside of business schools have grown in popularity. Furthermore, the entrepreneurial mindset focuses on developing the habits, behaviors, and attitudes of an entrepreneur so that they can be applied broadly to any endeavor (Gerhart and Melton 2016; Wheadon and Duval-Couetil 2015; Zappe et al. 2013), well beyond creating for-profit businesses.

16.4 IMMERSIVE EXPERIENCES WITH THE SDGS

This section explains a generic immersive challenge, grounded in the Sustainable Education Framework, that combines the following in a single integrated experience:

- A wicked problem that exercises systems thinking;
- A live case study that engages values thinking;
- A design challenge that focuses on strategic thinking;
- A social entrepreneurial venture that fosters future thinking.

Each section in the following contains the learning goals of a particular phase of the experience and an example or two of a pedagogical approach. Individual goals are supported by short presentations (~10–20 minutes), activities, reflections, and unstructured development time. Although the flow of the experience unfolds generally in the order presented, students often find that they need to return to previous steps (as will be discussed later). Several variations of this generic (detailed in the next section) have been offered, with some learning goals emphasized more than others.

16.4.1 Orientation and Problem Identification

The following learning goals support the problem ID phase:

- Articulate the importance (and difficulty) of identifying and defining a design problem;
- Perform background research on the sub-problems within one of the SDGs;
- Generate a list of viable sub-problems without coming up with a design solution;
- Identify several customer-appropriate value propositions (not solutions).

This phase begins with a pre-orientation during which students are placed in teams, are assigned one of the SDGs, engage in team-building exercises, and complete their first assignment.

A particularly powerful pre-assignment is to create a photo essay. For example, in one of the variations (K-WIDE, Section 16.5.1), students are challenged to spend at least three hours in a location (often their hometown), taking pictures of anything they feel intersects the SDG they are assigned. Their photo essay is five annotated slides highlighting their view of the issue, accompanied by a one-page reflective narrative. This pre-assignment is shared with their team at the start of the program. The goal is for students to see the problem with their own eyes in real environments.

Follow-up exercises vary depending upon the version but include first-hand conversations with those experiencing a particular problem or issue, generating a "live" list of potential problems to explore and a deep dive into background research. In particular, the SDG website contains helpful statistics, stakeholder viewpoints, progress reports, and international groups working on the problem. Various short lectures are delivered on teaming, interdisciplinary design, and methods of identifying problems.

This phase ends with a design review where students present their current view of the overall problem and stakeholders, sub-problems supported by background research, and existing solutions.

16.4.2 Decomposition

From their broad understanding, students are asked to decompose an SDG into progressively smaller tractable sub-problems. Learning goals of this phase are to:

- Narrow the scope of a large and complex problem to one that can be solved;
- Identify primary functions necessary for solving an open-ended problem;
- Decompose primary functions into supporting functions;
- Articulate the problem in a way that a non-technical expert can understand.

Students are introduced to the idea that problems and solutions are often entangled—considering possible solutions is a way to better understand the nature of a problem. Likewise, the process of "right sizing' a problem can point the way to scope solutions that are viable. Several working sessions engage students in generating "what-if" solution concepts for potential sub-problems, as well as functional deposition (primary and supporting functions) of these potential solutions.

Embedded within these workshops is further research and conversations with topical experts, regular (often several times a day) instructor check-in meetings, quick pitches to the entire group, and reflective prompts (described in Section 16.4.5).

This is typically the most difficult (and longest) phase for both students and the instructor. Instructors are used to "right-sizing" the projects and challenges we give our students. The SDGs flip the script—by giving a project that is intentionally too large to solve, it exercises the students' ability to right-size a project.

A particularly helpful pedagogical technique is for students to visually mind-map the interconnections between the high-level problem and smaller sub-problems (Figure 16.2A), using techniques such as DeBono's Provocation and Collaborative(C)-Sketch (Figures 16.2B and 16.2C). A Systems Canvas (Appendix A) is sometimes used to help groups as they struggle with the iterative push-pull between narrowing the problem and generating possible solution concepts. When students become stuck, it can help to focus on a particular stakeholder, a particular area of the world, or both.

A second technique is for students to fill out a Mad Lib of a Problem Statement. A Mad Lib is a story from which key words are removed, and then those who have no context of the story origin add in their own words (e.g., nouns, verbs, and adjectives), often resulting in a humorous version of the story. Pedagogically, a Mad Lib can be created that guides students to fill in a version of a story with their own information. These may start very simply such as:

> Did you know that______(catchy story/statistics here)_For our project we intend to _____(proposed final deliverable here)______which will contribute to the UN SDG # (# here)_______by______(explain sub goals and metrics here)

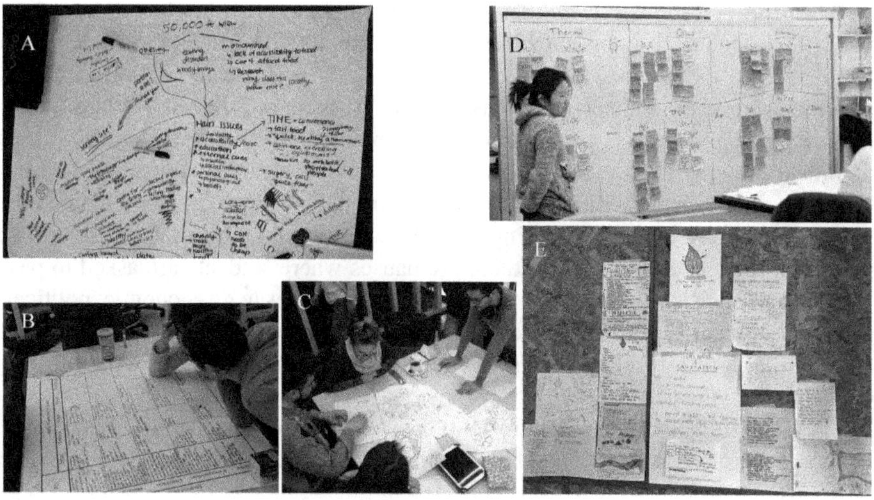

FIGURE 16.2 Summary of the decomposition and solution creation. A is a graphical decomposition of a problem. B is DeBono's Provocation exercise to explore possible solutions. C is a working session. D is an assessment of possible solutions. E is a summary of the problem and documentation of a solution decision

Simple Mad Libs can focus students, lead off design reviews, and quickly update a large group on the findings, intentions, and progress of individual teams. More complex Mad Libs can be created as the problem narrows and solutions emerge (Appendix B).

The deconstruction phase ends with a pitch and design review during which students must make a preliminary articulation of the sub-problem they have chosen, along with a high-level functional description of a solution.

16.4.3 From 10,000 to 1 m and Back Again

Once the SDG has been decomposed and a potential problem/solution pair has been identified, students are challenged to:

- Explain technical and non-technical dimensions of a problem, including economic, political, social, environmental, and ethical factors in selecting a sub-problem at a 10,000-m level;
- List the potential for positive (and negative) value at the 10,000-m level of implementing a solution concept;
- Articulate design decisions at the 1-m level;
- Move between intermedial levels between 1 and 10,000 m in iterating on a solution;
- Connect design decisions to the 10,000-m level.

The proposed solution from the decomposition phase is always flawed in several ways, both technical and non-technical. To iterate upon this solution, students are challenged to move rapidly between the large-scale problem (at 10,000 m) and a specific solution (at 1 meter). Previous techniques, such as C-Sketch (Figure 16.3A) and background research, are revisited and combined together with details such as technical drawing (Figure 16.3B) and the viability of obtaining parts and gaining access to prototyping facilities. Mini-lectures are delivered on the physical embodiment of functions, technical drawing, making decisions among alternative solutions, and feasibility. At each iteration, there are pauses where students are asked to pass their design decision through various non-technical lenses (e.g., economic, political, and environmental). In this process, students learn (with guidance) how to right-size a project—rarely a formal part of an engineering curriculum, but a hallmark of engaging with the SDGs.

The STEEPLED Canvas (Figure 16.4) is used at various points during this phase to further dissect the problem and as a reminder to think holistically about possible solutions.

This phase ends with a formal design review that serves as a gateway to prototyping.

16.4.4 Prototyping and Testing

Moving from an on-paper design to prototyping and testing is supported by the following learning objectives:

- Demonstrate the feasibility of a solution;
- Use engineering fabrication techniques to achieve functions and sub-functions;

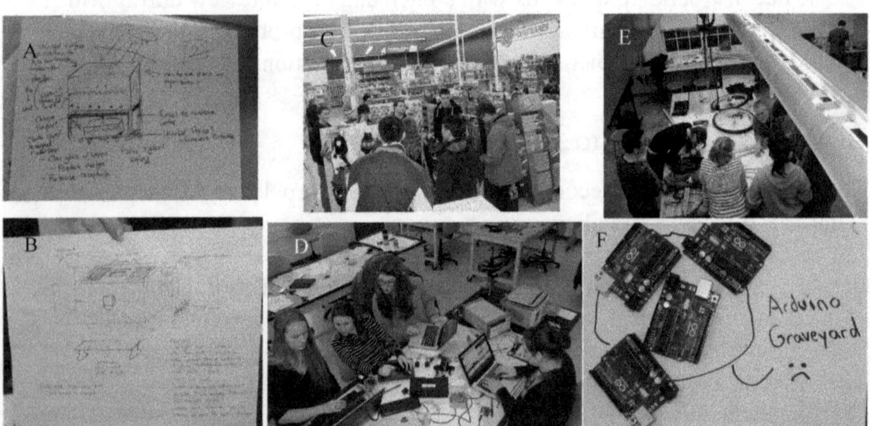

FIGURE 16.3 Summary of design and prototyping. A is an example of a C-sketch. B is an example draft solution. C is a scavenger hunt at a local hardware store. D is a group prototyping. E is a consultation with an expert machinist. F is an example of students celebrating learning from failure

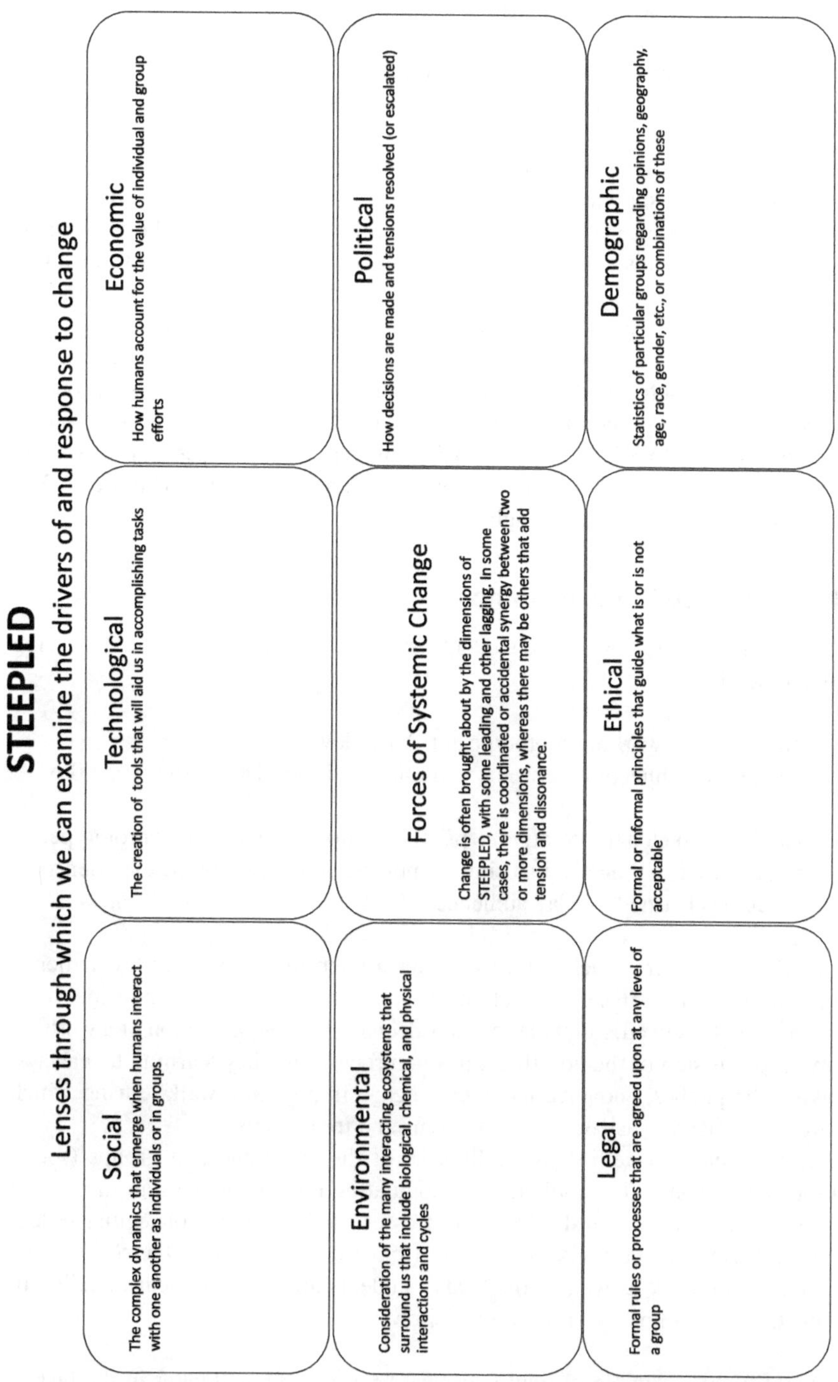

FIGURE 16.4 STEEPLED Canvas used for decomposition of a problem as well as navigating from 10,000 to 2 m

- Prepare and submit a materials order;
- Construct a functional prototype;
- Plan and conduct verification tests;
- Deliver a prototype/proof-of-concept presentation;
- Explain the manufacturability of the components of a future (final) solution.

Physical prototyping begins during orientation with the creation of a mascot (using basic crafting supplies) to "embody" the team name. Generally, during the previous two phases, at least one session is dedicated to learning about available resources (e.g., materials and fabrication techniques). A fun exercise is to turn this into a scavenger hunt on campus, but also at a local hardware store (Figure 16.3C). As part of the previous phase, there are times when a team is asked to build out the embodiment of a critical function to demonstrate the viability of the solution.

Students receive safety and basic shop training as well as mini-lectures on concept refinement and placing material orders. The majority of this phase is spent building (Figures 16.3D, 16.3E, 16.5A, and 16.5B), interspersed with design reviews and reflections. As there are many moments of failure and wrong turns (Figure 16.3F), instructors must keep motivation high.

16.4.5 Storytelling and Reflection

The final phase is a harvest of the students' hard work, supported by the following learning objectives:

- Demonstrate a working prototype at the 1-m level;
- Explain the connection between a solution and the SDGs at the 10,000-m level;
- Explain and sketch the iterative steps taken to arrive at the current prototype;
- Speak and write reflectively, using supporting stories, about the experience and lessons learned to a lay audience.

A final expo requires each team to deliver a pitch to an educated lay audience (Figures 16.5A and 16.5B). This pitch must include a clear articulation of the SDG, sub-problem to be solved, rationale for their decisions, a demonstration of a working prototype, discussion of the non-linear design process, and key learning takeaways. Following the pitches, audience members engage in a gallery walk, during which they are encouraged to ask questions of teams and individuals.

Reflection and storytelling are hallmarks of the experience, in groups (social dynamics on teams) and as individuals (modulating the emotions of an immersive experience). A workshop on the first day stresses the importance of regular reflection and storytelling. Prompts often draw from the four parts of the Sustainable Education Framework as well as the "hats" students are asked to wear (detailed in Section 16.6.4). Example prompts are as follows:

- Identify one example of how you have been a systems thinker in the last day?

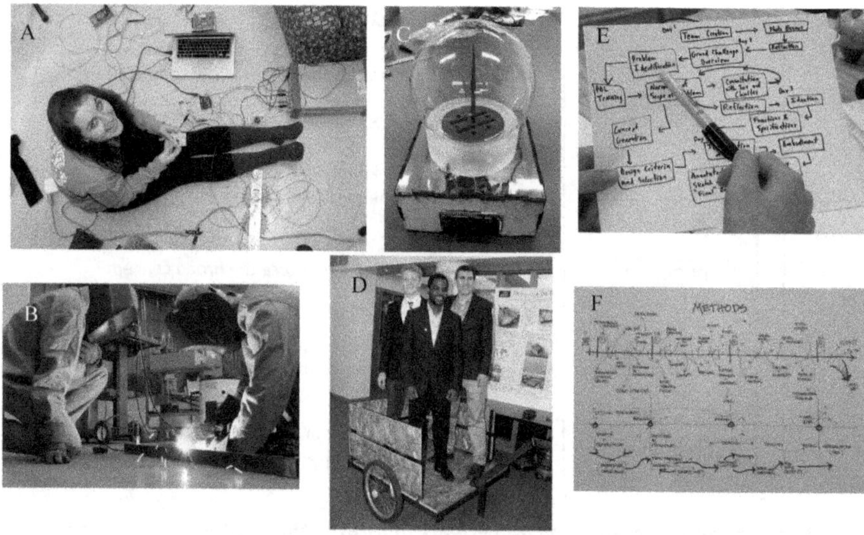

FIGURE 16.5 Summary of creating and presenting final deliverables. A is electrical prototyping. B is creating a final deliverable. C is an example of a final deliverable for the Signals and Systems course. D is an example of a final deliverable for the K-WIDE variation. E is an example of a non-linear design process sketch from the K-WIDE variation. F is an example of a non-linear design process from the Chile variation

- Which "Hat" do you feel most comfortable wearing? Which is your least comfortable?
- How have you grown in the last two days?
- What is the value proposition of this experience?
- What will you do to be uncomfortable in the next day?

Two techniques are particularly helpful in drawing our stories of growth. First is to ask the student to look over a set of words, such as:

Drive Grit Resourcefulness Integrity Decisiveness Generosity Daring Creativity Discipline Flexibility Empathy Playfulness Efficiency Inquisitiveness Vision

and choose one word they feel they expressed that day. They are then asked to write a vivid story about why they chose that word. More of these types of prompts can be found in the Reflection Collection (Tranquillo 2019a).

The second technique is to ask students to use the Reflection Ladder (Figure 16.6) in their verbal, written, and video reflections (Tranquillo 2016). A rich reflection has approximately one sentence at the bottom rung (summation—explain what happened), and then one sentence each for the higher rungs. The result is one paragraph (or one minute of talking) that abstracts an experience to extract learning that can be applied in other contexts.

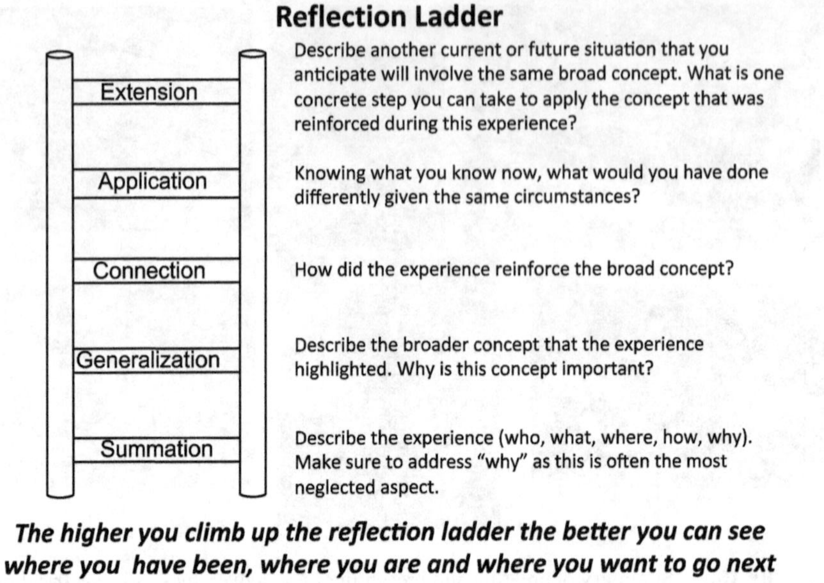

FIGURE 16.6 The Reflection Ladder used to guide verbal, written, and video reflection responses

16.4.6 Feedback to Learners

Such an ambitious and ambiguous endeavor requires significant and regular (both scheduled and impromptu) feedback. The majority of feedback is developmental and includes five-minute check-ins with teams (often at the tables where they were working), comments (usually verbal) on reflective prompts, and inviting guests to design reviews. In most of the variations (discussed in the next section), work is not graded. Even for the exceptions, grading by contract—students either complete the assignment to the instructor's satisfaction, allowing them to move on to the next step, or not.

There are, however, other forms of extrinsic accountability. Inviting the entire engineering college, Provost, and President to the final expo is a powerful motivator. A further advantage of inviting upper-level administrators is that they learn about the program. Audience members may also "invest" their venture capital using fake money on projects. In another voting scheme, there were categories (e.g., most innovative, most likely to success, best technical design)—teams that won a category received a gift certificate to a local shop.

16.5 FIVE VARIATIONS

This section outlines five variations on the generic immersive experience.

16.5.1 Winter Ten-Day Bootcamp

The KEEN (Kern Entrepreneurial Engineering Network) Winter Interdisciplinary Design Experience (K-WIDE) was a non-credit-bearing January design challenge that engaged sophomore students in developing solutions to wicked problems (Kim and Tranquillo 2014). It was built upon a first-year engineering design course that introduced the design process. Over the course of 10 days, and approximately 130 hours, students navigated the process in Section 16.4, culminating with an expo that was open to the entire Bucknell community. The program later spread to several other schools through faculty workshops (see Section 16.5.5).

16.5.2 Four-Day Design Challenge in Chile

In May 2016, the Engineering in a Global and Societal Context course was offered in Chile for 33 Bucknell University engineering students. The three-week trip involved 8 flights and 17 bus rides and focused on the impacts of engineering and science on natural, cultural, and designed environments. As part of the trip, the students and faculty stayed in a Ruka (a large round, traditional Chilean structure) where they engaged in an SDG Challenge over four days (Canziani et al. 2012). The format followed the process in Section 16.4, with one notable exception: the Ruka was out of cell phone range, did not have internet access, and the nearest town was 50 km away. Students were therefore required to design and build using only their own knowledge, skills, and local resources. The final deliverable was a pitch that was given in Ruka and again to faculty at the Universidad de Magallanes in Punta Arenas, Chile. Appendix C contains the pre-assignments used to prepare students for the challenge.

16.5.3 Biomedical Signals and Systems Course Project

The Biomedical Signals and Systems course has embedded within it a project with a theme that changes every year (Tranquillo 2018; Tranquillo and Cavanagh 2007). Examples of past themes have been the creation of real-time Bio-musical instruments, Interactive Fashion, Interactive Museum Exhibits, and Pet Technologies. The project serves as a pre-design course to the capstone, in that students have autonomy over the devices they build and navigate the design process. In Fall 2020, the course was taught in a hybrid format (to accommodate students who might be quarantined), and the project was based on the SDGs. Lectures were delivered by pre-recorded videos, team-based assignments were completed asynchronously or in lab shifts, and the expo was a poster and live video demonstration of the prototype. Faculty in the department reviewed materials asynchronously and provided developmental feedback to the teams. The project constituted 20% of the final grade, but individual assignments were graded by contract. Appendix D contains the assignments and worksheets used for this variation.

16.5.4 Two-Week Introduction to BME Senior Capstone Design

For 15 years, self-selected teams of two to three students engaged in a design sprint to kick off our two-semester senior capstone (Tranquillo and Cavanagh 2009). Rather than pass out a syllabus, the challenge served as an introduction to the complex non-linear design process that is a hallmark of our capstone experience. For four years, the challenge was driven by the SDGs, concluding with an expo at which faculty voted with venture capital. The project constituted 5% of the final grade, but individual assignments were graded by contract. Appendix E contains the assignments and worksheets used in this variation as well as a template of the final poster.

16.5.5 Half- to Full-Day Workshops (for Faculty)

With the success of K-WIDE, faculty at other universities requested being trained to offer a similar experience to their students. Train-the-trainer workshops shared much of the content of this chapter and actively engaged faculty in the process, leading up to but not including prototyping. Over the past decade, workshops were offered at Bucknell, the KEEN National Meeting, Trinity College (Hartford, CT), Worcester Polytechnic Institute, Universidad del Desarrollo (Chile), and Pontificia Universidad Catolica de Chile. Scaled-back versions were also offered to a Kindergarten class and a retirement community.

16.5.6 Possible Future Variations

The opportunities provided by the UN SDGs are vast, and only a small corner of the pedagogical space has been explored in the variations (Adams et al. 2003; Byrne et al. 2010; Huntzinger et al. 2007; Omenn 2006; Tillbury 2011). Entire courses could be offered, potentially where prototype revision and validation testing could be combined with stakeholder interviews, business model generation, impact statements, and grant writing. The deliverables could be expanded to include the design of social programs, policies, and marketing campaigns. Many high schools and middle schools are also including design and entrepreneurship in their curriculum or in socially oriented clubs in K-12 (Omenn 2006).

16.6 PEDAGOGICAL TECHNIQUES

This section is an overview of the pedagogical techniques and decisions employed that support design experiences based on the SDGs.

16.6.1 Immersive Experiences

A traditional course spreads an experience out over time by meeting periodically throughout a term. This is an effective format when the goal is for learners to become progressively better at the knowledge and skills associated with a particular domain, especially domains that are hierarchically organized. Breaks in the experience afford learners the opportunity to practice on their own and have "soak time" to process what they are learning.

A pedagogical decision was made for the SDG experiences to be as immersive as possible, even when embedded within a traditional course. For example, in both the Senior Capstone and Signals and Systems experiences, students were taking other courses, but no other work was assigned in these classes. Immersion helps minimize distractions. There are, however, at least two additional reasons why immersive experiences resonated with how humans have evolved to learn (Bransford et al. 2000).

First, immersive experiences facilitate learning complex processes by highlighting the inter-relationships between knowledge and skills across domains. We are spatiotemporal beings, meaning that we associate events and ideas that are experienced near one another in time and space. Immersive experiences naturally position different domains of knowledge, processes, and skills next to one another, with the benefit that they have the potential to form stable connections in one's mind. By encountering topics from different domains together, a learner does not silo the technical aspects of design from ethics, social and economic considerations, project management, and communicating with non-technical stakeholders. Rather, these topics are included in the design process. For example, the students in Chile quickly saw that a "perfect" technical solution that used expensive materials might, in fact, make the broader problem worse, not better. In other words, immersive experiences, following the analogy in the introduction, allow students to cross-train.

Second, immersive experiences are emotional. Emotions serve the evolutionary purpose of flagging important moments as worthy of remembering. This is known as the somatic marker hypothesis (Damasio 2008), and it applies to both positive and negative emotions. One cannot float through an immersive experience without there being highs and lows, often in a way that is more acute than in a traditional course—in an immersive experience, one must sit with emotions rather than compartmentalize them by going to the next class. This is the reason why most students, when asked (sometimes years later) to tell a significant story from their time in college, will choose an immersive trip, an intense project, or an emotionally charged event. Furthermore, learning that has taken place during emotional times, when coupled with reflection, has a better chance of being abstracted in a way that can be transferred to new situations.

16.6.2 Focus on Frameworks

A pedagogical dilemma arises when the instructor is not an expert, the process is non-linear, and the problem is super wicked—it can feel hopeless and unfair to students. The way forward is to use frameworks as guides (e.g., STEEPLED and MadLibs). The most effective frameworks will help:

- Communicate a shared vision, shape goals, and create action plans;
- Create a common language to use in conversation within and across groups;
- Seem obvious and is simple enough to keep in your mind all at once;
- Summarize a wide range of perspectives, stakeholders, constraints, and models;
- Expose gaps and helps diagnose problems;
- Provide a means of generating solutions, both top-down and bottom-up;
- Aid in determining which solutions have the greatest chance of succeeding;
- Aid in prioritizing how resources of all kinds are allocated;
- Predict how interventions and external events might interact in non-linear ways;
- Suggest measures that can assess progress.

Not every framework will serve all of these purposes, but the right framework at the right time can help students navigate ambiguity, encourage exploration, and guide their design process. When introducing the idea of a framework to students, it can be helpful to make an analogy to a children's playground—it is composed of structures that constrain what can be done, but allow for infinite possibilities for play. A framework is suggestive, not prescriptive.

16.6.3 The Adaptive Design Process (for Super Wicked Problems)

The design process is a framework that guides engineering designers. Dubberly (2004) cataloged over 100 unique design processes ranging from simple linear models (often used in introductory design courses), to feedback loops (similar to the FDA waterfall model), to spirals (similar to the Johns Hopkins BME Design Spiral), to helices, and even a 229-step process.

As expanded upon in Tranquillo (2019b), the processes that appear in textbooks and on corporate websites are rarely followed in practice. Rather, they are common pathways through an "action network." An action network is composed of the skills, resources, knowledge, and sub-processes that are required to navigate any process. What makes it an action network, however, is that parts of the network will be adaptively expressed to move a project forward. This is similar in spirit to how DNA is a collection of codes for possible proteins that perform functions:

- They are only expressed when needed. This is the reason for so many variations in the design processes.
- Master designers who work on different types of problems necessarily draw their abstracted design process differently.

To support the Sustainable Development Goal (SGD) design experience, no explicit design process is prescribed. Students are challenged to think of design as an inductive "action network" (Tranquillo 2019b)—one where the process emerges to suit the problem (Kim and Tranquillo 2014). This is in keeping with Szykman et al. (2005), who suggest that design pedagogy should move toward a more adaptive process that is grounded in collecting, synthesizing, and acting on relevant information.

This pedagogical approach is important for two reasons. First, wicked problems are by definition those that resist a formulaic approach. Trying to force solutions through a rigid process would send the wrong message to students. Second, introducing a more dynamic and adaptive design process returns agency to students as they make their own design decisions. Pedagogically, this is supported by a study by Crismond and Adams (2012), who described the developmental progression from a novice to an expert along nine design competencies. At any point in time, an individual may be a beginner at some competencies, developing at some, and advanced at others.

It is very rare for a student to be an expert in any of the competencies, as this usually requires experience with many projects of increasing complexity, typically in non-academic settings. An adaptive design process meets students where they are. If a student is a beginner at idea generation, engagement with the SDGs will allow them to practice. A student who is already well-versed in ideation, however, will still be challenged because the process of right-sizing will tune the scope of their project to be one that will encourage continued growth along this dimension.

16.6.4 Wearing Hats

The idea of a design action network is not explicitly shared with students. Rather, students are asked to wear six "hats" (the idea borrowed from DeBono's Six Thinking Hats). These hats are posted around the room as a reminder that members of the team are expected to selectively take on and off hats as appropriate. The six hats are described in the following.

1. The *designer* is concerned with delighting users by creating a high-value experience. They think about form (e.g., the user interface) and function (how a device works). A good designer will have internalized some version of Design Thinking—a broad term that includes technical engineering design, best exemplified by the Stanford d.school, MIT Media Lab, and design firms such as IDEO.
2. The *project manager* considers how to dynamically organize and allocate work, time, money, equipment, space, and other resources, as well as clearly communicate goals and tasks to the team and individuals.
3. The *maker* creates prototypes to think, prove, communicate, and gain information that will inform design decisions. A maker possesses the technical skills to create a prototype and a theoretical understanding that guides them in making choices before, during, and after building.
4. The *professional* expands (or contracts) their role to suit the needs of the team and project. They identify and communicate strengths and weaknesses in themselves and others, accept differences of opinions and goals, and aid in making timely decisions through strategic compromises and coordinated actions.
5. The *role model* searches for continuous growth in themselves and the team around them. They do not lead in the traditional sense but rather gain the respect of those around them through self-efficacy, a growth mindset, learning from failure, and intrinsic motivation.
6. The *value creator* identifies areas where value is lacking and then acts to fill the gaps. They apply this attitude to themselves, their team, the project, and the world around them.

A connection between these hats and the learning objectives is presented in Table 1 of Kim and Tranquillo (2014). For example, during the decomposition phase, the members of a team typically wear at least three hats—the designer considers the constraints and functions (and sub-functions) needed to achieve a solution concept; The project manager catalogs the resources that might be brought to the problem; the value creator considers the stakeholders and contexts that intersect the problem(s) and potential solutions. Each of these hats is needed to engage in a thorough decomposition of a larger problem into sub-problems. It is not usual for a student to wear more than one hat at a time. For example, all students are encouraged to wear the professional and role model hats nearly all of the time.

16.6.5 The Faculty Ulysses Contract

Every instructor has encountered the tension that occurs when a student asks a question. Answering the question is tempting in the moment and feels more efficient. Yet it can short-circuit deep learning in students who will not own the knowledge for themselves. Withholding the answer challenges the student to find the answer and is the basis for many forms of inductive learning, including PjBL and Flipped Classrooms. In reality, however, most PjBL and Flipped Classrooms are only flipped in terms of their delivery—the instructor is still the expert in the room. Students know that the instructor is intentionally not providing the answer, and if not handled carefully, this can lead to frustration with the instructor and an erosion of the learning environment.

No single person can be an expert in any of the SDGs, including the instructor. Tranquillo (2015) has called the assignment of such learning challenges a Faculty Ulysses Contract. In the Odyssey, Odysseus (Ulysses) wants to be the first human to hear the Sirens song and live to tell the story. He instructs his crew to tie him to the mast, plug their ears, and not listen to any of his pleading until they are clear of the islands. By taking action in the present, Ulysses limits his ability to make a bad choice in the future. The Ulysses Contract is often used in addiction programs—in a moment of clarity, the addict destroys their drink or drugs so that they cannot make a bad choice the next day.

For the instructor, engagement with the SDGs removes the temptation to be the sage-on-the-stage and quickly signals to students that they must find their own answers. There are certainly moments when the instructor plays the role of expert (such as suggesting a framework or resource), but for the majority of the experience, the instructor can only play the role of a guide.

16.7 PROGRAM ASSESSMENT

This section is an overview of the assessment of program effectiveness. Details of the protocols and more detailed results are discussed in the citations.

In Kim and Tranquillo (2014), two cohorts of the K-WIDE variation (42 students) were assessed in two ways. First, a pre/post-survey was administered to gauge students' perceptions of their own design abilities. Also included was a post-adjusted survey—asking students after the experience to give a more realistic (adjusted) score to their abilities before they began. This was to account for students over- (or under-) inflating their design abilities based on prior experience with a relatively simple linear design process. Many students ranked themselves highly in some competencies before the experience, only to mark their "past self" down significantly. Along some dimensions, students ranked themselves lower after the experience (post-survey) than their initial (pre-survey) but higher than their adjusted (post-adjusted score). In written comments, students explained this as due to becoming more conscious that engineering design encompasses much more than they originally imagined.

Second was a network analysis of pre- and post-experience drawings of the design processes. Pre-K-WIDE design process diagrams had many fewer actions, arranged linearly, with only a few feedback loops. Most were similar to diagrams in textbooks (Tranquillo, Goldberg, and Allen 2022) and the process followed in their introductory engineering course. Post-KWIDE diagrams, on the other hand, contained many more actions (Figures 16.5E and 16.5F), including economics, ethics, historical context, social and political impact, and reflection. All were tangled non-linear webs of activities—exactly what is needed to solve messy tangled problems, mirroring Conway's law (Conway 1967) and theories of organizational change (Senge 2006). Kim and Tranquillo (2014) quantified the changes in network structure through a variety of graph theory measures, including eigen-centrality, average node degree, and network diameter.

In Tranquillo (2018), assessment included a mixed methods analysis of 854 quotes from 95 student reflections from the Senior Capstone, K-WIDE, and Chile variations. Coding was based on the Sustainable Education Framework. During analysis, three additional codes were added in "Design Competence," "Mindset Growth," "Professional Development," and "Advice on Format."

With regard to Systems Thinking, 94 quotes supported growth, such as "think[ing] about designs through many people's points of view" as the key to "seeing the bigger picture in the project." Notably, 214 quotes supported growth in Values Thinking, for example, "how engineering could really make a difference in the world" by "us[ing] their engineering skills and knowledge to have a positive impact on the lives of others." A total of 105 quotes aligned with Strategic Thinking, such as "I found I could be resourceful, even when I didn't have many resources," "planning ahead is critical," and "the quest for the perfect can sometimes [be] the enemy of forward progress." Only 34 quotes were coded as Future Thinking, yet comments included, I "[would] look for ways in the future to keep addressing big problems like the UN Sustainable Development Goals" even though "the payoff might not be in [my] lifetime." A total of 153 quotes were coded for Design Competence, including students finding "a passion for engineering design," "surprise" by how much "a group of aspiring engineers could come up with" in a short time, and "moving through so many different design and prototypes [. . . we] can't even remember all the twists and turns."

Notably, 117 quotes were about perceived growth in attitude, behaviors, and mindsets. These included the need to "adapt and try new things," "being stretched," and that it felt easier to "learn something new, like a skill . . . from a peer [rather] than from a computer." Only 58 quotes were coded as pertaining to Professional Development. A representative quote is "I became much better at being a leader at some times and the follower at others." With regard to format, students scored the following highly: choosing their own problem, building a prototype, the final pitch at the expo, the length of time, real-world and complex nature of the challenge, regular assignments, and team size. Students were less receptive to the mini-lectures on design, development of specifications, and brainstorming.

In Boulanger and Tranquillo (2015), a linguistic analysis was conducted of 209 reflections during the experience from 45 students for the K-WIDE variation at Bucknell and Ohio Northern University. The sematic text mining package Leximancer (info.leximancer.com) was used to construct network maps of connected concepts.

This analysis is far more robust than "word clouds" created through online sources because concepts and themes, as well as connections, emerge as more reflections are added to create interactive visualizations. The entire body of two engineering design and two entrepreneurship texts was also analyzed to form "expert" networks, to which the student network maps were compared. Results demonstrated that students were very tightly linking "problem" and "solution," as well as deeply considering constraints in engineering design, such as "cost," "planning," and "value."

16.8 CONCLUSION

Education will always be a significant part of the solution to any complex problem. Training the future citizen-leaders of the world, especially those who will be creating next-generation technologies, is critical. Furthermore, both sustainability and education are inherently about hope for the future. For these reasons, the UN SDGs present the ultimate learning experience. They are as open-ended and complex as any problem a student will encounter in their career. They naturally exercise interdisciplinary thinking, innovation across disciplines, and an introduction to the large-scale problems the future generations will face. They encourage students to cross-train in systems thinking, values thinking, strategic thinking, and future thinking by wearing many hats while navigating a non-linear and adaptive design process. They generate personal stories of learning from failure, overcoming impossible challenges, confidence, and growth, in a way that matters to future employers. Faculty have no choice but to be a guide-on-the-side, placing the emphasis on learning rather than looking for the "right" answer or solution. The author has found these experiences to be the most satisfying pedagogical moments of his career. Finally, biomedical engineering students are particularly well-positioned to take on the challenges presented by the UN SDGs.

It is hoped that sharing the UN Sustainable Development Design Challenge will inspire other instructors to find ways to include sustainability in their own pedagogical environments.

ACKNOWLEDGMENTS

The author would like to acknowledge several collaborators who either helped offer versions of the design challenges described or aided in data analysis. They include James Baish, Katie Bieryla, Fernando Blanco, Dan Cavanagh, Trace Coats, Donna Ebenstein, Cory Hixson, Eric Kennedy, Charles Kim, Brian Boulanger, Ned Ladd, and Ann Marie Mullen.

REFERENCES

ABET. 2024. *ABET Engineering Accreditation Commission: Criteria for Accrediting Engineering Programs. Effective for Reviews During the 2025–2026 Accreditation Cycle. Incorporates All Changes Approved by the ABET Board of Delegates Engineering Area Delegation as of October 25, 2024.* https://www.abet.org/accreditation/accreditation-criteria/criteria-for-accrediting-engineering-programs-2025-2026/#1.

Adams, Robin S., Jennifer Turns, and Cynthia J. Atman. 2003. "Educating Effective Engineering Designers: The Role of Reflective Practice." *Design Studies* 24 (3): 275–94.

APL nextED. 2024. *Unlocking the Power of Accreditation: A Pathway to Academic Excellence.* https://aplnexted.com/accreditation-power/.

Azlina, Wan Asma K., Mohd S. Amran, Abdul B. Radiah, and A. Salmiaton. 2013. "Sustainable Development in Chemical and Biological Engineering Education." *Procedia—Social and Behavioral Sciences* 102: 490–8.

Bäckstrand, Karin. 2003. "Civic Science for Sustainability: Reframing the Role of Experts, Policy-Makers and Citizens in Environmental Governance." *Global Environmental Politics* 3 (4): 24–41.

Beaury, R., P. Boyer, and E. L. Kisenwether. 2010. "Using Live Cases in Problem-based Entrepreneurship Learning." In *VentureWell. Proceedings of Open, the Annual Conference.* National Collegiate Inventors & Innovators Alliance.

Bell, S. 2010. "Project-based Learning for the 21st Century: Skills for the Future." *The Clearing House* 83 (2): 39–43.

Blumenfeld, Phyllis C., Elliot Soloway, Ronald W. Marx, Joseph S. Krajcik, Mark Guzdial, and Annemarie Palincsar. 1991. "Motivating Project-Based Learning: Sustaining the Doing, Supporting the Learning." *Educational Psychologist* 26 (3–4): 369–98.

Bodnar, Cheryl A., Diane Anastasio, Julia A. Enszer, and David D. Burkey. 2016. "Engineers at Play: Games as Teaching Tools for Undergraduate Engineering Students." *Journal of Engineering Education* 105 (1): 147–200.

Bransford, John D., Ann L. Brown, and Rodney R. Cocking, eds. 2000. *How People Learn: Brain, Mind, Experience, and School.* Washington, DC: National Academy Press.

Brundtland, Gro Harlem, and Mansour Khalid. 1987. *Our Common Future: Report of the World Commission on Environment and Development.* New York: United Nations. http://www.un-documents.net/wced-ocf.htm.

Bybee, Rodger W. 2002. *Learning Science and the Science of Learning: Science Educators' Essay Collection.* Arlington, VA: National Science Teachers Association Press.

Byrne, Edmond P., Cheryl J. Desha, John J. Fitzpatrick, and Karlson Hargroves. 2010. "Engineering Education for Sustainable Development: A Review of International Progress." In *Proceedings of the 3rd International Symposium for Engineering Education ISEE2010: Educating Engineers for a Changing World: Leading Transformation from an Unsustainable Global Society.* Cork: International Symposium for Engineering Education. https://hdl.handle.net/10468/372.

Caine, Renate N., ed. 2009. *12 Brain/Mind Learning Principles in Action: Developing Executive Functions of the Human Brain.* Thousand Oaks, CA: Corwin Press.

Canziani, Bonnie F., Sevil Sönmez, Jinyoung Hsieh, and Eric T. Byrd. 2012. "A Learning Theory Framework for Sustainability Education in Tourism." *Journal of Teaching in Travel and Tourism* 12 (1): 3–20.

Casti, John, and Anders Karlqvist, eds. 1986. *Complexity, Language, and Life: Mathematical Approaches.* Berlin: Springer.

Condoor, Sridhar, and Greg Keogh. 2012. *Innovation Challenge: Mind Workouts for Teams.* iTunes, Apple Inc.

Conway, Melvin. 1967. *Conway's Law.* http://www.melconway.com/Home/Conways_Law.html.

Corburn, Jason. 2007. "Community Knowledge in Environmental Health Science: Co-Producing Policy Expertise." *Environmental Science & Policy* 10 (2): 150–61.

Costanza, R. 2012. "Needed: The Solutions Generation." *Solutions: For a Sustainable & Desirable Future* 3 (1): 29–30.

Crismond, David P., and Robin S. Adams. 2012. "The Informed Design Teaching and Learning Matrix." *Journal of Engineering Education* 101 (4): 738–97.

Damasio, Antonio R. 2008. *Descartes' Error: Emotion, Reason and the Human Brain.* New York: Random House.

Dolan, C. W. 2013. "The Engineering Design Challenge: A Creative Process." *Morgan and Claypool Synthesis Lectures on Engineering* 8 (1): 1–151.

Dubberly, H. 2004. *How Do You Design? A Compendium of Models.* Dubberly Design Office. https://www.dubberly.com/wp-content/uploads/2008/06/ddo_designprocess.pdf

Enderle, John D. 1999. "An Overview of the National Science Foundation Program on Senior Design Projects to Aid Persons with Disabilities." *International Journal of Engineering Education* 15 (4): 288–97.

Fischer, Frank. 1993. "Citizen Participation and the Democratization of Policy Expertise: From Theoretical Inquiry to Practical Cases." *Policy Sciences* 26 (3): 165–87.

Gagné, Marylène, and Edward L. Deci. 2005. "Self-Determination Theory and Work Motivation." *Journal of Organizational Behavior* 26 (4): 331–62.

Gerhart, Adam L., and David E. Melton. 2016. "Entrepreneurially Minded Learning: Incorporating Stakeholders, Discovery, Opportunity Identification, and Value Creation into Problem-Based Learning Modules with Examples and Assessment Specific to Fluid Mechanics." In *Proceedings of ASEE the 2016 ASEE Annual Conference & Exposition.* https://peer.asee.org/26724.

Gibson, H., and S. Venkateswar. 2015. "Anthropological Engagement with the Anthropocene: A Critical Review." *Environment and Society* 6 (1): 5–27.

Gibson, Robert B. 2006. "Sustainability Assessment: Basic Components of a Practical Approach." *Impact Assessment and Project Appraisal* 24 (3): 170–82.

Gibson, Robert B., Selim Hassan, and James Tansey. 2013. *Sustainability Assessment: Criteria and Processes.* London: Routledge.

Gimm, A., R. Goldberg, K. Caves, and R. Malkin. 2011. "Use of Simple Hands-On Design Challenges for Practicing Engineering Design Principles." In *Proceedings of the 2011 ASEE Annual Conference & Exposition*, Vancouver, BC. https://doi.org/10.18260/1-2--18359

Grunwald, Armin. 2004. "Strategic Knowledge for Sustainable Development: The Need for Reflexivity and Learning at the Interface Between Science and Society." *International Journal of Foresight and Innovation Policy* 1: 150–67.

Holifield, Ryan, Michael Porter, and Gordon Walker, eds. 2010. *Spaces of Environmental Justice.* Malden, MA: Wiley-Blackwell.

Huntzinger, Deborah N., Margot J. Hutchins, Jonathan S. Gierke, and John W. Sutherland. 2007. "Enabling Sustainable Thinking in Undergraduate Engineering Education." *International Journal of Engineering Education* 23 (2): 218–30.

Kelly, A. M., D. Jones, R. M. Hoy, E. Curtis, A. K. Pannier, and R. R. Stowell. 2013. "Implementation of a "Rapid Design Challenge" in a Cross-Disciplinary Senior Capstone Course and Evaluation of Device Performance." In *Proceedings* of the *2013 ASEE Annual Conference & Exposition*, Atlanta, Georgia. https://doi.org/10.18260/1-2--19709

Kim, Christine, and Joe Tranquillo. 2014. "K-WIDE: Synthesizing the Entrepreneurial Mindset and Engineering Design." In *Proceedings of ASEE of the 2014 ASEE Annual Conference & Exposition*, Indianapolis, Indiana. https://doi.org/10.18260/1-2--20728

Kuh, George D. 2008. *High-Impact Educational Practices: What They Are, Who Has Access to Them, and Why They Matter.* Washington, DC: Association of American Colleges and Universities.

Kuhlmann, Stefan. 2001. "Future Governance of Innovation Policy in Europe—Three Scenarios." *Research Policy* 30 (6): 953–76.

Lawrence, Elizabeth. 1999. *Strategic Thinking: A Discussion Paper.* Personnel Development and Resourcing Group, Public Service Commission of Canada. http://www.hrbartender.com/images/thinking.pdf.

Levin, Kelly, Benjamin Cashore, Steven Berstein, and Graeme Auld. 2012. "Overcoming the Tragedy of Super Wicked Problems: Constraining Our Future Selves to Ameliorate Global Climate Change." *Policy Sciences* 45: 123–52.

Loorbach, Derk A. 2007. *Transition Management: New Mode of Governance for Sustainable Development.* Utrecht: International Books.

Meadows, D. 2008. *Thinking in Systems: A Primer.* White River Junction, VT: Chelsea Green Publishing Company.

Mote, C. D., A. Dowling, and J. Zhou. 2016. "The Power of an Idea: The International Impacts of the Grand Challenges for Engineering." *Engineering* 2 (1): 4–7.

Murphy, C. F., D. Allen, B. Allenby, J. Crittenden, C. I. Davidson, C. Hendrickson, and H. S. Matthews. 2009. "Sustainability in Engineering Education and Research at U.S. Universities." *Environmental Science & Technology* 43 (15): 5558–64.

National Research Council. 2000. *How People Learn: Brain, Mind, Experience, and School: Expanded Edition.* Washington, DC: National Academies Press. https://doi.org/10.17226/9853

Newman, P., and I. Jennings. 2008. *Cities as Sustainable Ecosystems: Principles and Practices.* Washington, DC: Island Press.

Omenn, G. S. 2006. "Grand Challenges and Great Opportunities in Science, Technology, and Public Policy." *Science* 314: 1696–1704. https://doi.org/10.1126/science.1135003

Ostrom, E. 1990. *Governing the Commons: The Evolution of Institutions for Collective Action.* Cambridge, MA: Cambridge University Press.

Prince, M. 2004. "Does Active Learning Work? A Review of the Research." *Journal of Engineering Education* 93 (3): 223–31.

Prince, M., and R. Felder. 2007. "The Many Faces of Inductive Teaching and Learning." *Journal of College Science Teaching* 36 (5): 14.

Rawls, John. 1985. "Justice as Fairness: Political Not Metaphysical." *Philosophy & Public Affairs* 14 (3): 223–51.

Rittel, Horst W. J., and Melvin M. Webber. 1973. "Dilemmas in a General Theory of Planning." *Policy Sciences* 4 (2): 155–69.

Robinson, John, Sarah Burch, Simin Talwar, Meg O'Shea, and Mark Walsh. 2011. "Envisioning Sustainability: Recent Progress in the Use of Participatory Backcasting Approaches for Sustainability Research." *Technological Forecasting and Social Change* 78: 756–68.

Rockström, Johan, Will Steffen, Kevin Noone, Åsa Persson, F. Stuart Chapin III, Eric Lambin, Timothy M. Lenton, et al. 2009. "Planetary Boundaries: Exploring the Safe Operating Space for Humanity." *Ecology and Society* 14, no. 2: 32. https://doi.org/10.5751/ES-03180-140232

Sarasvathy, Saras D. 2001. "Causation and Effectuation: Toward a Theoretical Shift from Economic Inevitability to Entrepreneurial Contingency." *Academy of Management Review* 26 (2): 243–63.

Selin, Cynthia. 2007. "Scenarios for Success: Turning Insights into Action." In *Scenarios for Success: Insights from International Case Studies*, edited by Kees van der Heijden and George Wright, 27–52. Cheltenham: Edward Elgar.

Senge, Peter. 2006. *The Fifth Discipline: The Art and Practice of the Learning Organization.* New York: Broadway Business.

Sipos, Yona, Brian Battisti, and Kurt Grimm. 2008. "Achieving Transformative Sustainability Learning: Engaging Head, Hands and Heart." *International Journal of Sustainability in Higher Education* 9 (1): 68–86.

Stibbe, Arran, and Horacio Luna. 2009. *The Handbook of Sustainability Literacy: Skills for a Changing World.* Cornwall: Green Books.

Szykman, S., S. J. Fenves, W. Keirouz, and S. B. Shooter. 2005. "A Foundation for Interoperability in Next-generation Product Development Systems." *The Most Influential CIE Papers*: 1980–2000, ASME.

Tillbury, Daniella. 2011. *Education for Sustainable Development.* Paris: UNESCO. http://unesdoc.unesco.org/images/0019/001914/191442e.pdf.

Tranquillo, Joe. 2008. "Kinesthetic Learning in the Classroom." In *Proceedings of ASEE, Annual Conference & Exposition*, Pittsburgh, Pennsylvania. https://doi.org/10.18260/1-2--3389.

Tranquillo, Joe, and D. Cavanagh. 2007. *A Project Driven Approach To Biomedical Signals And Systems.* In: *Proceedings of 2007 ASEE Annual Conference & Exposition*, Honolulu, Hawaii. https://doi.org/10.18260/1-2--2136

Tranquillo, Joe, and D. Cavanagh. 2009. "Preparing Students for Senior Design with a Rapid Design Challenge." In *Proceedings of the 2009 ASEE Annual Conference & Exposition*, Austin, Texas. https://doi.org/10.18260/1-2--5619

Tranquillo, Joe. 2012. *How to Run a Design Bootcamp.* Stanford Epicenter Archive. http://epicenter.stanford.edu/resource/design-bootcamp-joe-tranquillo-bucknell-university.html.

Tranquillo, Joe. 2014. "Moving Analogies." In *Proceedings of NCIIA OPEN, the National Collegiate Inventors & Innovators Alliance (NCIIA) 18th Annual Conference*, San Jose. https://www.proquest.com/openview/485e88e3115d24b8ebc9b9054bad6199/1?pq-origsite=gscholar&cbl=38283

Tranquillo, Joe. 2015. "The Faculty Ulysses Contract." In *Proceedings of ASEE Annual Conference & Exposition*, Seattle, Washington. https://doi.org/10.18260/p.24870

Tranquillo, Joe. 2016. "Mirror Mirror: Reflection and the Building of Mindsets." In *Proceedings of ASEE Annual Conference & Exposition*, New Orleans, Louisiana. https://doi.org/10.18260/p.25724

Tranquillo, Joe. 2017a. "The T-Shaped Engineer." *Journal of Engineering Education Transformations* 30 (4): 12–24.

Tranquillo, Joe. 2017b. "The Benefits to Integrating Entrepreneurship and Sustainability Programs in Higher Ed." *LinkedIn*, September 7. https://www.linkedin.com/pulse/benefits-integrating-entrepreneurship-sustainability-keller-jackson.

Tranquillo, Joe. 2018. "Signals and Systems Without Control." *ASEE Prism* 28 (1): 40–3. https://www.jstor.org/stable/26820092

Tranquillo, Joe. 2019a. *Reflection Collection*™. http://joetranquillo.com/reflectioncollection.

Tranquillo, Joe. 2019b. *An Introduction to Complex Systems: Making Sense of a Changing World.* Cham: Springer Nature.

Tranquillo, Joe. n.d. *BME Program Survey.* Unpublished manuscript.

Tranquillo, Joe, Jay Goldberg, and Robyn Allen. 2022. *Biomedical Engineering Design.* Amsterdam: Elsevier Academic Press.

UNESCO. 2010. *Engineering: Issues, Challenges and Opportunities for Development.* http://unesdoc.unesco.org/images/0018/001897/189753e.pdf.

United Nations Educational, Scientific, and Cultural Organization (UNESCO). 2004. *United Nations Decade of Education for Sustainable Development: Draft International Implementation Scheme.* http://portal.unesco.org/education/en/ev.php-URL_ID=36025&URL_DO=DO_TOPIC&URL_SECTION=201.html.

U.S. Bureau of Labor Statistics. 2024. *Occupational Outlook Handbook: Bioengineers and Biomedical Engineers.* https://www.bls.gov/ooh/architecture-and-engineering/biomedical-engineers.htm.

Veugelers, Wiel. 2000. "Different Ways of Teaching Values." *Educational Review* 52 (1): 37–46.

Warren, Aaron, Leanna Archambault, and Reid W. Foley. 2014. "Sustainability Education Framework for Teachers: Developing Sustainability Literacy Through Futures, Values, Systems, and Strategic Thinking." *Journal of Sustainability Education* 6 (special issue): 1–14.

Wheadon, Jason D., and Nathalie Duval-Couetil. 2015. "Using an Intention-Uncertainty Matrix to Categorize Entrepreneurship Education Offerings." In *Proceedings of ASEE Annual Conference & Exposition*, Seattle, Washington. https://doi.org/10.18260/p.24994

Wheeler, George. 2014. "Core and Essential to Education for Sustainability." *Journal of Sustainability Education* 6: 1–4.

Wiek, Arnim, Lauren Withycombe, and Charles L. Redman. 2011. "Key Competencies in Sustainability: A Reference Framework for Academic Program Development." *Sustainability Science* 6 (2): 203–18.

Zappe, Sarah, Kathryn Hochstedt, Elizabeth Kisenwether, and Amy Shartrand. 2013. "Teaching to Innovate: Beliefs and Perceptions of Instructors Who Teach Entrepreneurship to Engineering Students." *International Journal of Engineering Education* 29 (1): 45–62.

Appendix A: Systems Canvas (Understanding the Problem)

Network Map What other problems are related? Are there any hubs or densely connected sub-problems?	**Critical Stakeholders** Who are the stakeholders? Who has power and influence? Who is impacted most? Least?	**Feedback Loops** What negative feedback loops may be used to control or limit the problem? What positive feedback loops might accelerate change?
Immunities to Change What aspects of the current ways (status quo) will fight against change? What are they hoping to preserve? What are the path dependencies?	**Value Proposition** What is the system disease? What changes when advances are made toward a solution? Who feels this change? Where? In what ways?	**Levers** What small changes might initiate change? Are their network hubs that can be captured? Are there bottlenecks? Non-linearities?
Information Flow Are there policies/procedures that could be added or changed? Are there communication/distribution/PR channels that could be used?	**Partners** Who is already working in this space who might become a partner? Who doesn't care now but might be convinced to become a partner?	**Bright Spots** Are there some ideas that already show promise and could be amplified as levers? Who is working on them? What difference have they made?

Appendix B: Mad Lib for Sustainable Development Challenge

The Hook

Did you know that ____
(Catchy Stat, Story or Bit of Information)

In this ____________________, we will focus on____________________________
(class or experience) (Name of UN Goal)

Goal #___ of the 17 UN Sustainable Development Goals. As a group we will follow the

work of ________________, an organization working on ___________________
(Organization) (mission of organization)

This aligns with the sub-goal of ___________________________ in ______________.
(sub goal or metric to improve) (country or region)

This is critical because ____
(Value Proposition Here)

Details

Over the course of ________________, we will work _____________________________
(Time Period) (Individual/Team/Collaboration)

to create__________________, by ____
(Target/ Final Deliverable) (Techniques/ Resources)

Along the way we will complete __________________and _____________________
(Task 1) (Task 2)

Learning

By working on this project, we will be able to:

____

____

____

Assessment

And demonstrate growth in the follow:

____(Rubric item 1)

____(Rubric Item 2)

____(Rubric Item 3)

Appendix C: Pre-Assignment for Chilean Ruka Project

To be completed in country (Chile)

Spend 10–15 minutes on your own (quietly) exploring the 17 UN SDGs at: https://sustainabledevelopment.un.org/sdgs

On a sheet of paper, write down your name and the top three topics you would like to explore while in Chile (not counting Goal 17). You are not committing yourself to any one topic at this point. This is the first step to identifying potential problems to solve.

Once we are in Chile, we will assign you to two of your three choices. As we explore Chile during the first week of our trip, you will create two photo essays (of your own photos) that show challenges and opportunities that exist with regard to your two assigned UN goals. You are expected to find stats, cite sources, and use text to supplement your photos.

Your photo essay should capture the following dimensions of your problem:
Who are the stakeholders (broadly) (*)
Economics (micro and macro)
Socio-political impacts
Geographic/climate considerations
Cultural/historical perspectives
Ethical concerns
Technical solutions, either existing or possible (*)

You must do the ones that are * and then pick at least two others (or come up with one on your own).

Appendix D: BMEG 350 Assignments and Assessment

DESIGN CHALLENGE ASSIGNMENT #1: POTENTIAL PROBLEMS

Due August 28, 2020, by 8:30 am

Turn the filled template to your group folder

The first step in any design process is to narrow the problem to one that can be solved with the time and resources available. The UN SDGs are so high-level that progress will only be made by working on sub-problems. In this first assignment, you will narrow the scope of your design project. The following steps may look daunting but should be achievable in two to three hours (likely separated into several short sessions spaced out in time).

Step 1: Download the template Google Doc to document the following steps.
Step 2: Visit sdgs.un.org/goals, and each individual should come up with two or three goals that resonate with you.
Step 3: Discuss which three goals might be suitable for your project. Keep in mind that your project must intersect (directly or indirectly) healthcare in some way. At this phase, the problem is very high level, and so you cannot yet know what your solution will be. However, be mindful that you will need to build a technical solution.
Step 4: Split up and research your possible topics. A helpful place to start is to click on the goal, which will bring you to a page with a description. You will find various videos, infographics, and other helpful information here. Scrolling down, you will see a menu (with the options "Overview," "Targets and Indicators," and "Progress and Info"). In particular, the Targets and Indicators further break down goals into sub-problems that have more concrete deadlines and measures of success.
Step 5: Discuss the positives and negatives of having your remaining goals become the basis for your project.
Step 6: Discuss how you might focus on a particular sub-problem and try to narrow to two to four possibilities.
Step 7: Perform more research (as individuals) of possible sub-problems, again using the lenses of healthcare and technology, but now also add in if you think this is a sub-problem you can make progress on.
Step 8: Repeat the steps above until you feel you have narrowed down to a problem you would like to have become the focus of your project.

Please have a copy of this assignment handy for the next class period

UN Sustainable Development Problem Narrowing Template

After copying this document, remember to rename it and place it in the group folder

Names:

Step 2:

Each list three goals that resonate with you

Step 3:

Note from team discussion of your top three goals

Step 4:

Research findings from the top three goals

Goal 1 Notes

Goal 2 Notes

Goal 3 Notes

Step 5:

Goal #	Pros	Cons

Step 6:

General notes on possible sub-problems

Narrowed Sub-Problem 1

Narrowed Sub-Problem 2

Narrowed Sub-Problem 3

Narrowed Sub-Problem 4

Step 7:

Research on Sub-Problems

Research for Sub-Problem 1

Research for Sub-Problem 2

Research for Sub-Problem 3

Research for Sub-Problem 4

Step 8:

Short description of the narrowed problem

DESIGN CHALLENGE ASSIGNMENT #2: GENERATING A PROJECT STATEMENT

Due September 2, 2020, by 8:30 am in your group folder

Based upon your narrowed problem, you will generate a project statement that contains the following information and flow:

A project statement generally begins with a statement of the ***medical need*** as it is experienced by users. Often, the specific population impacted, incidence rate, and severity are included to demonstrate both urgency and clarify the scope of the problem. For this project, you should also declare a country (or region of the world) where your work will have the most impact. The aim of discussing the medical need is to convince a reader that your project will focus on an important healthcare problem.

The ***current solutions*** are the means by which users are currently satisfying their needs. When the need is known, a variety of solutions may be available that include procedures, guidelines, technologies, or policies. Often, there is a "gold standard" solution. On the other hand, if the need has gone unrecognized, there may be no solutions or only ad hoc "work-arounds." The aim of writing about current solutions is to convince a reader that there is an opportunity to add value to the healthcare ecosystem.

The ***technical barriers*** in meeting the need typically derive from biological, clinical, regulatory, ethical, financial, technological, or other constraints. These technical barriers will later be translated into technical specifications. Within a project statement, only the highest-level barriers or constraints will be discussed with the aim of convincing a reader that the need can be solved through a technological solution.

Measurable goals are metrics that, if met, will indicate that value has been added to the healthcare ecosystem. Declaring measurable goals will capture what will change when the problem is solved.

A ***project objective*** is a clear definition of the scope of your project. It is typically one sentence that declares your intended endpoint along with critical project constraints such as timeline or budget. For example, you may make it clear that your endpoint will be a functional prototype that has undergone benchtop testing, and the project will be completed in three weeks. The goal is to define what will count as success for your project, noting that your project objective may be a step toward the real-world measurable goal.

The following guidelines will help you craft your statement:

The statement must be one self-contained in one (or at most two) paragraphs.
No graphics (figures or tables) are allowed.
Any statistics/numbers you have to support your claims are encouraged.
The writing style should be understood by an educated lay audience.
No particular design solution should be stated or implied.
You must focus on a particular developing country, but you may also point to other countries or areas that have a similar problem.

Please have a copy of this assignment handy for the next class period

DESIGN CHALLENGE ASSIGNMENT #3: FUNCTIONS AND SPECIFICATIONS

Due September 4, 2020, by 10 am in your group folder

The *design input* is defined as the functions and specifications that, if met, will meet the needs of the user/customer. Record your work in the template provided.

Step 1: Using assignments 1 and 2 as inputs, identify at least five attributes of a device that would solve the problem. You are encouraged to frame these attributes as functions.

Step 2: Develop at least eight project specifications that should be met and can be measured.

Please have a copy of this assignment handy for the next class period

FUNCTIONS AND SPECIFICATIONS

After copying this document, remember to rename it and place it in the group folder.

Names:

Step 1:

What are the five attributes (functions) of a device that would solve the problem?

Step 2:

Specification	How might you create a test to measure whether or not the spec has been met

DESIGN CHALLENGE ASSIGNMENT #4: POSSIBLE SOLUTIONS

Due September 7, 2020, by 10 am

Generating potential solutions is one of the most creative (and challenging) parts of the design process. The following are some steps to follow along with the deliverables you will share in the template provided.

Step 1: Engaged in a C-Sketch session. You may need to do this virtually and share your diagrams using photos that you share online. You may wish to engage in multiple sessions at different times to generate several ideas. The more ideas (and the wilder the better). Take a picture of each of your annotated ideas and upload them to your Google folder.
Step 2: Have a discussion about the pros and cons of each idea with the aim of narrowing to approximately three general ideas.
Step 3: Use functional decomposition (or another method of your choosing) to develop variations and refine your ideas.
Step 4: Create a sketch of three ideas for a solution that will address the problem stated in your project statement and meet the design inputs.

You will be asked to share your alternative solutions at a meeting on August 31.

Please have a copy of this assignment handy for the next class period

Possible Solutions

After copying this document, remember to rename it and place it in the group folder.

Names:

Step 1:

Place snapshots of your sketches below.

Steps 2 and 3:

Take notes on your discussions of these three steps, including images as needed to document your process.

Step 4:

Share three sketches below (with descriptive captions).

DESIGN CHALLENGE ASSIGNMENT #5: UPDATE MEMO AND MEETING

Due September 10, 2020, at 9 am

Meetings starting at 12:50 pm in the lab

Please place a copy of your memo in your group folder

Write a memo (two pages or less) outlining the following items:

A solution chosen from the list of possible solutions along with justification. Your solution should include a sketch of your intended design. Justification should be tied directly to how your device will solve the problem as stated in your project statement by meeting all of the specifications.

Timeline for building and testing the chosen solution by the design challenge contest.

A list of materials (for building and testing your device) with associated costs. This includes any requested additional funds, with justification.

Tests you may conduct to demonstrate the functionality of your device.

Conduct a meeting with the instructor during the lab. The meeting should be no longer than 15 minutes and address the points in the memo. The team should drive the meeting forward using questions that are prepared ahead of time.

DESIGN CHALLENGE ASSIGNMENT #6: FINAL MATERIALS

Due September 17, 2020, by midnight

Upload files to your group folder

Create a two-minute video (mp4 format please) that explains:

The problem you are trying to solve and why it is important;

The potential value that could be gained;

Show your prototype working;

The results of any testing that you completed to demonstrate that your device will work;

Any other key technical features or selling points.

Imagine that you are making these for someone who is interested in funding your idea.

Create a poster using the poster template. You may adjust sizes and add or modify as needed, but please do not cut the second page, as this is where our judges will make their comments.

You are encouraged to balance creativity and professionalism in your presentation.

FINAL POSTER TEMPLATE

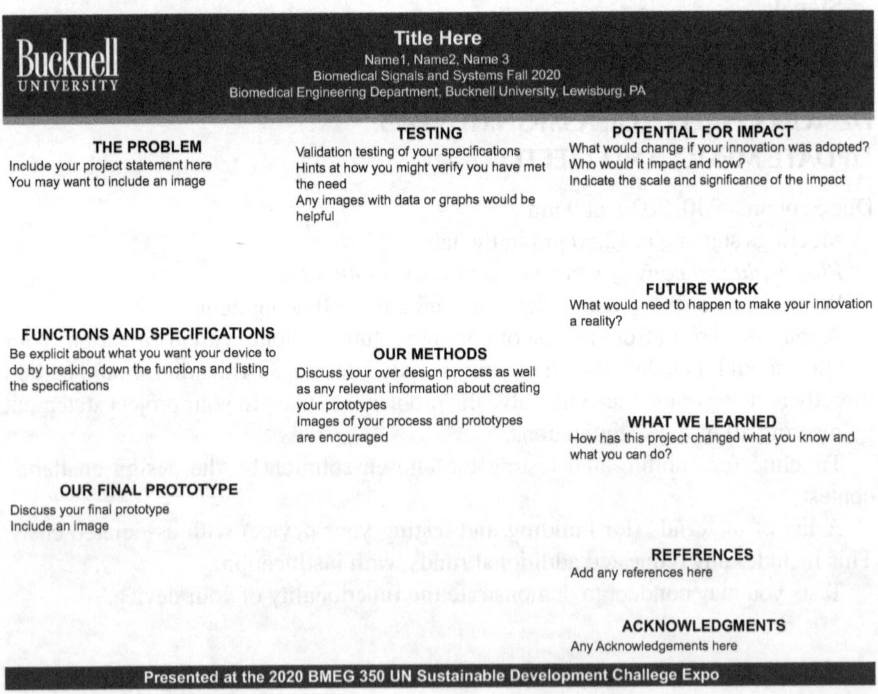

Faculty Scoring Worksheet

Comments from Judges	
Value Proposition Comments:	**Innovation** Comments:
Functionality and Usability Comments:	**Design and Fabrication** Comments:
Presented at the 2020 BMEG 350 UN Sustainable Development Challenge Expo	

BMEG 350 Final Presentation Directions and Links

Friday, September 18, from 8:50 to 9:42

Zoom Link

We will use this Google Doc to coordinate the flow of this class period.

Flow of the Session

The goal of this class period is to mimic a live expo, which is composed of (formal) presentations followed by (less formal) Q&A. The following is a general flow of the session.

We will all log in to the zoom link above before 8:50 am.
There will be a short introduction at 8:50 am.
We will play all of the videos in the order listed below (~16 minutes).
We will break out into separate breakout rooms (one room per team).
Faculty will rotate in and out of rooms to ask questions (~30 minutes).
There will be a short conclusion.

For Students

Step 1: Please review the assignment requirements and have everything turned in to your team folder no later than midnight the day before the presentations.

Step 2: Please change the permissions of your poster (make it editable) and video (make it viewable) by the following:
FACULTY NAMES AND EMAILS REDACTED

Step 3: Please add your project title and link your poster/video in the following table. I will download your videos from this link to play on my laptop during the session. Faculty will be using these links to find your posters when they go into breakout sessions.

No.	Title	Names	Poster Link	Video Link
1	Safe Drinking Water: pH Detector for Home Use	Student Names	Poster	Video
2	Turbidity Testing and Improvement of Hand Washing Techniques in Chad	Student Names	Poster	Video
3	Sterilization of Surgical Tools in Myanmar	Student Names	Poster	Video
4	Auto-Angle Rehabilitation Device	Student Names	Poster	Video
5	Food For You: Connecting Women Through Agriculture	Student Names	Poster	Video
6	Filter for Clean Water at Remote Healthcare Facilities in Tanzania	Student Names	Poster	Video
7	Testing Nutritional Content in Breast Milk to Prevent and Treat Malnutrition in Infants in South Sudan	Student Names	Poster	Video
8	Remote Diagnosis Device for ADHD Children	Student Names	Poster	Video

Step 4: Agree where your team will be (virtual? In the lab? Outside? Some hybrid?) for the breakout sessions. You will need to have at least one laptop and an internet connection.

Step 5: Log in at least five minutes early to the Zoom link above and rename yourself to begin your name with the corresponding number (e.g., "8 Joe Tranquillo"). This will allow me to quickly put you all into breakout rooms.

Step 6: After the videos are played, you will host any faculty who enter into your breakout room. You should be ready to post the link to your poster in the chat window. Please direct the faculty to your poster, which you can use to further explain your project.

For Faculty

Step 1: Join us some time before 8:50 at this **Zoom Link**.

Step 2: View the videos from each of the eight teams (they will be played through the Zoom link) and enter any comments you have into the second slide in the poster. You may also want to generate some questions for the teams.

Step 3: Enter into your first assigned breakout session and ask any questions you might have.

Step 4: Come back to the main room (anytime you want) and let me know what room you would like to move to next. You may wish to also enter more comments for the teams.

Step 5: Continue visiting the rooms to ask questions.

Step 6: During (or after) the session, please enter some comments into the posters. This is not a competition. Rather, you will be asked to give evaluative feedback on four areas:

Value Proposition: How well is the device matched to the end goal as stated by the team? Would scaling and distribution of a refined device have the intended impact?

Functionality and Usability: Does the device do what it is supposed to? Are the tests well-designed and executed? Are the results convincing such that the functionality of the device is sound? Is the device designed with the user in mind?

Design and Fabrication: Is the quality of the design and construction such that the team has made good use of their technical skills? Have they followed a design process?

Innovation: Is the device unique? Does it have a chance in a global marketplace?

DESIGN CHALLENGE ASSIGNMENT #7: MEDITATION

Due September 18, 2020, by 5 pm

This is an INDIVIDUAL ASSIGNMENT

Uploaded to your Meditation Folder

The design process is THE defining characteristic (an unifying concept) of the engineering profession and one of the primary modes of systems thinking. You have just spent several weeks immersed in this process. It is therefore time to reflect on what you have taken away from your experience that you can abstract and apply to the next time you encounter a design process.

You must summarize your reflection in a one-page (single-spaced, 12 pt font) first-person narrative style. You are "graded" not by what you say you got out of (or did not get out of) the design challenge, but by how in-depth you have looked at new skills, knowledge, or attitudes that you may have gained, or where you have identified shortcomings that you would like to address.

Some questions to consider are the following:

What do you feel were the strengths/weaknesses of your team's effort?

What do you feel were your own strengths/weaknesses?

What would you do differently when you encounter design again?

What skills from the design challenge do you hope will carry over to other projects?

What technical experiences and skills did you gain?

How might you describe these technical and soft skills to a potential employer?

Please contact Dr. Tranquillo for further clarification

Appendix E: Capstone Timeline and Assignments

It is important that students receive scaffolding to navigate the open-ended nature of the challenge. Below is a

Project Introduction

You will work in teams of two or three to identify and construct a device that will address one of the specific Sustainable Development targets listed in the bottom section of https://sustainabledevelopment.un.org/focussdgs.html. Regardless of the topic chosen, the impact must have some tie to improving health and well-being. You are encouraged to think and build creatively, while also letting you show off your technical talents. While you will only build one functional prototype, you should be able to explain how scaling and distribution will make an impact.

Process and Grading

The overall purpose of the design challenge is to familiarize you with the design process, from problem identification through prototype testing. Class and lab time will be utilized for discussion of design topics and for work on projects. While teams will have frequent written assignments to turn in throughout the process, these assignments will be brief and, therefore, allow teams to focus most of their time on the identification and construction of their design solution. The design challenge will account for 10% of your overall grade for BMEG 401 and will be based upon your process and performance at the expo, as evaluated only by the instructor.

Design Constraints

The instructor will verify that the constraints below have been met at the expo.

Cost less than or equal to the total budget allocated to the team (see below).

Demonstrate the functionality of the prototype in five minutes or less.

Directly or indirectly provide a value to healthcare.

Directly address one of the first 16 SDGs (see above).

The device should be scalable and relatively easy to construct.

Show evidence of a quantitative performance assessment of your final prototype.

Contain no more than two 3D printed parts.

Supplies and Budget

Each team will have a guaranteed budget of \$25 and will be provided access to an additional \$25 following the submission and approval of your memo (8/30). If teams need a cash advance to make purchases, they should contact the instructor. As teams are expected to go through multiple construction phases, you should plan your budget carefully. Teams are allowed to utilize tools and materials in the BME labs as long as they are returned when the challenge is over. Turning in receipts for your parts will allow you to be reimbursed for your expenses. Any grey areas in policy should be passed by the instructor before a team utilizes a questionable supply.

Final Exposition

The final expo will consist of a one-minute pitch from each team, followed by a 45-minute open expo. You may use any materials or aids that you feel will help you in communicating your device, but purchased materials will come out of your budget. Each team will be assessed by those present (potential funders) at the expo. Each funder will have $100 (fake money in $20 increments) that they may invest in a project. The overall winner will be the team that has raised the most start-up funds. Funders may request a demonstration, evidence of testing, details on the technical design, or further clarification of the value proposition. In addition to investing, each funder will indicate their top three teams (ranked 1, 2, and 3) in the following four categories:

Value Proposition: How well is the device matched to the end goal as stated by the team? Would scaling and distribution of a refined device have the intended impact?

Functionality and Usability: Does the device do what it is supposed to? Are the tests well designed an executed? Are the results convincing, such that the functionality of the device is sound? Is the device designed with the user in mind?

Design and Fabrication: Is the quality of the design and construction such that the team has made good use of their technical skills? Have they followed a design process?

Innovation: Is the device unique? Does it have a chance in a global marketplace?

Timeline

As indicated in the following schedule, teams will be required to achieve specific milestones as the design challenge progresses. The final prototype will be evaluated in the final Design Challenge Exposition.

Tentative Design Challenge Schedule

Date	Day	Topic/Event	Assignment Due
8/21	M	Design Intro, Users, and Objectives	
8/23	W	Functions and Problem Statements	
8/23	W	Design Doc, Memos, Specifications	Problem, Users, and Objectives
8/25	F	Alt Solutions	Functions and Specifications
8/28	M	Sketches, Design Decisions	Alternative Solutions
8/30	W	Prototypes, Validation, and Testing	
8/30	W	Memo Meetings	Solution, Memo, and Meeting
9/1	F	Build—Test—Refine	
9/4	M	Build—Test—Refine, Presentations	
9/6	W	Build—Test—Refine	
9/6	W	Design Competition, Capstone Teams	Design Challenge
9/8	F	First Day of Capstone Project	Design Challenge Reflection

ASSIGNMENT #1: PROBLEM, USERS, AND OBJECTIVES

Based upon your research, you must generate a problem statement for your device. The following guidelines will help you craft your statement:

The statement must be one self-contained paragraph.
No graphics (figures or tables) are allowed.
The writing style should be understood by a lay audience.
No particular design solution should be stated or implied.
The last line of the statement should be in bold and give a one-sentence summary of the problem.
You must focus on a particular developing country, but you may also point to other countries or areas that have a similar problem.
Based upon our discussion of users and needs,
Create a list of the people you would contact to discuss the needs for your device.
Create a list of the multiple types of users of your device.
Create a list of known and anticipated needs and wants for each of the users identified earlier (thoughtful work here is key to success in the rest of the assignment).
Identify which needs are objectives and create an Objectives Tree of at least four levels.

ASSIGNMENT #2: FUNCTIONS AND SPECIFICATIONS

Based upon your problem, you must report the functions and specifications that should guide your solution generation and later validation testing.

Functions

Using the user needs and objectives you identified in assignment #1, identify up to ten desired functions of your device. Recall that functions are derived from users' needs and are intended to describe what the artifact must do. Identify each function as basic or secondary.

Specifications

For at least five of the functions identified:

Determine (or estimate) the appropriate design specifications. Recall that the specifications must be measurable and indicate how well the artifact performs each function.

Indicate the type of specification (as outlined in class) next to each specification.

ASSIGNMENT #3: ALTERNATIVE SOLUTIONS

Generate a list of preliminary solution ideas for the design challenge. Do not constrain yourself as to what seems reasonable or doable. In your team brainstorming, generate as many ideas as possible, no matter how farfetched. You must submit a list of all solutions generated. Solution ideas may be presented in graphical form (i.e., a sketch). You will be asked to share your alternative solutions at a meeting on August 31.

ASSIGNMENT #4: UPDATE MEMO AND MEETING

As an interim check-in, you must submit a one-page memo and run a meeting.

Write a formal one-page memo outlining the following items:

A solution chosen from the list of alternative solutions along with justification. Your solution should include a sketch of your intended design. Justification should be tied directly to how your device will solve the problem as stated in your problem statement by meeting all of the specifications.

Timeline for building and testing the chosen solution by the design challenge contest.

A list of materials (for building and testing your device) with associated costs. This includes any requested additional funds, with justification.

Tests you may conduct to demonstrate the functionality of your device.

The memo must be placed in Dr. Tranquillo's dropbox

Conduct a meeting with Dr. Tranquillo on August 30. The meeting should be no longer than 15 minutes and address the points in the memo. The team should drive the meeting forward using questions that are prepared ahead of time.

ASSIGNMENT #5: REFLECTION

The design process is THE defining characteristic of the engineering profession. You have just spent two and a half weeks confronting the process, and will continue on with a new project for the next year. The purpose of this reflection is for you to take an hour or two to look back over your notes, assignments, and final project.

You must summarize your reflection in a one-page (single-spaced, 12 pt font) first-person narrative style. You are "graded" not by what you say you got out of (or did not get out of) the design challenge, but by how in-depth you have looked at new skills, knowledge, or attitudes that you may have gained, or where you have identified shortcomings that you would like to address. You are encouraged to use the reflection ladder to help you go deeper.

Some questions to consider are the following:

What do you feel were the strengths/weaknesses of your team's effort?
What do you feel were your own strengths/weaknesses?
What would you do differently when you encounter design again?
What skills from the design challenge will you carry over to your design project?
What technical experiences and skills did you gain?
How might you describe these technical and soft skills to a potential employer?

Index

www.ingramcontent.com/pod-product-compliance
Lightning Source LLC
LaVergne TN
LVHW021957280826
846781LV00022B/197
* 9 7 8 1 0 3 2 8 5 8 8 4 5 *